ABC of
Rheumatology

Fifth Edition

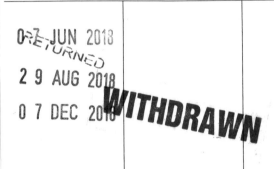

ABC series

An outstanding collection of resources for everyone in primary care

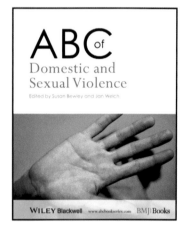

ABC of Domestic and Sexual Violence
Edited by Susan Bewley and Jan Welch

WILEY Blackwell   www.abcbookseries.com   BMJ|Books

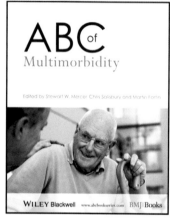

ABC of Multimorbidity
Edited by Stewart W. Mercer, Chris Salisbury and Martin Fortin

WILEY Blackwell   www.abcbookseries.com   BMJ|Books

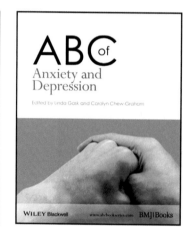

ABC of Anxiety and Depression
Edited by Linda Gask and Carolyn Chew-Graham

WILEY Blackwell   www.abcbookseries.com   BMJ|Books

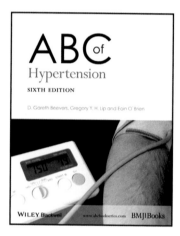

ABC of Hypertension
SIXTH EDITION
D. Gareth Beevers, Gregory Y. H. Lip and Eoin O'Brien

WILEY Blackwell   www.abcbookseries.com   BMJ|Books

The *ABC* Series contains a wealth of indispensable resources for GPs, GP registrars, junior doctors, and all those in primary care

- **Highly illustrated, informative, and practical**

- **Covers the symptoms, investigations, and treatment and management of conditions presenting in daily practice**

- **Full colour photographs and illustrations aid diagnosis and patient understanding**

For more information on all books in the ABC series, including links to further information, references and links to the latest official guidelines, please visit:

www.abcbookseries.com

BMJ|Books

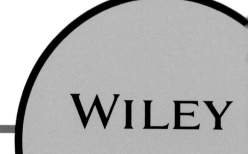

WILEY

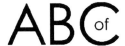

ABC of

Rheumatology

Fifth Edition

EDITED BY

Ade Adebajo

Associate Director of Teaching, University of Sheffield Medical School,
Honorary Professor and Consultant Rheumatologist/Director of Undergraduate
Medical Education, Faculty of Medicine, Dentistry and Health,
University of Sheffield and Barnsley Hospital,
South Yorkshire, UK

Lisa Dunkley

Consultant Rheumatologist and TPD Rheumatology (S Yorks),
Royal Hallamshire Hospital,
Sheffield, UK

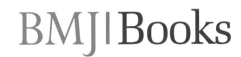

Registered Office(s)
John Wiley & Sons, Inc., 111 River Street, Hoboken, NJ 07030, USA
John Wiley & Sons Ltd, The Atrium, Southern Gate, Chichester, West Sussex, PO19 8SQ, UK

Editorial Office
9600 Garsington Road, Oxford, OX4 2DQ, UK
For details of our global editorial offices, customer services, and more information about Wiley products visit us at www.wiley.com.
Wiley also publishes its books in a variety of electronic formats and by print-on-demand.
Some content that appears in standard print versions of this book may not be available in other formats.

Library of Congress Cataloging-in-Publication Data

Names: Adebajo, Ade, editor. | Dunkley, Lisa, editor.
Title: ABC of rheumatology / edited by Dr Ade Adebajo, Dr Lisa Dunkley.
Description: Fifth edition. | Hoboken, NJ : John Wiley & Sons, Inc., 2018. |
  Series: ABC series | Includes bibliographical references and index. |
  Identifiers: LCCN 2017055315 (print) | LCCN 2017056755 (ebook) | ISBN
  9781118793183 (pdf) | ISBN 9781118793206 (epub) | ISBN 9781118793213 (pbk.)
Subjects: | MESH: Rheumatic Diseases
Classification: LCC RC927 (ebook) | LCC RC927 (print) | NLM WE 544 | DDC
  616.7/23–dc23
LC record available at https://lccn.loc.gov/2017055315

Cover Design: Wiley
Cover Image: © Science Photo Library/GettyImages

Set in 9.25/12pt MinionPro by SPi Global, Pondicherry, India

Printed and bound in Spain by Graphycems

10 9 8 7 6 5 4 3 2 1

Contents

Preface

This edition of *ABC of Rheumatology* welcomes a new co-editor, Dr Lisa Dunkley. Lisa has a strong pedigree in medical education, having previously worked at the Department of Medical Education at University College in London, subsequently at the Leeds Rheumatology Department and now in Sheffield Teaching Hospitals and Sheffield Medical School. Her extensive expertise and experience have substantially enriched this new edition.

We have built on the earlier successful editions of the book and added new chapters on radiology and immunology. These new chapters reflect areas in which the field of rheumatology has experienced phenomenal growth in recent years. Musculoskeletal ultrasound is now a well-established tool in the diagnosis of rheumatoid arthritis, whilst biological agents such as anti-tumour necrosis factor drugs are commonly used in the treatment of several rheumatic conditions.

I thank all authors, old and new, for their excellent chapters. I also thank the publishers for their ongoing support for this book. It is our hope that this authoritative, up-to-date, yet easy-to-read book will continue to benefit students and healthcare professionals across the world and enable them to better understand rheumatic diseases as well as to appropriately treat patients with these conditions.

Ade Adebajo
Lisa Dunkley

Contributors

A. Abhishek

Clinical Associate Professor of Rheumatology and Honorary
Consultant Rheumatologist
Academic Rheumatology
University of Nottingham;
Nottingham University Hospitals Trust, Nottingham, UK

Ade Adebajo

Associate Director of Teaching
University of Sheffield Medical School
Honorary Professor and Consultant Rheumatologist/Director of
Undergraduate Medical Education
Faculty of Medicine, Dentistry and Health
University of Sheffield and Barnsley Hospital
South Yorkshire, UK

Mohammed Akil

Consultant Rheumatologist
Sheffield Teaching Hospitals NHS Foundation Trust
Sheffield, UK

Carol M. Black

Emeritus Professor of Rheumatology
Royal Free Hospital and UCL Medical School
London, UK

Edwin S.L. Chan

Adjunct Associate Professor of Medicine
Department of Medicine
New York University
New York, USA

Bruce N. Cronstein

Paul R. Esserman Professor of Medicine
Department of Medicine
New York University
New York, USA

Paul Davis

Emeritus Professor of Medicine
University of Alberta
Edmonton, Canada

David D'Cruz

Professor and Consultant Rheumatologist
Louise Coote Lupus Unit
Guys and St Thomas' Hospitals
London, UK

Chris Deighton

Consultant Rheumatologist
Derbyshire Royal Infirmary
Derby, UK

Elaine M. Dennison

Professor of Musculoskeletal Epidemiology and Honorary Consultant
MRC Lifecourse Epidemiology Unit, University of Southampton
Southampton General Hospital
Southampton, UK

Christopher P. Denton

Professor of Experimental Rheumatology and Consultant
Rheumatologist
Royal Free Hospital and UCL Medical School
London, UK

John Dickson

Community Specialist in Rheumatology
Honorary Senior Lecturer
University of Bradford, Bradford, UK

Rajiv K. Dixit

Clinical Professor of Medicine
University of California
San Francisco;
Director
Northern California Arthritis Center
Walnut Creek, USA

Michael Doherty

Clinical Associate Professor of Rheumatology and Honorary Consultant
Rheumatologist
Academic Rheumatology
University of Nottingham;
Nottingham University Hospitals Trust, Nottingham, UK

Adrian Dunbar

General Practitioner with a special interest in musculoskeletal medicine and chronic pain management
Skipton, North Yorkshire, UK

Richard Eastell

Northern General Hospital;
Professor of Bone Metabolism
Academic Unit of Bone Metabolism
Mellanby Centre for Bone Research
Department of Oncology & Metabolism
University of Sheffield, Sheffield, UK

Helen Foster

Professor of Paediatric Rheumatology, Newcastle University;
Honorary Consultant, Great North Children's Hospital
Newcastle upon Tyne Hospitals NHS Foundation Trust
Newcastle upon Tyne; UK

Caroline Gordon

Professor of Rheumatology and Consultant Rheumatologist
University of Birmingham;
Department of Rheumatology
Sandwell and West Birmingham Hospitals NHS Trust
Birmingham, UK

William R. Grant

Consultant Rheumatologist and Honorary Senior Lecturer
Department of Rheumatology
Royal Hallamshire Hospital
Sheffield, UK

Andrew Hamer

Consultant Orthopaedic Surgeon
Department of Orthopaedic Surgery
Sheffield Teaching Hospitals NHS Foundation Trust
Sheffield, UK

Andrew Hassell

Consultant Rheumatologist
Staffordshire and Stoke on Trent Partnership NHS Trust;
Keele University School of Medicine
Keele, UK

Philip S. Helliwell

Senior Lecturer and Consultant Rheumatologist
Leeds Institute of Rheumatic and Musculoskeletal Medicine
University of Leeds, Leeds, UK

Samantha L. Hider

Senior Lecturer and Honorary Consultant Rheumatologist
Arthritis Research UK Primary Care Centre
Keele University
Keele, UK

Robert Inman

Professor and Director of Spondylitis Program
Toronto Hospital –Western Division
Toronto, Canada

Rajendra Vara Prasad Irlapati

Associate Professor
Department of Rheumatology
Nizams Institute of Medical Sciences
Hyderabad, India

John Isaacs

Professor of Clinical Rheumatology and Honorary Consultant Rheumatologist
Newcastle University and Newcastle upon Tyne Hospitals NHS Trust
Newcastle, UK

David Isenberg

Professor of Rheumatology
Centre For Rheumatology, Department of Medicine
University College London
London, UK

Jeffry Katz

Professor of Medicine
Case Western Reserve University School of Medicine
Cleveland, USA

Andrew Keat

Consultant Rheumatologist
Arthritis Centre
Northwick Park Hospital
Harrow, UK

Anna E. Litwic

Clinical Research Fellow
MRC Lifecourse Epidemiology Unit, University of Southampton
Southampton General Hospital
Southampton, UK

Christian D. Mallen

Deputy Director
Institute for Primary Care and Health Sciences
NIHR Research Professor in General Practice
NIHR CLAHRC West Midlands;
Deputy Director
NIHR School for Primary Care Research Training Lead
Honorary Professor in Rheumatology, University of Birmingham;
Arthritis Research UK Primary Care Centre
Research Institute for Primary Care & Health Sciences
Keele University
Keele UK

Eric L. Matteson

Professor of Medicine
Division of Rheumatology
Department of Internal Medicine and Department of Health Sciences Research
Mayo Clinic College of Medicine
Rochester, USA

Eugene McCloskey

Northern General Hospital; Academic Unit of Bone Metabolism
Mellanby Centre for Bone Research
Department of Oncology & Metabolism
University of Sheffield, Sheffield, UK

Anne-Marie McMahon
Consultant in Paediatric and Adolescent Rheumatology;
Honorary Senior Clinical Lecturer
Sheffield Children's Hospital
Sheffield, UK

Caroline Mitchell
General Practitioner and Senior Clinical Lecturer
Academic Unit of Primary Medical Care
University of Sheffield
Sheffield, UK

Robert Moots
Professor of Rheumatology
University of Liverpool
Honorary Consultant Rheumatologist
Aintree University Hospital
Liverpool, UK

Marisa Fernandes das Neves
Clinical Immunologist
Medicine IV Department
Fernando Fonseca Hospital, Amadora;
CEDOC – Chronic Diseases, Faculty of Medical Sciences
New University of Lisbon
Lisbon, Portugal

Voon H. Ong
Senior Clinical Lecturer and Honorary
Consultant Rheumatologist
Royal Free Hospital and UCL Medical School
London, UK

Nicola Peel
Clinical Lead
Metabolic Bone Centre
Northern General Hospital (Sheffield Teaching Hospitals Foundation Trust)
Sheffield, UK

Rosalind Ramsey-Goldman
Solovy Arthritis Research Society Research, Professor of Medicine
Northwestern University Feinberg School of Medicine
Chicago, USA

Vijay Rao
University of Birmingham;
Department of Rheumatology
Sandwell and West Birmingham Hospitals NHS Trust
Birmingham, UK

Sarah Ryan
Nurse Consultant Rheumatology
Staffordshire and Stoke on Trent Partnership NHS Trust
Haywood Hospital
Stoke on Trent
UK

Evdoxia Sapountzi
Clinical Fellow in Paediatric Rheumatology
Sheffield Children's Hospital
Sheffield, UK

David G.I. Scott
Professor and Consultant Rheumatologist
Norfolk and Norwich University Hospital NHS Trust;
Norwich Medical School
Norwich, UK

Michael Shipley
Honorary Consultant Rheumatologist
University College London Hospitals
London, UK

Heidi J. Siddle
Associate Professor and NIHR Clinical Lecturer
Leeds Institute of Rheumatic and Musculoskeletal Medicine
University of Leeds, Leeds;
Foot Health Department
Leeds Teaching Hospitals NHS Trust, Leeds, UK

Simon Somerville
GP Researcher
Arthritis Research UK Primary Care Centre
Keele University
Keele, UK

Cathy Speed
Professor of Sports and Exercise Medicine
University of St Mark and St John
Plymouth;
Consultant Rheumatologist, Sports and Exercise Medicine
Centre for Health and Perfomance
Cambridge, UK

David Stanley
Consultant Shoulder and Elbow Surgeon
BMI Thornbury Hospital
Sheffield, UK

Kay Stevenson
Consultant Physiotherapist and NIHR Knowledge
Mobilisation Fellow
Arthritis Research UK Primary Care Centre
Keele University
Keele; Haywood Hospital, Burslem, UK

Nishanthi Thalayasingam
Clinical Research Fellow
Institute of Cellular Medicine
Newcastle University
Newcastle, UK

Mohammed Tikly
Professor of Rheumatology
Chris Hani Baragwanath Academic Hospital and University of the Witwatersrand, Johannesburg, South Africa

Lori Tucker
Professor of Paediatric Rheumatology
British Columbia's Children's Hospital
Vancouver, Canada

Martin Underwood

Professor of Primary Care Research
Warwick Clinical Trials Unit
Warwick Medical School
The University of Warwick Coventry
Warwick, UK;
Adjunct Monash Warwick Professor,
Department of Epidemiology and Preventive Medicine Monash University
Clayton, Australia

Richard J. Wakefield

Senior Lecturer and Honorary Consultant in Rheumatology
Leeds Institute of Rheumatic and Rehabilitation Medicine
Chapel Allerton Hospital
Leeds, UK

Jennifer Walsh

Northern General Hospital;
Senior Clinical Lecturer
Academic Unit of Bone Metabolism
Mellanby Centre for Bone Research
Department of Oncology & Metabolism
University of Sheffield, Sheffield, UK

Louise Warburton

Clinical Lead for Telford MSK Service (TEMS)
Associate Medical Director, Shropshire Community NHS Trust;
Senior Lecturer, Keele University
Keele, UK

Richard A. Watts

Consultant Rheumatologist
Department of Rheumatology
Ipswich Hospital NHS Trust
Ipswich;
Honorary Professor
Norwich Medical School
Norwich, UK

Mark Wilkinson

Professor of Orthopaedic Surgery
University of Sheffield
Sheffield; Honorary Consultant Orthopaedic Surgeon, Sheffield Teaching
Hospitals NHS Foundation Trust
President British Orthopaedic Research Society, UK

Anthony G. Wilson

Professor of Rheumatology
EULAR Centre of Excellence/UCD Centre for Arthritis Research
Conway Institute of Biomolecular & Biomedical Research
University College Dublin
Dublin, Ireland

List of Abbreviations

AAV	ANCA-associated vasculitis
ACD	anaemia of chronic disease
ACE	angiotensin-converting enzyme
ACR	American College of Rheumatology
ACTH	adrenocorticotrophic hormone
ADCC	antibody-dependent cellular cytotoxicity
AIHA	autoimmune haemolytic anaemia
ANA	antinuclear antibody
ANCA	antineutrophil cytoplasmic antibody
APC	antigen-presenting cell
APS	antiphospholipid syndrome
AS	ankylosing spondylitis
AST	aspartate aminotransferase
BAFF	B-cell activating factor
BASDAI	Bath Ankylosing Spondylitis Disease Activity Index
BASFI	Bath Ankylosing Spondylitis Functional Index
BASMI	Bath Ankylosing Spondylitis Metrology Index
BLyS	B-lymphocyte stimulator
BMD	bone mineral density
BMI	body mass index
CCP	cyclic citrullinated peptide
CDC	complement-dependent cytotoxicity
CDH	congenital dislocation of the hip
CHB	congenital heart block
CI	confidence interval
CK	creatine phosphokinase
CKD	chronic kidney disease
COX	cyclo-oxygenase
CRP	C-reactive protein
CT	computed tomography
CTGF	connective tissue growth factor
DDH	developmental dysplasia of the hip
DEXA	dual-energy X-ray absorptiometry
DIC	disseminated intravascular coagulation
DIPJ	distal interphalangeal joint
DMARD	disease-modifying drug
ELISA	enzyme-linked immunosorbent assay
ERA	enthesitis-related arthritis
ESR	erythrocyte sedimentation rate
ESWT	extracorporeal shock wave therapy
EULAR	European League against Rheumatism
FAI	femoro-acetabular impingement
FMF	familial Mediterranean fever
FMS	fibromyalgia syndrome
GCA	giant cell arteritis
GFR	glomerular filtration rate
GI	gastrointestinal
GIO	glucocorticoid-induced osteoporosis
GU	genitourinary
GWAS	genome-wide association
HCPC	Health and Care Professions Council
HFCS	high fructose corn syrup
HIV	human immunodeficiency virus
HLA	human leucocyte antigen
HLH	haemophagocytic lymphohistiocytosis
HRCT	high-resolution computed tomography
HSP	Henoch–Schönlein purpura
IAI	intra-articular steroid injection
IBD	inflammatory bowel disease
IFN	interferon
IL	interleukin
INR	international normalized ratio
JAK-STAT	Janus kinase-signal transducer and activator of transcription
JDM	juvenile dermatomyositis
JIA	juvenile idiopathic arthritis
JPsA	juvenile psoriatic arthritis
LBP	low back pain
LDG	low-density granulocyte
LDH	lactate dehydrogenase
MAS	macrophage activation syndrome
MCP	metacarpophalangeal
MDT	multidisciplinary team
MHC	major histocompatibility complex
MIF	macrophage inhibitor factor
MMF	mycophenolate mofetil
MMP	matrix metalloproteinase
MRI	magnetic resonance imaging
mSASSS	modified Stoke AS Spinal Score
MSK	musculoskeletal
MTP	metatarsophalangeal
NET	neutrophil extracellular trap
NICE	National Institute for Health and Care Excellence
NSAID	non-steroidal anti-inflammatory drug

OA	osteoarthritis	SI	sacroiliac
OT	occupational therapist	SLE	systemic lupus erythematosus
PAH	pulmonary artery hypertension	SoJIA	systemic-onset JIA
PAWP	pulmonary artery wedge pressure	SpA	spondyloarthritides
PET	positron emission tomography	SPECT	single-photon emission computed tomography
PDB	Paget's disease of bone	SRC	scleroderma renal crisis
PH	pulmonary hypertension	SSc	systemic sclerosis
PIP	proximal interphalangeal	SUFE	slipped upper femoral epiphysis
PMR	polymyalgia rheumatica	TGF	transforming growth factor
PRP	platelet-rich plasma	TJR	total joint replacement
PUO	pyrexia of unknown origin	TNF	tumour necrosis factor
RA	rheumatoid arthritis	TRAPS	tumour necrosis factor receptor-associated periodic syndrome
RANKL	receptor activator of nuclear factor kappa-B ligand		
RCT	randomized controlled trial	TTP	thrombotic thrombocytopaenic purpura
ReA	reactive arthritis	UI	uncertainty interval
RF	rheumatoid factor	US	ultrasound
RNS	rheumatology nurse specialist	WBC	white blood cell
RP	Raynaud's phenomenon		
RSD	reflex sympathetic dystrophy		

CHAPTER 1

Delivering Musculoskeletal Care Across Boundaries

Samantha L. Hider[1,2], Simon Somerville[1] and Kay Stevenson[1,2]

[1]Arthritis Research UK Primary Care Centre, Keele University, Keele, UK
[2]Haywood Hospital, Burslem, UK

OVERVIEW

- The burden of musculoskeletal disease is increasing and the importance of a multidisciplinary care pathway in the management of these patients is well established.

- A community-wide approach encompassing the involvement and education of both patient and primary care physician will lead to earlier diagnosis, speedier and more appropriate secondary care referrals, and quicker treatment and ultimately improved clinical outcomes.

- Innovative models of care have been developed within primary/secondary care interface services for patients with musculoskeletal disease.

- Identifying patients with inflammatory arthritis for rapid secondary care referral remains a key challenge for primary care.

Introduction

The ever-increasing demand upon acute hospitals to deliver emergency medicine means that the management of long-term chronic conditions is being delivered in a number of different settings rather than the traditional acute hospital. This chapter discusses different ways of working to try to ensure that patients with musculoskeletal conditions receive timely, appropriate treatments with the 'right person, right place and right time'.

One way of transferring rheumatological expertise to the community, without increasing the burden on the primary care team, is to develop the roles of the wider multidisciplinary team such as nurses, physiotherapists and occupational therapists. Such practitioners, working in an extended role, operate at a high level of clinical practice and cross traditional professional boundaries. This is particularly evident within musculoskeletal interface services.

Rheumatology in the community: the impact on primary care

Musculoskeletal problems are common in primary care, representing about 20% of all consultations, although these disorders often are not given the same priority as conditions such as cancer or cardiovascular disease. More years are lived with a musculoskeletal disability than any other condition. These patients often have other co-morbidities such as depression and cardiovascular disease. Increasing life expectancy and risk factors such as obesity mean that larger numbers of patients with musculoskeletal problems will require help from health and social services in the future. The challenge is to fill gaps and improve co-ordination of care within existing resources.

Who should be referred to secondary care?

The GP is often viewed as the gatekeeper to secondary care. A more modern and helpful approach is to consider both vertical (with secondary care) and horizontal integration of care, involving primary care-based agencies such as physiotherapy and social care working together rather than in isolation to deliver individualized care.

Waiting times for new rheumatology appointments vary widely and depend on local resources but also, to some extent, on how clinicians triage referrals from GPs. The majority of patients seen in primary care will have non-inflammatory problems such as osteoarthritis or back pain and most can be managed in primary care with appropriate advice and education or referral to primary care physiotherapy.

Effective triage depends largely upon the information contained in the referral letter. The GP is well placed to give an overall picture of the patient, particularly including psychosocial as well as biomedical issues. Recognizing and dealing with them is known to

---

ABC of Rheumatology, Fifth Edition. Edited by Ade Adebajo and Lisa Dunkley.
© 2018 John Wiley & Sons Ltd. Published 2018 by John Wiley & Sons Ltd.

improve patient outcomes, reduce costs and increase efficiency. Helpful information to include in a referral letter is given in Box 1.1.

A number of simple tools, such as the STarTBack tool for low back pain (Hill *et al.*, 2011), are starting to be employed in primary care to quickly screen patients to identify which are at low risk of poor outcome and require minimal intervention and which may benefit from onward referral so that matched packages based on need can be implemented. The STarTBack tool is highlighted in Box 1.2.

A key challenge for the GP is how to spot the small number of patients with early inflammatory arthritis who will benefit from early secondary care and prompt treatment with disease-modifying drugs (DMARDs). There are no specific examination or investigation findings that are diagnostic for rheumatoid arthritis (RA). Normal blood test results or a negative rheumatoid factor do not rule out RA but a positive test is not diagnostic of it either. Box 1.3 gives some clinical features that may be suggestive of inflammatory

arthritis. The recent NICE standards of care emphasize the importance of rapid secondary care referral for *all* patients suspected of having rheumatoid arthritis (NICE, 2013).

Given that the diagnosis of early inflammatory arthritis can be difficult, it is a good idea to refer too many rather than too few patients. Many rheumatology services operate an interface service or early synovitis clinic so access to early triage and diagnosis is facilitated.

An alternative method when considering secondary care referral, which may be useful in primary care, involves using the 'red flag' approach to identify patients with potentially serious pathology. Red flags are highlighted in Box 1.4 and may prompt consideration of further investigation or referral.

Patients with 'red flags' and certain other patients with specific diagnoses, including suspected inflammatory arthritis or connective tissue disorders, should be considered for referral to secondary care for further investigation and management. The next step is to decide how best to manage the remainder (the majority) of patients consulting with musculoskeletal problems. Many can be managed in primary care or may be referred to musculoskeletal interface services.

Box 1.1 Important information to include in a referral letter

- Length of history
- Pattern of joint involvement
- The presence of joint swelling and/or stiffness
- Referrals for and response to previous treatments
- Results of investigations
- Distress or disability – results of screening tools such as STarT Back
- Significant co-morbidity and risk factors
- Other medical and psychosocial issues

Box 1.2 The STarTBack tool for back pain

Questions 1–8: tick box for agree/disagree	No	Yes
1 My back pain has spread down my leg(s) at some time in the last 2 weeks	☐	☐
2 I have had pain in the shoulder or neck at some time in the last 2 weeks	☐	☐
3 I have only walked short distances because of my back pain	☐	☐
4 In the last 2 weeks, I have dressed more slowly than usual because of back pain	☐	☐
5 It's not really safe for a person with a condition like mine to be physically active	☐	☐
6 Worrying thoughts have been going through my mind a lot of the time	☐	☐
7 I feel that my back pain is terrible and it's never going to get any better	☐	☐
8 In general, I have not enjoyed all the things I used to enjoy	☐	☐
9 Overall, how bothersome has your back pain been in the last 2 weeks? (Not at all/Slightly/Moderately/Very much/Extremely) (score 1 for 'very much/ extremely')	☐	☐

A total score of <3=low risk, total score ≥4=medium/high risk. (medium risk=scores from items 5–9 of ≤3, high risk=scores from items 5–9 of 4 or more).

Source: www.keele.ac.uk/sbst

Box 1.3 Features suggestive of inflammatory arthritis

- **Stiffness** of joints – especially early morning stiffness for >30 minutes.
- **Swelling** (synovitis) of any joints – especially wrists and/or metocarpophalangeal (MCP) joints and/or proximal interphalangeal (PIP) joints.
- **Squeezing** the affected joints is painful.

Box 1.4 'Red flags' for regional pain syndromes

History of significant trauma

- Fracture
- Major soft tissue injury

Localized joint swelling and/or redness

- Septic arthritis
- Inflammatory arthritis
- Haemarthrosis

Unremitting night pain

- Malignancy
- Inflammation/infection

Bone tenderness

- Fracture
- Malignancy
- Infection

Systemic disturbance

- Weight loss
- Fever

Significant co-morbidity

- Previous malignancy

Musculoskeletal interface services

These services have been established across the UK and designed and commissioned in a range of formats, varying from physiotherapy-led services to those where expertise is gained from a variety of professional backgrounds including physiotherapy, GP and rheumatology. The aim of these services is to improve the management of patients with musculoskeletal pain problems whilst reducing the numbers of patients referred to secondary care. Common to most models is the notion that patients will be seen quickly, assessed, investigated and managed in a 'one stop shop' approach, with minimal follow-up.

Commissioned services vary depending on their population needs. Initially, services were commissioned assuming that most patients would have a single site of pain, with a short duration and would require appropriate assessment but minimal intervention. However, a recent study of interface clinic consulters (Roddy *et al.*, 2013) identified that over half of those presenting had pain for more than 1 year, and co-existent anxiety and depression and work disability were common, highlighting that these patients have more complex physical and psychological needs than anticipated. Clinicians who work in the interface setting need to have a broad range of skills to assess and manage these patients. They need to be able to assess single joint disease but also be able to spot those with serious pathology or inflammatory arthritis and refer accordingly. They also need to understand the surgical thresholds for appropriate referral where indicated.

Physiotherapists with extended skills have been a consistent feature in interface services. These highly trained clinicians have additional skills in differential diagnosis, clinical assessment, and prescribing or injection therapy. They bring their knowledge of physical rehabilitation, pain management and motivation to such services. Designs of these services vary, but an effective interface service should draw on the skills of the multidisciplinary workface and maximize the skills of the clinicians involved to address the broad range of conditions. Individual clinicians may not treat depression, anxiety, low mood or poor exercise tolerance, but they need to know how to spot them and who/where to refer on to for further input. Box 1.5 highlights key factors for a successful interface service.

Box 1.5 **Key factors for a successful interface service**

- Multidisciplinary
- Strong clinical leadership and governance framework
- Competency based
- Education and research embedded in practice

Further management

The large numbers of patients and the burden of musculoskeletal disease require a more planned and co-ordinated approach, as is used in other long-term conditions such as diabetes. Many patients with musculoskeletal disease have additional co-morbidity or are at higher risk of vascular disease such as those with rheumatoid arthritis or gout. Screening for vascular risk factors such as hypertension, diabetes and hyperlipidaemia is key as they are often not optimally managed within this population.

Within primary care, there is a vital role to be played by practice and district nurses who are well placed to lead on these issues. This includes holistic assessment, supplying advice and education, provision of treatments, appropriate referrals and, most importantly, overall care co-ordination.

For patients managed within secondary care, the shared management of (often multiple) disease-modifying drugs and co-morbidity is increasingly important. Specialist nurses based in secondary care have a key role in helping co-ordinate this care, providing additional expertise and extended role procedures such as joint injection and as a link with hospital consultants.

Conclusion

Musculoskeletal problems are extremely common and many can be successfully managed in primary care. Screening tools such as those for red flags or STarTBack can be useful to identify patients most likely to benefit from onward referral or additional interventions. Prompt referral to secondary care for patients with suspected inflammatory arthritis is key to allow rapid institution of disease-modifying agents shown to improve prognosis. Co-ordination of care between primary and secondary care teams is important in providing ongoing effective management of musculoskeletal disease and its common associated co-morbidities.

References

Hill JC, Whitehurst DG, Lewis M *et al.* Comparison of stratified primary care management for low back pain with current best practice (STarT Back): a randomised controlled trial. *Lancet* 2011; **378**(9802): 1560–1571.

NICE. *Quality Standard 33. Rheumatoid Arthritis in Over 16s.* Available at: www.nice.org.uk/guidance/QS33 (accessed 3 November 2017)

Roddy E, Zwierska I, Jordan KP *et al.* Musculoskeletal clinical assessment and treatment services at the primary–secondary care interface: an observational study. *British Journal of General Practice* 2013; **63**(607): e141–148.

CHAPTER 2

Pain in the Wrist and Hand

Michael Shipley

University College London Hospitals, London, UK

OVERVIEW

- Nodal osteoarthritis affecting the distal interphalangeal joints is very common and generally each joint is painful for a few months.
- If a patient presents with swollen and painful joints in the hand, consider inflammatory arthritis as a diagnosis.
- The hand and wrist are common sites for overuse and injury. Remember to ask about precipitating factors, especially work/occupation and hobbies.
- Carpal tunnel syndrome is a common peripheral nerve entrapment syndrome and has a typical presentation.
- Raynaud's syndrome generally requires symptomatic treatment only, but consider secondary causes if seen in older people.

Hand or wrist pain and resultant impaired function are often the cause of great anxiety for patients. Hands give us a great deal of information about the world in which we live. They are capable of performing fine and delicate movements and are essential for work, sport, hobbies and social interaction.

Functional anatomy

The wrist is a complex structure comprising three groups of joints: the radiocarpal joints, which allow flexion, extension, abduction, adduction and circumduction; the inferior radioulnar joint, which allows pronation and supination; and the intercarpal joints (Figure 2.1).

The eight carpal bones, in two rows of four, form a bony gutter and are the base of the carpal tunnel. The flexor retinaculum, a strong fascial band, forms the palmar side of the tunnel. Running through the carpal tunnel are the deep and superficial flexor tendons, the tendons of flexor pollicis longus, flexor carpi radialis and the median nerve. The ulnar nerve lies superficial to the flexor retinaculum but deep to the transverse carpal ligament in Guyon's canal. The extensor tendons are held in position on the extensor surface of the wrist by the extensor retinaculum. Fibrous septa divide the extensor compartment into six. All the flexor tendons are encased in a common synovial tendon sheath, which extends from a position just proximal to the wrist to the middle of the palm. Flexor pollicis longus and flexor carpi ulnaris have their own individual sheaths, as do each of the six extensor tendons.

The hand bones are the metacarpals, proximal phalanges, middle phalanges, distal phalanges and sesamoid bones. A sesamoid bone lies at the base of the thumb in the tendons of flexor pollicis brevis. The first metacarpal bone of the thumb is the shortest and most mobile of the metacarpals and lies in a different plane to the others. This is important to allow opposition, i.e. pincer actions to grasp objects. The carpometacarpal and trapezoscaphoid joints are prone to osteoarthritis.

Individual tendon sheaths for the deep and superficial flexor tendons start at the level of the distal transverse crease of the palm and end at the bases of the distal phalanxes. The sheath for flexor pollicis longus continues from the carpal tunnel to the distal phalanx. During flexion, five fibrous bands, or pulleys, hold the flexor sheaths in position.

The second to fifth metacarpophalangeal joints flex to about 90°. Active extension is rarely more than 30°. Passive extension varies from 60° to more than 100° in people with hypermobility. The proximal and distal interphalangeal joints are hinge joints. The lumbrical and interossei muscles produce complex movements that involve extension of the interphalangeal joints and flexion at the metacarpophalangeal joints and are essential to fine hand functions, such as writing.

There are many possible causes of pain in the wrist and hand (Table 2.1).

Tendon problems

Flexor tenosynovitis

Unaccustomed or repetitive use of the fingers or inflammatory arthritis can cause flexor tenosynovitis (Figure 2.2). This is inflammation of the synovial sheath of the finger flexor tendons, which leads to volar swelling and tenderness just proximal and

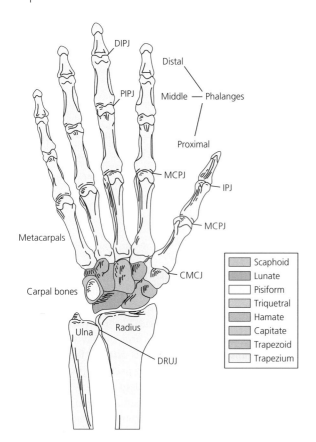

Figure 2.1 The bones of the hand. CMCJ = carpometacarpal joint; DIPJ = distal interphalangeal joint; DRUJ = distal radioulnar joint; IPJ = interphalangeal joint; MCPJ = metacarpophalangeal joint; PIPJ = proximal interphalangeal joint

Table 2.1 Causes of pain in the wrist and hand

At all ages	In older patients
• Trauma	• Nodal osteoarthritis
	○ Distal interphalangeal joints
	(Heberden's nodes)
	○ First carpometacarpal joints
	○ Proximal interphalangeal joints
	(Bouchard's nodes)
• Flexor tenosynovitis	• Scaphoid fracture
○ Carpal tunnel syndrome	
• Flexor tendonosis	• Pseudogout
○ Trigger finger or thumb	
• De Quervain's tenosynovitis	• Gout
	○ Acute
	○ Chronic tophaceous
• Extensor tenosynovitis	• Dupuytren's contracture
• Ganglion	• Diabetic stiff hand
• Mallet finger	• Septic arthritis
• Cubital tunnel syndrome	
• Inflammatory arthritis	
• Raynaud's syndrome	
• Writer's cramp	
• Chronic upper limb pain	
• complex regional pain syndrome (Type I)	
• Scaphoid fracture	
• Osteonecrosis	

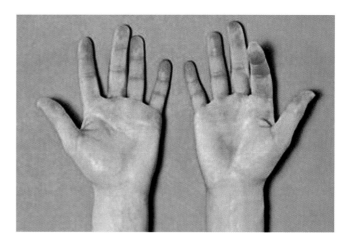

Figure 2.2 Flexor tenosynovitis

distal to the wrist. The flexor tendon sheaths in the palm or finger may also be affected. The hand feels stiff, painful and swollen, particularly in the morning. Rest helps. Injection is sometimes needed. Local anaesthetic helps introduce the needle alongside the tendon in the palm just proximal to the metacarpophalangeal joint.

Finger flexor tendonosis and trigger finger

Gripping and hard manual work cause palpable thickening and nodularity of the finger flexor tendons; tendon sheath synovitis may also be present. The affected fingers are stiff in the morning, when the patient also has pain in the palm and along the dorsum of the finger(s). The pain is reproduced by passive extension of the finger. This is common in rheumatoid arthritis and in dactylitis caused by seronegative arthritis. Nodular flexor tenosynovitis is more common and less responsive to treatment in patients with diabetes than in other patients.

Trigger finger is caused by a nodule catching at the pulley that overlies the metacarpophalangeal joint in the palm. The patient wakens with the finger flexed and has to force it straight with a painful or painless click. Triggering also occurs after gripping. The nodule and the 'catch' in movement are felt in the palm.

Management and injection technique – A low-pressure injection of local anaesthetic followed by a locally acting steroid preparation alongside the tendon nodule in the palm helps (Figure 2.3) (Schubert *et al.*, 2013). If symptoms are persistent or recurrent, surgical release is needed.

Overuse and local injury (e.g. after opening a tight jar) are the most common causes of thumb flexor tenosynovitis and trigger thumb. Either the interphalangeal joint cannot be flexed or it sticks in flexion and snaps straight. The sesamoid bone in the flexor pollicis brevis tendon is tender on the volar surface of the thumb's metacarpophalangeal joint. Corticosteroid injection next to the sesamoid bone at the site of maximal tenderness helps.

De Quervain's tenosynovitis

De Quervain's stenosing tenosynovitis affects the tendon sheath of abductor pollicis longus and extensor pollicis brevis at the radial styloid. It causes pain at or just proximal or distal to the styloid (in

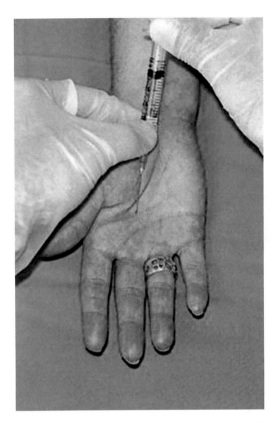

Figure 2.3 Injection technique for flexor tenosynovitis and trigger finger

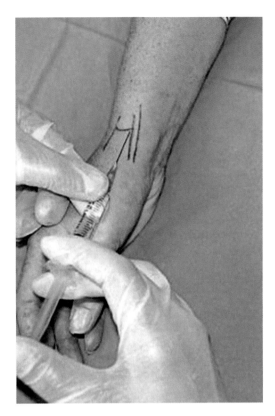

Figure 2.4 Injection technique for de Quervain's tenosynovitis

contrast with first carpometacarpal osteoarthritis, which causes pain at the base of the thumb). There is tenderness, and swelling and pushing the thumb into the palm while holding the wrist in ulnar deviation increases the pain. A tendon nodule may cause triggering.

Management and injection technique – Rest is essential, with avoidance of thumb extension and pinching, but immobilization splints are inconvenient. Therapeutic ultrasound or local anti-inflammatory gels help; injection of local anaesthetic, then a locally acting steroid preparation alongside the tendon under low pressure at the point of maximum tenderness rapidly relieves the pain (Figure 2.4). A second injection may be needed. Surgery is rarely necessary, unless stenosis or nodule formation develops (Peters-Veluthamaningal *et al.*, 2009).

Extensor tenosynovitis

Inflammation of the common extensor (fourth) compartment causes well-defined swelling that extends from the back of the hand to just proximal to the wrist. The extensor retinaculum causes a typical 'hourglass' shape proximal and distal to the wrist. This contrasts with wrist synovitis, which causes diffuse swelling distal to the radius and ulna. Repetitive wrist and finger movements, especially with the wrist in dorsiflexion, are the cause, and this is one of the several causes of forearm and wrist pain seen in keyboard workers and pianists. It is also common in rheumatoid arthritis. Rest helps extensor tenosynovitis, but often a corticosteroid injection into the tendon sheath is needed. Workplace reviews

and wrist supports for those who use a keyboard and mouse help prevent recurrences.

Mallet finger

This is a flexion deformity affecting the distal interphalangeal joint of the finger and is due to either distal extensor tendon rupture or avulsion with a bony fragment after traumatic forced flexion of the extended fingertip. The resultant weakness is often painless and presents with an inability to actively extend the fingertip. Treatment is usually by splinting the distal interphalangeal joint in extension or, rarely, surgery.

Dupuytren's contracture

Dupuytren's contracture (Figure 2.5) is a relatively common and painless condition associated with palpable fibrosis of the palmar aponeurosis, usually in the palm but occasionally at the base of a digit. It is more common in white people, men, heavy drinkers, smokers and patients with diabetes mellitus. The cause is unknown, but repeated trauma may be important. Fibroblast proliferation starts in the superficial fascia and invades the dermis. An early sign is skin pitting or puckering. The contraction eventually causes flexion of the digit(s), most often the ring finger of the dominant hand, but disability is often minimal. Disabling and progressive flexion is more common in the familial form. Specialist hand clinics use magnetic resonance imaging to assess the lesion.

The role of local corticosteroid or a new *Clostridium histolyticum*-derived collagenase injection and radiotherapy in early disease is unclear, although placebo controlled studies of collagenase indicate

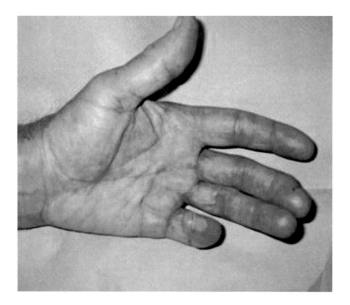

Figure 2.5 Dupuytren's contracture

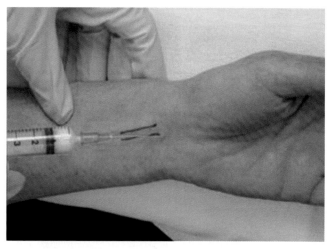

Figure 2.6 Injection technique for carpal tunnel syndrome

a high success rate, but with a significant incidence of complications. Percutaneous fasciotomy or open fasciectomy are helpful but recurrence is common. No controlled studies exist. Nodular fibromatosis also affects the sole of the foot, the knuckle pads (Garrod's pads) and the penis (Peyronie's disease), and these conditions may co-exist.

Peripheral nerve entrapment syndromes

Carpal tunnel syndrome

Carpal tunnel syndrome is a peripheral nerve entrapment syndrome of the median nerve, often caused by flexor tenosynovitis or arthritis. It can occur in the third trimester of pregnancy. Repetitive use of the hand increases the risk of developing carpal tunnel syndrome but its status as a 'work injury' is controversial (Yagev *et al.*, 2001).

A ganglion, or very rarely amyloidosis or myxoedema, can cause carpal tunnel syndrome. Pain, tingling and numbness in a median nerve distribution (thumb, index finger, middle and radial side of ring finger) are typically present on waking or can wake the patient. The patient feels the fingers are more swollen than they look and intense aching is felt in the forearm. The symptoms may appear when the patient holds a newspaper or a car steering wheel. Permanent numbness and wasting of the thenar eminence (flexor pollicis and opponens pollicis) cause clumsiness. The patient's description often indicates the diagnosis

Tests and investigations – Tinel's sign (tapping the median nerve in the carpal tunnel) or Phalen's test (holding the wrist in forced dorsiflexion) may provoke symptoms. Weakness of abduction of the thumb distal phalanx with the thumb adducted towards the fifth digit is typical. The carpal tunnel and median nerve are seen on ultrasonic images, although ultrasound and MRI are not usually needed. Nerve conduction studies can confirm the diagnosis, but are often not required if the history and examination are typical.

Management and injection technique – A splint worn on the wrist at night relieves or reduces the symptoms of carpal tunnel syndrome.

This is diagnostic and may be curative. A corticosteroid injection into the carpal tunnel (Figure 2.6) may also be considered, as this often helps rapidly, although recurrence is common. The needle is inserted at the distal wrist skin crease, just to the ulnar side of the palmaris longus tendon, or about 0.5 cm to the ulnar side of flexor carpi radialis at an angle of 45° towards the middle finger. The local anaesthetic is injected superficially. If a small test injection of corticosteroid causes finger pain, the needle is in the nerve and needs to be repositioned. An injection often exacerbates the symptoms briefly, but it is effective and non-toxic (Huisstede *et al.*, 2010a).

Recurrent daytime symptoms, unrelieved by splints, warrant nerve conduction studies. Slowing of median nerve conduction at the wrist suggests demyelination due to local compression. The action potential is reduced or absent due to nerve fibre loss if the lesion is severe or prolonged. Needle electromyography is unpleasant but detects denervation.

Decompression surgery should be considered for recurrent symptoms not eased by splints or injection; significant nerve damage; muscle wasting; and/or permanent numbness (Huisstede *et al.*, 2010b). Pins and needles often increase briefly postoperatively while the nerve recovers. Recovery of sensation or strength, or both, may be limited or non-existent if the lesion is severe and longstanding. See also https://cks.nice.org.uk/carpal-tunnel-syndrome.

Cubital tunnel syndrome

Ulnar nerve compression at the elbow can be caused by direct pressure from leaning on the elbow, stretching the nerve with the elbow in prolonged flexion at night, or holding a telephone. It causes pins and needles in an ulnar distribution (little finger and the ulnar side of the ring finger). Prolonged entrapment causes hypothenar wasting and weakness of the hand's intrinsic muscles. The nerve is tender and sensitive at the elbow, where Tinel's sign is positive. Nerve conduction studies are normal in around 50% of cases. Avoidance of direct pressure and prolonged elbow flexion help. Surgical anterior transposition of the nerve is occasionally needed. In some cases, the ulnar nerve is compressed in Guyon's canal at the wrist (Townley *et al.*, 2006).

Osteoarthritis

Nodal osteoarthritis

Nodal osteoarthritis most commonly involves the distal interphalangeal joints and is familial. The joint swells and becomes inflamed and painful, but the pain subsides over a few weeks or months and leaves bony swellings (Heberden's nodes) (Figure 2.7). Most patients manage with local anti-inflammatory gels or no treatment once they know the prognosis is good. The appearance sometimes causes distress. Occasionally, the joint becomes unstable and limits pinch gripping. Surgical fusion of the index distal interphalangeal joints or thumb interphalangeal joint in slight flexion improves grip, although this is rarely necessary. Involvement of the proximal interphalangeal joints (Bouchard's nodes) is less common and may be mistaken for early rheumatoid arthritis (Figure 2.8). Stiffness and pain of the proximal joints impair hand function significantly.

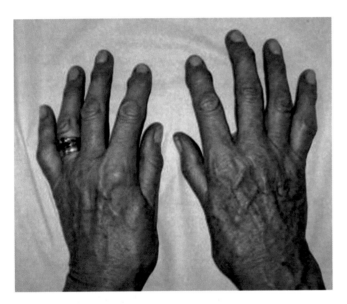

Figure 2.7 Nodal osteoarthritis (Heberden's nodes) and first carpometacarpal osteoarthritis

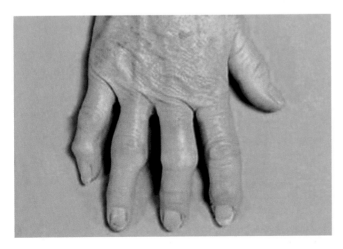

Figure 2.8 Nodal osteoarthritis with Bouchard's nodes

First carpometacarpal osteoarthritis

Pain at the base of the thumb in the early phase of first carpometacarpal osteoarthritis (see Figure 2.7) is disabling, but with time the joint stiffens and adducts, and pain and disability decrease. The hand becomes 'squared'. Management is usually conservative, but a corticosteroid injection helps severe pain associated with local inflammation. Surgical replacement is rarely warranted, although the outcome is good. Some find a splint helpful (Anakwe and Middleton, 2011).

Systemic disorders causing hand pain

Inflammatory arthritis

The hands are often affected early in rheumatoid arthritis, with symmetrical swelling of the metacarpophalangeal joints, proximal interphalangeal joints and wrists. The feet and other joints are usually also affected. Psoriatic and other forms of seronegative arthritis are less common, are more likely to be asymmetrical, and may be associated with marked skin and tendon changes that produce a 'sausage' finger (dactylitis). The distal interphalangeal joints and adjacent nails may also be affected in psoriasis. Morning pain and stiffness are typical. Intra-articular steroids are often useful adjuncts to systemic medication. Early referral to a specialist for inflammatory arthritis is recommended

Acute pseudogout and chondrocalcinosis of the wrist

Sudden wrist pain in an older patient may be due to calcium pyrophosphate arthritis (pseudogout). Marked swelling and inflammation are observed – the joint feels hot and infection may need to be excluded. Chondrocalcinosis (Figure 2.9), although often asymptomatic, is usually seen in the triangular fibrocartilage of the wrist on X-ray. The joint aspirate is turbid and contains weakly positively birefringent crystals under polarized light. Steroid

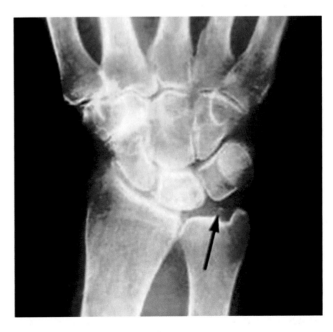

Figure 2.9 Chondrocalcinosis in wrist

injection or a short course of a non-steroidal anti-inflammatory drug or colchicine usually helps; regular use of non-steroidal anti-inflammatory drugs or colchicine can be used to manage frequent attacks.

Acute gout and chronic tophaceous gout

Acute urate gout rarely affects the hands. Tophaceous deposits in individuals with renal failure or who have been on long-term diuretic treatment are initially painless, chalky subcutaneous deposits. The tophi can ulcerate and a few such patients also develop acute gout in the hand and elsewhere.

Diabetic stiff hand (cheiroarthropathy – limited joint mobility syndrome)

Stiff hands are seen in 5–10% of patients with type 1 diabetes. This is more common in those with poor diabetic control and is associated with limited shoulder mobility, diabetic nephropathy and retinopathy. Patients develop waxy, tight skin and a so-called positive prayer sign — inability to hold the fingers and palms together (Figure 2.10). However, limited joint mobility in diabetes is multifactorial, and may also be due to flexor tenosynovitis, Dupuytren's contracture or nodal osteoarthritis. Good diabetic control is essential. Injection for symptomatic flexor tenosynovitis helps. No specific treatment exists for the skin changes.

Raynaud's phenomenon

This disorder, which results from severe vasospasm in response to a temperature change, causes marked and typically sharply demarcated pallor of one or more digits. As circulation recovers, the digit becomes blue (cyanotic) and then bright red because of rebound hyperaemia – the 'triphasic colour change'. Raynaud's is more common in females than males. In young women, the condition is often

a harmless nuisance, requiring warm gloves and sometimes vasodilators. Its onset for the first time in older people warrants investigation. Raynaud's may also be part of a systemic autoimmune disorder (rheumatoid arthritis, systemic lupus erythematosus or systemic sclerosis), and it occasionally leads to necrosis. Autoimmune-associated Raynaud's can be extremely severe and requires specialist referral (Herrick, 2012). Vibration white finger is a compensationable industrial disease in people who use vibrating tools. It can be clinically similar to Raynaud's but the patient's occupational history will usually distinguish the difference Primary Raynaud's phenomenon may resolve spontaneously.

Other disorders

Ganglion

A ganglion is a cystic swelling in continuity with a joint or tendon sheath through a fault in the capsule. It is filled with clear, viscous fluid rich in hyaluronan. Ganglia are common on the dorsal wrist, are often painless and resolve spontaneously (50% at 6 years). Often, reassurance of the patient is all that is required. Wrist splints relieve the pain. Aspiration and injection are rarely effective, and surgical excision is best if the ganglion is persistent and painful.

Chronic (work-related) upper limb pain

The main symptom of chronic (work-related) upper limb disorder is pain (Box 2.1). A local cause (carpal tunnel syndrome, flexor or extensor tenosynovitis or tennis elbow) may be the initial trigger. The patient develops widespread pain that is often disproportionate to the findings but causes great distress. A prior change in work pattern may exist, and often disharmony is found at the workplace. The cause is unclear, but neurophysiological and psychosocial factors are probably involved. The phenomenon of central 'wind-up' of pain seen in many chronic pain syndromes probably plays a role. It is easy for the doctor to find the problem exasperating and difficult to understand, but it is best managed non-judgementally. Early reductions in work activities and pain control measures are important, but it is best not to ask the person to take too much time off. Advice to the employer to review work practices reduces the risk of litigation. Referral to a specialist pain clinic should be considered (Barr et al., 2004).

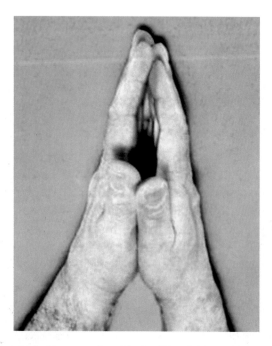

Figure 2.10 Positive prayer sign: diabetic stiff hands (also nodal osteoarthritis and flexor tenosynovitis)

Box 2.1 **Characteristics of chronic upper limb pain syndrome**

- Often starts as carpal tunnel syndrome, flexor tenosynovitis or tennis elbow
- Spreads to affect the upper arm more diffusely
- Physical signs may be minimal
- Often associated with:
  - use of keyboards
  - sudden changes in work practices
  - disharmony at work
  - anxiety and sleeplessness
- Neurophysiological and psychosocial mechanisms involved
- Best dealt with non-judgementally

Osteonecrosis (rare)

Kienböck's disease is the late result of a dorsiflexion wrist injury often seen in manual labourers. Fragmentation and collapse of the lunate cause shortening of the carpus and secondary osteoarthritis. Osteonecrosis takes up to 18 months to appear on X-ray radiography.

Scaphoid bone fracture

Pain in the anatomical snuffbox after a fall onto an outstretched hand requires an immediate X-ray examination, although a fracture is not always visible immediately. Any severe wrist injury should be managed as a potential scaphoid fracture with a plaster, and a further X-ray should be taken 3 weeks later. Unrecognized scaphoid fracture leads to pain associated with failed union, osteonecrosis and secondary osteoarthritis.

Writer's cramp

Writer's cramp is the most common type of focal dystonia and occurs during complex hand activities such as writing or playing a musical instrument. Clumsiness and painful tightness in the hand and forearm occur during writing or playing, and abnormal tension and strange posturing develop. They are task specific, i.e. related to writing, typing or playing an instrument, and don't occur with other activities. Focal dystonias are often inappropriately described as 'psychological'. Local botulinum toxin injection produces temporary relief. Retraining and learning new techniques help some patients, but the outlook is poor and the condition may lead to the end of a musician's career.

Septic arthritis

Septic arthritis or tenosynovitis of the hand or wrist are rare. It is an important differential diagnosis of acute pseudogout of the wrist. If septic arthritis is suspected, it should be treated as a medical emergency and referred to accident and emergency or a specialist unit for investigation and appropriate intravenous antibiotic treatment. The patient is usually febrile and unwell. It is essential not to start antibiotics before all the necessary samples have been taken for culture. Non-steroidal anti-inflammatory drugs and analgesics can be given for pain, which is often severe.

Complex regional pain syndrome

This poorly understood syndrome causes persistent burning pain and stiffness in the hand, usually after a minor injury. The pain is out of proportion to the original injury and this is a useful clue to the diagnosis. There is swelling initially with increased skin sensitivity. Later, the skin becomes atrophic. Early recognition and referral to a pain management centre may reduce the risk of long-term pain and disability.

Local corticosteroid injection technique

During local corticosteroid injections (Box 2.2), an injection of local (or topical) anaesthetic is followed by 0.2–1 mL of a suitable insoluble steroid preparation, such as hydrocortisone acetate 25 mg/mL, depot methylprednisolone 40 mg/mL or triamcinolone acetate 40 mg/mL. Methylprednisolone and triamcinolone are about five times as powerful as hydrocortisone on a milligram per milligram basis.

Box 2.2 **Local corticosteroid injection technique**

- Hand and arm well supported
- Equipment readily to hand
- Clean skin thoroughly
- Use small-bore needle
- Inject small volume of local anaesthetic
- Inject corticosteroid through same needle
- Always inject under low pressure

It is best first to introduce the needle with local anaesthetic and then to inject the steroid under low pressure through the same needle. Patients should be warned that the pain might increase for a day or two after injection. Superficial injections or leakage of the corticosteroid along the needle track cause local skin depigmentation and atrophy of subcutaneous fat; this is more likely with depot injections of steroid. Ultrasound-guided injections in superficial lesions may reduce the risk of steroid-induced skin thinning and depigmentation.

Consent from the patient should always be obtained.

References

Anakwe RE, Middleton SD. Osteoarthritis at the base of the thumb. *BMJ* 2011; **343**: d7122.

Barr AE, Barbe MF, Clark BD. Work-related musculoskeletal disorders of the hand and wrist: epidemiology, pathophysiology, and sensorimotor changes. *Journal of Orthopaedic and Sports Physical Therapy*, 2004; **34**: 610–627.

Herrick AL.The pathogenesis, diagnosis and treatment of Raynaud phenomenon. *Nature Reviews Rheumatology* 2012; **8**: 469–479.

Huisstede BM, Hoogvliet P, Randsdorp MS, Glerum S, van Middlekoop M, Koes BW. Carpal tunnel syndrome. Part I: effectiveness of nonsurgical treatments – a systematic review. *Archives of Physical Medicine and Rehabilitation* 2010a; **91**: 981–1004.

Huisstede BM, Randsdorp MS, Coert JH, Glerum S, van Middelkoop M, Koes BW. Carpal tunnel syndrome. Part II: effectiveness of surgical treatments – a systematic review. *Archives of Physical Medicine and Rehabilitation* 2010b; **91**: 1005–1024.

Peters-Veluthamaningal C, Winters JC, Groenier KH, Meyboom-DeJong B. Randomised controlled trial of local corticosteroid injections for de Quervain's tenosynovitis in general practice. *BMC Musculoskeletal Disorders* 2009; **10**: 131.

Schubert C, Hui-Chou HG, See AP, Deune EG. Corticosteroid injection therapy for trigger finger or thumb: a retrospective review of 577 digits. *Hand* 2013; **8**: 439–444.

Townley WA, Baker R, Sheppard N, Grobbelaar AO. Dupuytren's contracture unfolded. *BMJ* 2006; **332**: 397.

Yagev Y, Carel RS, Yagev R. Assessment of work-related risk factors for carpal tunnel syndrome. *Israel Medical Association Journal* 2001; **3**: 569–571.

Further reading

Bland JDP. Carpal tunnel syndrome. *BMJ* 2007; **335**: 343–346.

Zhang W, Doherty M, Leeb BF *et al.* EULAR evidence based recommendations for the management of hand osteoarthritis: report of a Task Force of the EULAR Standing Committee for International Clinical Studies Including Therapeutics (ESCISIT). *Annals of the Rheumatic Diseases* 2007; **66**: 377–388.

CHAPTER 3

Pain in the Neck, Shoulder and Arm

Caroline Mitchell[1] and David Stanley[2]

[1] Academic Unit of Primary Medical Care, University of Sheffield, Sheffield, UK
[2] BMI Thornbury Hospital, Sheffield, UK

OVERVIEW

- Neck, shoulder and elbow pain are common musculoskeletal problems for which patients seek healthcare.

- Non-specific neck pain is often acute, self-limiting and attributed to a mechanical cause. Persistence or recurrence, however, is common. For most patients with acute neck pain and no 'red flags', further investigation is not normally necessary.

- Neck pain usually responds to analgesia and simple mobilization exercises. High-quality evidence for the effectiveness of many treatment modalities is limited and often contradictory.

- For patients presenting with shoulder pain, the diagnosis can usually be made clinically. Treatment aims to control pain and restore movement and function of the shoulder.

- Most shoulder complaints are due to rotator cuff disease, which is increasingly prevalent with advancing age. Adhesive capsulitis, or 'frozen shoulder', is a significantly disabling condition, occurring usually in middle age. It can be distinguished from rotator cuff disease by the presence of global restriction of shoulder movements. It is also more common in people with diabetes and following periods of immobility, for example after stroke, fracture or surgery.

- The most common elbow disorder is lateral epicondylitis. This is thought to be an overload injury at the origin of the common extensors at the lateral epicondyle. Patients present with pain and tenderness over the lateral epicondyle and pain with resisted movements. Prognosis is generally favourable, with 80% recovery within a year. Management is directed towards controlling pain, avoiding aggravating activities and maintaining movement.

The neck and shoulder are two of the most common sources of musculoskeletal pain. Neck pain has a self-reported point prevalence of between 10% and 20%. The majority of neck pain is acute and self-limiting and can be attributed to a mechanical or postural cause. However, moderate or severe symptoms may persist in up to 30% of patients.

Shoulder pain has a self-reported point prevalence of between 14% and 26% in the general population. The incidence of shoulder pain increases with age, as does its functional impact. About one-quarter of all new episodes presenting for care resolve fully within 1 month, and nearly half have resolved within 3 months of onset. However, persistence or recurrence of shoulder symptoms within a year of initial presentation is common (in up to 50% of people).

Anatomy and function of the neck and shoulder joint

By the actions of the surrounding muscles, the neck moves almost constantly during waking hours through flexion, extension and rotation at the intervertebral and facet joints of the seven cervical vertebrae.

The shoulder is a series of articulations. It includes the glenohumeral joint, acromioclavicular joint and scapulothoracic articulation which allows the scapula to slide on the ribcage (Figure 3.1). Soft tissue structures – capsules, ligaments, muscles, tendons, bursae and neurovascular elements – complete the framework and allow remarkable mobility to be achieved. Instability problems involving the glenohumeral joint usually occur in young men and are most often the result of trauma. Infrequently, instability is associated with congenital laxity. With increasing age, rotator cuff disease results in shoulder pain and limited shoulder function.

The elbow is a compound synovial joint composed of a complex of two closely related articulations between the humerus and both the ulna and radius. It is supported by ligaments and muscles.

Clinical evaluation

Neck and arm pain have a wide differential diagnosis, making it hard at times to distinguish between pain arising from the neck or the shoulder (Figure 3.2). Pain proximal to the shoulder, in the shoulder girdle or over the scapula indicates referred pain from the neck.

It is always important when taking a history to assess the patient's concerns, expectations, functional disability and any psychosocial and occupational issues. Details of hand dominance, trauma, hobbies, sporting activities and previous similar symptoms should be

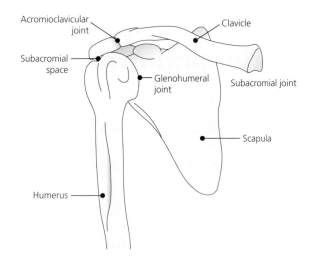

Figure 3.1 The shoulder 'complex' of joints. This includes the scapulothoracic articulation, where the scapula slides on the ribcage. Source: Adapted from Speed *et al.* (2000)

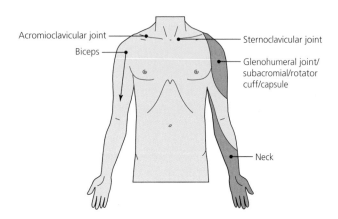

Figure 3.2 Sites and radiation of pain in the shoulder, arm and neck. Source: Adapted from Speed *et al.* (2000)

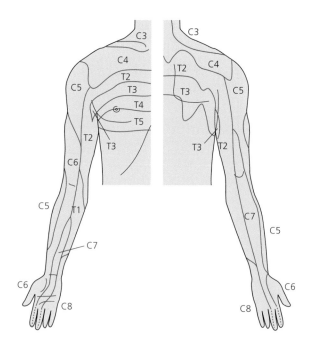

Figure 3.3 Features of cervical nerve root lesions

noted together with all treatments that have been undertaken. Significant past and current medical history – including prescribed drugs and adverse reactions – should be recorded. The history must also elicit the presence of any clinical features that indicate potentially serious systemic and musculoskeletal pathology.

The clinician should determine the mode of onset and duration of the pain, its nature, site, radiation, temporal characteristics, exacerbating and relieving features, and associated symptoms. Disturbed sleep is common with both neck and shoulder pain. However, nocturnal pain should raise suspicion of nerve root pain, bony pathology or underlying malignancy, particularly if there is a history of cancer and/or systemic symptoms.

Radiation of pain distally from the upper arm or elbow suggests referred pain from the neck or peripheral neurological lesions (see Figure 3.2). Neurological symptoms should be sought and their distribution ascertained (Figure 3.3).

Joint swelling around the shoulder or elbow can occur in relation to arthropathy, infection or trauma. Other notable symptoms of arthropathy include stiffness, clicking, clunking or locking. It is important to enquire about proximal muscle pain and weakness in the upper and lower limbs as this may represent

a neurological disorder. Systemic symptoms, such as fevers, night sweats, weight loss, generalized joint pains, new 'lumps' (lympadenopathy, mass lesions) and new respiratory symptoms, should be specifically sought and recorded.

A structured examination must define the source of the pain and the degree of functional deficit and co-existing pathologies. It includes careful inspection, palpation, movement, special clinical tests and a neurological assessment. Depending on the findings, appropriate further investigations should then be undertaken.

Neck pain

Pain in the neck usually occurs due to poorly defined mechanical influences but may result from pathology within the spine or be referred from elsewhere. A list of the differential diagnoses of neck pain is shown in Box 3.1. When considering the diagnosis, it is important to look for specific 'red flags' as these indicate that there might be a serious underlying cause of the complaint (Table 3.1).

Restricted cervical movements and local tenderness help to confirm the local origin of neck pain. Risk factors include manual jobs, heavy workload, increasing age and depression. Chronicity is weakly predicted by the presence of concomitant low back pain, older age and previous episodes of neck pain.

Simple mechanical neck pain describes a common, usually self-limiting, clinical presentation of pain with or without restricted movement, but without neurological or 'red flag' features. Onset may be acute (acute torticollis, or 'wry neck') or gradual, and, like low back pain, tends to be recurrent. It usually responds to conservative treatment with analgesics and simple exercise regimes. Patients should be instructed to return for further assessment if symptoms persist or change in quality. Neck pain may be accompanied by myofascial or diffuse regional pain often involving the shoulder girdle and reproduced by palpation of trigger points ('knots' within muscle).

Box 3.1 **Differential diagnosis of neck pain**

Structural
- Mechanical or non-specific
- Prolapsed intervertebral disc
- Cervical myelopathy

Neoplasm
- Primary or secondary

Inflammatory
- Rheumatoid arthritis
- Polymyalgia rheumatica and giant cell or temporal arteritis
- Spondyloarthropathies

Infection
- Discitis
- Osteomyelitis
- Paraspinal abscess

Metabolic
- Paget's disease

Myofascial
- Myofascial syndromes, fibromyalgia

Table 3.1 "Red flags" or clinical features indicative of potentially serious pathology in the neck and/or shoulder

'Red flags'	Potential pathology
History of cancer, symptoms and signs of cancer, unexplained deformity, mass or swelling	Malignancy
Fever, systemically unwell, redness and swelling	Infection
Trauma, epileptic fit. electric shock, loss of rotation and normal shape	Unreduced shoulder dislocation
Recent trauma, acute disabling pain and significant weakness, positive 'drop arm' sign	Acute rotator cuff tear
Diffuse poorly localized pain and/or abnormal sensation, unexplained wasting, loss of power or altered reflexes	Neurological lesion, cervical radiculopathy, myelopathy
Referred pain: neck pain, myocardial ischaemia, referred diaphragmatic pain, apical lung cancer, metastases	Pain arising from elsewhere
Bilateral shoulder pain with or without neck pain, early morning stiffness	Polymyalgia rheumatic, rheumatoid arthritis, giant cell arteritis
Rapid swelling after trauma	Haemarthrosis of the shoulder

Radicular pain, due to compression of a nerve root from herniation of a cervical disc, or as a result of local infection or tumour, refers to neck pain that radiates into the shoulder girdle and/or arm with paraesthesia or numbness in a root distribution. Subjective weakness is less common. Examination may not reveal the nerve root level because of the extensive overlap of dermatomes (Table 3.2). Motor involvement and/or objective sensory loss warrant urgent referral for specialist assessment. In general, 40–80% of

Table 3.2 Arm dermatomes

Nerve root	Weakness	Reflex change
C5	Shoulder abduction	Biceps
C6	Wrist extension, supination, elbow flexion	Radial
C7	Elbow extension, wrist flexion	Triceps
C8	Finger flexors	NA
T1	Finger abductors	NA

NA = not applicable

people with compressive cervical radiculopathy will have complete resolution of their symptoms over time with conservative treatment. Patients should, however, be specifically advised about 'red flag' symptoms and told to return if there are concerning changes or persistence of symptoms.

Cervical myelopathy (compression of the spinal cord), which may arise due to midline disc herniation, is suggested by a history of difficulty in walking and bladder and bowel dysfunction. Signs of myelopathy below the level of spinal cord involvement may include motor weakness with increased reflexes and tone (upper motor neurone signs), decreased pinprick sensation and loss of position and/or vibration sense. These symptoms warrant urgent referral for specialist assessment.

Whiplash injury, an abrupt flexion/extension movement of the cervical spine as a result of sudden acceleration-deceleration, may occur in road traffic or sporting accidents. It is characterized by neck and arm pain with muscle spasm, and limited neck movements. Symptoms may be persistent, although 50% of patients recover within 3 months and 80% within 12 months. Risk factors for chronicity after whiplash include the severity of the initial symptoms and psychological disturbance. Neurological sensory and/or motor deficit warrants immobilization of the cervical spine and urgent specialist assessment.

Neck pain is common in inflammatory arthritis, and atlantoaxial and subaxial subluxation may develop, particularly in rheumatoid arthritis. Consequently, special care is needed when rheumatoid patients with cervical spine involvement require a general anaesthetic. Osteophytic linking of vertebrae may be seen in ankylosing spondylitis, resulting in reduced or absent cervical spine movement.

Investigation of neck pain

For most patients with acute neck pain and no 'red flags', further investigation (radiographs, blood tests) is not necessary. Due to the high prevalence of asymptomatic degenerative changes in the cervical spine, plain radiographs are rarely diagnostic, and pain severity correlates poorly with radiographic abnormalities.

Magnetic resonance imaging (MRI) is highly sensitive in detecting disc and cord abnormalities if these are suspected, whereas computed tomography is better for evaluation of bone.

Treatment of neck pain

Patients should be informed of the generally favourable prognosis of neck pain and the fact that serious underlying conditions are very unlikely. Pertinent psychosocial and occupational issues may need to be explored in order to tailor the management plan.

Neck pain usually responds to simple analgesia and advice on self-care, including simple mobilization and exercises. High-quality evidence for the effectiveness of many treatment modalities is limited and often contradictory.

Advise to stay active – Encourage patients to persist with their normal activities. There is no evidence that collars reduce pain or improve function, nor is there evidence about special pillows. In general, patients are advised to sleep on their side with a single pillow supporting the neck. Early mobilization and return to normal activity may reduce pain in people with acute whiplash injury more than immobilization or rest with a collar.

Drug therapy – There is limited evidence about the relative benefits of paracetamol, opioid analgesics, non-steroidal anti-inflammatory drugs (NSAIDs) and antidepressants. Potential benefits versus the risks of NSAIDs should be considered, particularly in high-risk patients (consider potential drug interactions, the elderly, co-existing asthma, past history of peptic ulceration, renal impairment and whether co-prescription of a gastroprotective drug is required). All patients on regular analgesia should be reviewed for both efficacy and potential adverse effects. If there is significant nocturnal pain, a tricyclic drug at night may be helpful (e.g. amitriptyline 10–50 mg orally).

Exercises – Gentle neck exercises may be a useful and effective treatment for acute neck pain. The best type and mix of exercise have not been defined, but include stretching and strengthening exercises. Proprioceptive retraining exercises are usually prescribed by a physiotherapist. Patients should either be provided with exercise self-care leaflets or directed to an appropriate online resource (www.arthritisresearchuk.org/). Exercises for cervical radiculopathy are unproven. Exercise therapy is contraindicated in the presence of myelopathy.

Mobilization or manipulative techniques – However, unproven mobilization or manipulative techniques for both acute and chronic pain (typically performed by physiotherapists, chiropractors or osteopaths), either alone or in combination with other physical interventions, may have only a modest effect.

Multidisciplinary biopsychosocial rehabilitation – The principle underlying multidisciplinary rehabilitation for chronic neck pain is to simultaneously address all components (physical, psychological and social) of the patient's pain experience. Cognitive behavioural therapy has been shown to decrease time off work and other behavioural manifestations of pain but not to change the degree of pain.

Other non-operative treatments – The efficacy of most passive non-manipulative therapies (heat, massage, transcutaneous electrical nerve stimulation, pulsed electromagnetic field treatment) is not supported by evidence. Acupuncture may provide short-term pain relief in people with chronic neck pain, but evidence is limited. There is also limited evidence about the effectiveness of massage for neck pain. Similarly, myofascial trigger-point injections using local

anaesthetic into tender points have not been shown to be beneficial in reducing chronic neck pain. There is inconclusive evidence about the effectiveness of traction for neck pain which in any case should not be performed before imaging to exclude spinal cord compression or a large disc protrusion. A short course of oral glucocorticoids prescribed by a specialist, and after appropriate investigation, may be of benefit for cervical radiculopathy but is unproven. Facet joint injections, medial branch blocks and percutaneous radiofrequency denervation are performed under the premise that pain arises from the facet joint; however, the evidence to support these procedures is very limited. Botulinum A intramuscular injections have been shown to be ineffective for neck pain with or without radiculopathy.

Surgery – Surgery is not indicated for patients with neck pain in the absence of neurological symptoms of radiculopathy or myelopathy. When appropriate, an anterior cervical discectomy with or without fusion is the most commonly used procedure.

Shoulder pain

The differential diagnosis of shoulder pain is summarized in Box 3.2. Pain may also arise in the scapulothoracic region, and a list of differential diagnoses is shown in Box 3.3. 'Red flags' or clinical features suggestive of serious underlying pathology in people who present with shoulder pain are shown in Table 3.1.

Box 3.2 **Differential diagnosis of shoulder pain**

Pain arising from the shoulder
- Rotator cuff disease or associated with the rotator cuff
  - Tendinitis, partial- and full-thickness tears
  - Calcific tendonitis
  - Complete rotator cuff tear
  - Rupture of the origin of the long head of biceps
  - Subacromial bursitis
- Adhesive capsulitis ('frozen shoulder')
- Glenohumeral joint
  - Osteoarthritis
  - Rheumatoid arthritis
  - Septic arthritis
  - Instability and dislocation
  - Traumatic labral tears
- Acromioclavicular and sternoclavicular disorders
- Malignancy – myeloma, bony metastases

Pain arising from elsewhere
- Polymyalgia rheumatic
- Referred pain from the neck
- Myocardial ischaemia, referred diaphragmatic pain
- Lesions of axillary, suprascapular, long thoracic, radial, musculocutaneous nerves, brachial plexus, referred pain
- Malignancy – apical lung cancer

Regional or diffuse pain
- Myofascial pain syndromes, fibromyalgia

Box 3.3 **Differential diagnosis of scapulothoracic pain**

- Local muscle injury
- Myofascial pain syndrome
- Subscapular bursitis
- Snapping scapula
- Suprascapular nerve palsy
- Referred pain from cervical or thoracic spine
- Bone injury, e.g. fracture or metastatic deposit in scapula

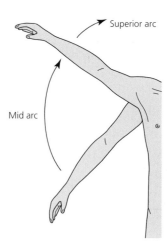

Figure 3.5 Mid or superior painful arcs of abduction represent subacromial impingement or acromioclavicular pathology, respectively

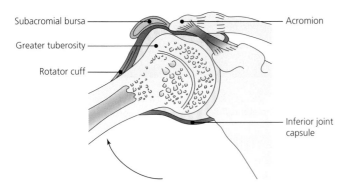

Figure 3.4 Subacromial impingement of the rotator cuff can occur with abduction of the arm. Source: Adapted from Speed *et al.* (2000)

Rotator cuff disease

Most shoulder complaints (60–70%) are due to rotator cuff disease, a broad term that includes a wide array of diagnostic labels. Some labels derive from clinical features (e.g. painful arc syndrome); some from assumed pathophysiology (e.g. impingement syndrome – impingement upon the cuff tendons between the acromion and head of the humerus) (Figure 3.4) and some from the imaging appearance (e.g. calcific tendinitis, rotator cuff tendinitis or tendinopathy, subacromial bursitis and partial- or full-thickness tears).

Based upon MRI scans, asymptomatic cuff tears are common. The incidence increases with age and it has been shown that more than 50% of normal subjects aged over 60 years have tears, suggesting that it may be part of the normal ageing process combined with repetitive microtrauma. A significant number of asymptomatic tears will become symptomatic over time, and long-standing tears can result in glenohumeral arthritis. Rotator cuff disorders may occasionally occur in young people engaged in overhead sports activities but are most common in middle and older age. Occupational associations include repetitive movements, working with vibrating tools, working in awkward and/or overhead postures and performing similar work for a prolonged period.

The patient typically complains of pain felt in the shoulder and/or lateral aspect of the upper arm that is worse with overhead activities and at night, particularly when lying on the affected side.

Characteristic features of the examination include pain in the midrange of active abduction (Figure 3.5) and on resisted shoulder abduction with or without external rotation. Impingement pain is produced if the arm is flexed forwards to 90°, adducted and internally rotated. In contrast to adhesive capsulitis, which causes global restriction of both active and passive movements, passive range of

motion is often normal in rotator cuff disease, although certain movements may be restricted by pain. It is therefore important to assess both active (patient moves the shoulder) and passive (the examiner moves the shoulder) movements to distinguish apparent from true restriction of shoulder motion.

Painful weakness and muscle atrophy suggest significant rotator cuff tears. The 'drop arm' test suggests a complete or large rotator cuff tear.

Calcific tendinitis usually affects women aged 30–50 years and is associated with the formation and resorption of calcific deposits within the cuff. The patient typically presents with acute onset of severe pain and severe limitation of shoulder movements due to pain. In the more chronic stages, pain and catching are reported, and signs of impingement may be noted.

Diagnosis – The diagnosis of rotator cuff disease can usually be made clinically. Blood tests and plain radiographs are not necessary in the absence of 'red flags' unless there is a failure to respond to treatment. Plain radiographs may exclude other causes of shoulder pain, such as significant glenohumeral osteoarthritis. If calcific tendinitis is suspected, there may be fluffy calcific deposits, situated just proximal to the rotator cuff insertion (Figure 3.6), and the erythrocyte sedimentation rate and white cell count may also be raised. Ultrasound and MRI will detect full-thickness rotator cuff tears but have less accuracy for detecting partial-thickness tears. These investigations are useful in patients who fail to respond to conservative treatment regimes.

Treatment – The aims of treatment of rotator cuff disease are to control pain and restore movement and function of the shoulder. Paracetamol is suitable as a first-line therapy and may be supplemented by short-term mild opioids such as codeine phosphate. NSAIDs (alongside gastroprotective therapy if indicated) may provide short-term pain relief if there are no contraindications to their use. Initially, patients may need to modify their activities and address occupational factors.

Subacromial injection of depot corticosteroid and local anaesthetic may provide rapid relief of pain, but its effect may be limited and not maintained beyond a few weeks. If the initial response is

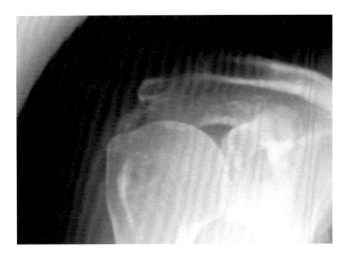

Figure 3.6 Plain X-ray showing calcific tendinitis. Source: Adapted from Speed *et al.* (2000)

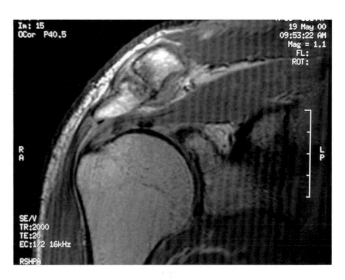

Figure 3.7 MRI scan of shoulder, showing acromioclavicular osteophytes and underlying rotator cuff tendinitis

good, injections may be repeated up to two or three times at 6-weekly intervals. There is insufficient evidence to prove whether injections performed under fluoroscopy or ultrasound whilst increasing the accuracy of needle placement significantly produce better outcomes.

For disabling persistent symptoms, physiotherapy comprising a combination of mobilization techniques and directed exercises designed to strengthen and stabilize the cuff and scapular muscles can be used alone or combined with other measures. Global strengthening and proprioception training may reduce instability and minimize impingement in those with glenohumeral joint hypermobility.

The benefits of heat or ice packs, low-power laser, ultrasound and pulsed electromagnetic field therapy are unproven. Acupuncture and suprascapular nerve blockade may provide short-term pain relief but the evidence for these treatments is limited. Trials have failed to establish the efficacy of extracorporeal shock wave therapy (ESWT) for rotator cuff disease.

Surgery is indicated when symptoms fail to respond to conservative management. Operative treatment involves decompression of the subacromial space, with or without rotator cuff repair. MRI may be useful to plan surgery (Figure 3.7). Observational studies have reported good outcomes of surgery, although three randomized controlled trials found that surgery was not superior to treatment with supervised exercises.

Subacromial steroid injections, needling of calcific deposits under fluoroscopic guidance and percutaneous needle aspiration and lavage by ultrasound guidance have all been advocated to relieve pain in calcific tendinitis. There is, however, no data from controlled trials to show that these techniques are effective. Ultrasound can provide short-term pain relief and, like ESWT, may improve the radiological appearance of calcific deposits but if symptoms persist, surgical excision of the calcific deposit is normally required.

Adhesive capsulitis

Adhesive capsulitis ('frozen shoulder' or painful stiff shoulder) affects 2–5% of the population, women slightly more often than men, and 10–36% of people with diabetes, in whom it is more severe. It occurs most commonly in the fifth and sixth decades of life and is rare before the age of 40 years. The cause is poorly understood. It is usually idiopathic, although it may occur in the context of prolonged shoulder immobility (e.g. following a stroke or cardiac, breast or shoulder surgery).

Three phases have been described:

- initial gradual development of diffuse and severe shoulder pain, typically worse at night with an inability to lie on the affected side – this usually lasts between 2 and 9 months
- a stiff phase with less severe pain present at the end range of movement, characterized by global stiffness and severe loss of shoulder movement – this lasts between 4 and 12 months
- and finally a recovery phase characterized by a gradual return of movement over 5 to 24 months.

Severe disability may result in absence from work and an inability to perform leisure activities. Although generally thought to run a self-limiting course over 2–3 years, some studies have found that up to 40% of patients have persistent symptoms and restricted movement beyond 3 years.

Diagnosis – The diagnosis can be made clinically, as the restriction of both active and passive movement in all planes of movement, especially external rotation, distinguishes it from other causes of shoulder pain. Plain radiographs are normal and therefore exclude a diagnosis of glenohumeral arthritis.

Treatment – Treatment is needed to control severe pain, improve range of movement and promote function. Patients should be informed of the generally favourable prognosis. Treatment with analgesia and NSAIDS is the same as for rotator cuff disease.

Intra-articular injection of corticosteroid combined with local anaesthetic using either an anterior or posterior approach may provide rapid pain relief, but the effect is rarely sustained beyond 6–7 weeks.

Alternative treatments for patients who are struggling to work or continue social activities include arthrodilatation, manipulation under anaesthesia and arthroscopic capsular release.

Arthrodilatation of the glenohumeral joint (or hydrodilatation) is performed under radiological guidance, usually using a combination of local anaesthetic, corticosteroid and saline to a mean volume of 20–45 mL. It has been demonstrated to have a sustained beneficial effect on pain, function and range of movement and is the preferred treatment option of some clinicians. It may be more effective in the intermediate (stiff) and recovery stages and may also be repeated if the effect wanes over time.

Manipulation under anaesthesia can also be a very effective treatment. It is normally combined with an intra-articular steroid and local anaesthetic injection. Postoperatively, the patient must perform regular physiotherapy exercises to maximize the improvement achieved by the procedure. If the technique is not performed carefully, there is a small risk of fracturing the proximal humerus as the shoulder is manipulated and for this reason the patient must be advised of this potential complication when consent is taken.

An arthroscopic capsular release is an alternative to manipulation under anaesthesia. The procedure is performed either under general anaesthesia or by using a suprascapular nerve block. The arthroscope is inserted into the glenohumeral joint and then via a separate arthroscopic portal instruments are introduced into the shoulder to allow division of the thickened capsule. A gentle shoulder manipulation is normally performed at the end of the procedure. Postoperatively, physiotherapy is undertaken to assist with rehabilitation and speed recovery.

Other shoulder disorders

Acromioclavicular and sternoclavicular joint disorders – Osteoarthritis of the acromioclavicular joint is common and presents with well-localized pain and tenderness over the joint. Examination may reveal a superior painful arc of abduction (see Figure 3.5) and restriction of passive horizontal adduction of the shoulder. It can be managed symptomatically with analgesics, and local corticosteroid injections may also provide relief. Surgery in the form of excision of the distal 5 mm of the clavicle can be effective in resistant cases.

The acromioclavicular joint can also be strained or dislocated as a result of trauma or sports injuries. This can be managed with taping and analgesia and, in severe cases, surgery may be required.

The sternoclavicular joint can be the presenting site of an inflammatory arthritis, but it is frequently overlooked. Rarely, the sternoclavicular and/or acromioclavicular joints can be involved in the rare SAPHO syndrome (synovitis, acne, pustulosis, hyperostosis, osteomyelitis).

Glenohumeral joint arthritides – Isolated osteoarthritis of the shoulder is rare but may occur following fractures of the humeral head or neck, large rotator cuff tears, or as an end-result of rheumatoid arthritis. It may be suspected, particularly in the older age group, if there is a limited range of painful movement sometimes accompanied by crepitus. Plain radiographs will confirm the diagnosis.

Milwaukee shoulder, which mainly affects elderly women, is a severe destructive apatite-associated arthropathy that presents with shoulder pain, limited movements and a large joint effusion. Aspiration reveals a large amount of blood-tinged synovial fluid, which contains calcium phosphate crystals.

New onset of bilateral shoulder pain and stiffness should prompt consideration of polymyalgia rheumatica in those over 50 years of age. Polymyalgia rheumatica commonly presents with proximal pain and weakness of the upper limbs although, occasionally, there is initial asymmetry/unilateral symptoms. The patient may report stiffness, fatigue-associated disability and also proximal lower limb/pelvic girdle symptoms. A raised ESR and CRP are used to confirm the diagnosis and a rapid response to steroids is pathognomonic of the condition. It is important to exclude co-existing symptoms and signs of temporal arthritis such as headache, jaw claudication, visual disturbance and tenderness of the scalp which warrant urgent (same-day) specialist discussion and/or assessment. Treatment must be urgently started with initiation of higher dose steroids in order to prevent irreversible visual loss.

Biceps tendinitis/rupture – The long head of the biceps tendon passes through the bicipital groove of the anterior proximal humerus and is often involved in rotator cuff disease but can present as an isolated problem. It causes anterior shoulder pain, aggravated by lifting, carrying objects and overhead reaching. If the tendon becomes severely frayed, it may rupture, giving rise to a 'popeye' sign with the biceps muscle appearing more distal in the arm compared to the contralateral side. It is important to distinguish this condition, which usually doesn't require treatment, from a distal biceps rupture. Distal biceps ruptures usually occur after heavy lifting and are usually associated with antecubital fossa bruising. The biceps muscle after this injury appears more proximal in the arm when compared to the contralateral side. Distal biceps tendon ruptures should be referred urgently for consideration of surgical repair.

Shoulder instability – General glenohumeral instability or looseness may be seen in young women with weak shoulder muscles, in young athletes (especially swimmers and throwers) and following large rotator cuff tendon tears, especially in the elderly. There may be diffuse shoulder pain, and instability may be multi- or unidirectional. The majority of patients with unidirectional instability are young and have a clear history of traumatic dislocation of the shoulder. If the shoulder recurrently dislocates, referral for stabilization is appropriate.

Glenoid labrum (cartilage) injuries – These can cause persistent shoulder pain and instability, and usually occur after an episode of trauma or dislocation or with overuse. Diagnosis can be difficult, requiring magnetic resonance arthrography or arthroscopy. Management involves pain control and rehabilitation, which is followed by surgery if necessary.

Neurological causes – Shoulder pain may result from neurological causes, including nerve root entrapment at the neck, brachial plexus lesions or peripheral nerve lesions, including the axillary, long thoracic, suprascapular, radial or musculocutaneous nerves. Brachial neuritis can affect one or more components of the brachial plexus. Often idiopathic, some cases occur after a viral infection, immunizations or mechanical trauma. A sudden onset of diffuse pain in the shoulder, upper arm and occasionally forearm is accompanied by weakness, wasting, scapular winging and variable sensory loss of the affected neuromuscular structures. Electromyographic studies may be confirmatory. Tricyclic agents, carbamazepine, gabapentin or pregabalin may be helpful. Rehabilitation is started early to prevent stiffness and improve function.

Thoracic outlet syndrome – Compression of the neurovascular structures of the thoracic outlet, brachial plexus and subclavian artery may occur due to local masses, a high first or cervical rib or fibrous bands. Symptoms depend on the structures compressed, but are usually exacerbated by heavy manual work. Neurogenic symptoms usually predominate, including aching in the arm, paraesthesia and weakness. Vascular symptoms are usually intermittent cyanosis and trophic skin changes can occur. A causative structure is rarely identified, and management is symptomatic.

Elbow and forearm pain

Lateral and medial epicondylitis

The 12-month period prevalence of elbow pain has been estimated to be 11.2%. Box 3.4 displays a list of differential diagnoses of elbow pain. Most complaints of elbow pain are due to lateral epicondylitis ('tennis elbow' or lateral elbow pain), which has an estimated annual incidence in general practice of 4–7 per 1000 patients. People aged between 40 and 50 years are most commonly affected. Lateral epicondylitis is thought to be an overload injury at the origin of the common extensors at the lateral epicondyle, and typically follows minor and often unrecognized trauma of the extensor muscles of the forearm. In spite of the term 'tennis elbow', tennis is a direct cause in only 5% of cases. Risk factors include repetitive wrist turning or hand gripping. Medial epicondylitis, or 'golfer's elbow', is a similar but less common condition involving the common flexors at their origin at the medial epicondyle.

Both conditions are characterized by pain and tenderness over the respective epicondyle, and pain on resisted movements: resisted dorsiflexion of the wrist, middle finger, or both, in lateral epicondylitis (Figure 3.8), and resisted flexion of the wrist in medial epicondylitis. Both may be aggravated by repetitive movements and lifting. There

may be night pain, early morning stiffness and stiffness after periods of inactivity. Pain referred from the neck or shoulder is distinguishable by less localized symptoms, associated neurological symptoms and the lack of local signs. Pain arising from the elbow joint is usually more posterior and less well localized and may be associated with an elbow effusion, making it difficult to straighten the elbow.

Lateral and medial epicondylitis are generally self-limiting and patients should be informed of the generally favourable prognosis. In a general practice trial, 80% of patients with elbow pain of already greater than 4 weeks' duration were recovered after 1 year, simply following an expectant policy without any specific treatment. Prognostic factors found to be at least moderately associated with a poorer outcome at 1 year include previous occurrence, high physical strain at work, manual jobs, high baseline levels of pain and/or distress, passive coping and less social support.

Treatment – Interventions have mainly been tested for lateral epicondylitis, but the results are probably generalizable to medial epicondylitis. Treatment in the acute stage involves relative rest and avoidance of specific activities that aggravate the discomfort. Ice may be applied, but there is no data about its effectiveness. Use of a tennis elbow brace or strap is common and may provide short-term pain relief while worn, allowing some return to activity.

Topical and oral NSAIDs may provide short-term relief of pain, although evidence is limited. Local skin reactions may occur with topical treatment and eccentric exercises have been shown to be superior to steroid injection in a single RCT. These may be self-taught using an online video resource or by a physiotherapist.

Stretching and strengthening exercises may be helpful. Most studies have assessed their effect as part of multimodal interventions involving mobilization techniques at the elbow and other physical therapies, with mixed results.

Corticosteroid injection with local anaesthetic in some individuals may provide short-term pain relief (less than 3 months), although over the long term there is no evidence that this is more

---

Box 3.4 **Differential diagnosis of elbow pain**

- Lateral epicondylitis ('tennis elbow' or lateral elbow pain)
- Medial epicondylitis ('golfer's elbow' or medial elbow pain)
- Olecranon bursitis
- Elbow joint
  - Rheumatoid arthritis
  - Septic arthritis
  - Osteoarthritis (rare)
- Cervical radiculopathy
- Tendinopathies
  - Biceps tendinopathy (anterior elbow pain)
  - Triceps tendinopathy, avulsion (posterior elbow pain)
- Nerve compression, entrapment
  - Ulnar neuropathy
  - Median nerve
  - Anterior interosseous nerve
  - Cubital tunnel syndrome

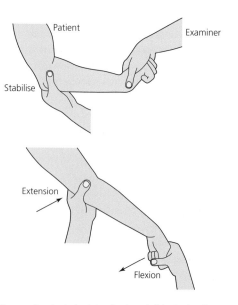

Figure 3.8 Provocation tests for lateral epicondylitis. Resisted extension of the middle finger also elicits pain

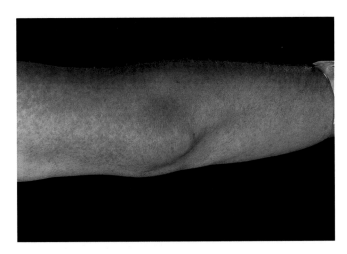

Figure 3.9 Olecranon bursitis, e.g. tophaceous gout at the elbow

effective than no treatment or physiotherapy incorporating 'eccentric' exercises. It is important to consider the close proximity of the ulnar nerve when performing steroid injection for medial epicondylitis. Patients should be advised that the adverse effects of injection are generally mild and include postinjection pain, depigmentation and local skin and subcutaneous atrophy.

Trials of ultrasound have reported marginal or no benefit, while laser therapy trials and trials of various other physical therapies have consistently been negative. There is no strong and consistent evidence that ESWT provides benefits in terms of pain and function in lateral epicondylitis. Acupuncture (needle, laser or electroacupuncture) may provide short-term pain relief. Botulinum toxin injection and topical glyceryl trinitrate have recently been proposed as treatments for lateral epicondylitis, but further research is required before these therapies can be recommended.

Surgery is reserved for patients with recalcitrant symptoms, although evidence of benefit from controlled trials is limited. The most common operations are open excision, debridement and release and/or repair of the extensor or flexor tendon origins at the lateral or medical epicondyle. Percutaneous and arthroscopic procedures have also been described.

Other elbow disorders

Arthritis of the elbow joint may be due to systemic inflammatory arthritides, including rheumatoid and seronegative arthritis, crystal-induced synovitis (gout or pseudogout) and, rarely, septic arthritis. *Neisseria* gonococcus arthritis is rare but should be suspected in at-risk individuals. Osteoarthritis of the elbow is rare and usually relates to previous trauma.

Olecranon bursitis presents with discrete swelling, pain and inflammation at the posterior aspect of the elbow. It may be caused by acute or repetitive trauma, crystals or sepsis (Figure 3.9, Box 3.5). The presence of nodules suggests either rheumatoid arthritis (seen in active disease or as a side effect of methotrexate) or gout (tophi). Infection may follow an abrasion or initial cellulitis and the most common causative organism is *Staphylococcus aureus*. Systemic symptoms such as fever, leucocytosis and elevated inflammatory markers occur with sepsis and crystals. If superimposed infection of an olecranon bursitis is suspected, referral for blood cultures and aspiration for crystals, Gram stain, and culture is warranted.

Box 3.5 **Causes of olecranon bursitis**

- Trauma (acute or chronic)
- Sepsis
- Metabolic or crystals
- Inflammatory arthritis
- Uraemia
- Calcific deposits
- Idiopathic

Broad-spectrum antibiotics and possibly open drainage and lavage are used when sepsis is present.

Steroid injection is often helpful for olecranon bursitis due to inflammatory or crystal arthritis.

The simple, most common form of olecranon bursitis subacute painless mobile swelling over the olecranon process may be conservatively managed with a tubular bandage to protect the bursa. The bursa would normally resolve spontaneously within 4–6 weeks.

Entrapment or inflammation of the ulnar, radial and median nerves can cause neurological disturbances involving the elbow and forearm. Paraesthesia and numbness involving the fourth and fifth fingers accompanied by weakness of the interossei is caused by ulnar neuropathy, the most common compression neuropathy affecting the elbow. Tapping over the ulnar groove may reproduce pain or numbness in the fourth and fifth fingers (Tinel's sign). Nerve conduction studies are helpful in diagnosis. Management depends on the severity of the disorder. Mild cases will often resolve spontaneously but if neurological signs are progressive, referral for possible nerve decompression should be considered.

Reference

Speed C, Hazleman B, Dalton S. *Fast Facts: Soft Tissue Rheumatology*. Health Press, Oxford, 2000.

Further reading

Arthritis Research Campaign. *The Painful Shoulder*. Arthritis Research Campaign, York, 2009. Available at: www.arthritisresearchuk.org/arthritis-information/daily-life/pain-and-arthritis/common-aches-and-pains/shoulder-pain.aspx

Binder A. Neck pain. *Clinical Evidence* 2006; **15**: 1654–1675.

Bjelle A. Epidemiology of shoulder problems. *Baillière's Clinical Rheumatology* 1989; **3**: 437–451.

Buchbinder R, Green S, Struijs P. Tennis elbow. *Clinical Evidence* 2008. Available at: http://clinicalevidence.bmj.com

Dalton S. Clinical examination of the painful shoulder. *Baillière's Clinical Rheumatology* 1989; **3**: 453–474.

Hadler NM. Coping with arm pain in the workplace. *Clinical Orthopaedics and Related Research* 1998; **351**: 57–62.

McClune T, Burton AK, Waddell G. Whiplash associated disorders: a review of the literature to guide patient information and advice. *Emergency Medicine Journal* 2002; **19**: 499–506.

Mitchell C, Adebajo AO, Hay E, Carr A. Shoulder pain: diagnosis and management in primary care. *BMJ* 2005; **331**: 1124–1128.

Royal College of Radiologists. *Making the Best Use of a Department of Clinical Radiology: Guidelines for Doctors*. Royal College of Radiologists, London, 1999.

Speed C. Shoulder pain. *Clinical Evidence* 2005; **14**: 1543–1560.

CHAPTER 4

Low Back Pain

Rajiv K. Dixit[1] and John Dickson[2]

[1] University of California, San Francisco; Northern California Arthritis Center, Walnut Creek, USA
[2] University of Bradford, Bradford, UK

OVERVIEW

- Ninety percent of patients with acute low back pain improve within 6 weeks.
- Degenerative change (osteoarthritis) in the lumbar spine is the most commonly identified cause of pain.
- Early imaging is rarely indicated in the absence of trauma, significant neurological involvement or suspicion of systemic disease (infection, malignancy or spondyloarthritis).
- Imaging abnormalities should be carefully interpreted as they are frequently present in asymptomatic people.
- Most patients respond to a programme that includes analgesia, education, back exercises, aerobic conditioning and weight control.
- Surgery is indicated for severe or progressive neurological deficit and is rarely needed.

Box 4.1 **Causes of LBP**

Mechanical
- Lumbar spondylosis*
- Disc herniation*
- Spondylolisthesis*
- Spinal stenosis*
- Fractures (mostly osteoporotic)
- Idiopathic ('non-specific')

Neoplastic
- Primary
- Metastatic

Inflammatory
- Spondyloarthritides

Infectious
- Vertebral osteomyelitis
- Epidural abscess
- Septic discitis
- Herpes zoster

Metabolic
- Osteoporotic compression fractures
- Paget's disease

Referred pain to spine
- From major viscera, retroperitoneal structures, urogenital system, aorta or hip

*Related to degenerative changes

Low back pain (LBP) is the most common musculoskeletal symptom and represents a major socioeconomic burden. An estimated 80% of the population will experience back pain during their lifetime; 90% of these patients will be largely pain free within 6 weeks. Recurrence, also generally self-limited, is common.

Sciatica is the result of nerve root impingement and occurs in <1% of patients. The pain is radicular (and almost invariably radiates below the level of the knee) in the distribution of a lumbosacral nerve root, sometimes accompanied by sensory and motor deficits. Sciatica should be differentiated from non-neurogenic sclerotomal pain, which arises from pathology within the disc, facet joint or paraspinal muscles and ligaments. Sclerotomal pain is non-dermatomal in distribution and often radiates into the lower extremities but rarely below the knee or with associated paraesthesiae as with sciatica.

Causes of low back pain

Low back pain usually originates from the lumbar spine (Figure 4.1); pain is occasionally referred to the spine from other structures (Box 4.1). Over 95% of LBP is mechanical. Mechanical pain is due to an anatomical abnormality, generally the result of degenerative change, in the lumbar spine that increases with physical activity and is relieved by rest and recumbency. Systemic disease (infection, neoplasm and spondyloarthritis) accounts for only 1–2% of LBP.

Lumbar spondylosis

The most common cause of mechanical LBP is degenerative change. In lumbar spondylosis (lumbar osteoarthritis), degenerative changes occur in the intervertebral disc and facet joint. Imaging

---

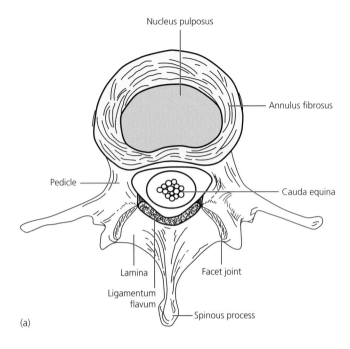

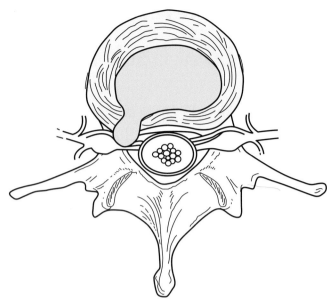

Figure 4.2 Posterolateral disc herniation resulting in nerve root impingement

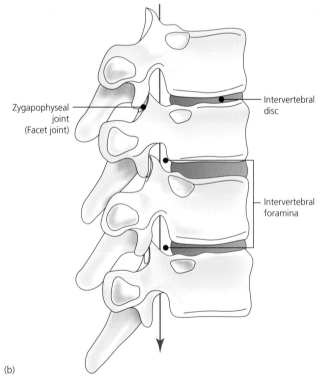

Figure 4.1 Basic anatomy of the lumbar spine; (a) cross-sectional view through a normal lumbar vertebra; (b) lateral view of the lumbar spine

---

> Box 4.2 **Spectrum of symptoms of cauda equina syndrome**
>
> The patient will develop some or all of the following:
>
> - Altered/ reduced urinary sensation
> - Loss of desire to void or poor stream
> - Sexual dysfunction
> - Saddle area anaesthesia
> - Bilateral (or unilateral) sciatica
> - Motor weakness of lower extremities
> - Urinary and faecal incontinence

---

evidence of lumbar spondylosis (disc space and facet joint narrowing, osteophytes and subchondral sclerosis) is common, increases with age and is often asymptomatic.

The clinical spectrum of mechanical LBP secondary to lumbar spondylosis is wide. Patients may present with self-limited acute LBP (with recurrent episodes in some), whereas chronic LBP (often with periods of acute exacerbation) may develop in others. Some patients may develop sclerotomal pain that radiates into the buttocks and lower extremities. Lumbar spondylosis predisposes patients to intervertebral disc herniation, spondylolisthesis and spinal stenosis.

Disc herniation

The nucleus pulposus in a degenerated disc may prolapse and push out from the weakened annulus, usually posterolaterally. Imaging evidence of disc herniation is common even in asymptomatic adults. Occasionally, disc herniation may result in nerve root impingement (Figure 4.2), causing sciatica. Of all clinically significant herniations, 95% involve the L4–5 or L5–S1 disc. Generally, the more caudal nerve root is impinged; that is, the L5 nerve root with L4–5 herniation and S1 nerve root with L5–S1 herniation. In most patients the sciatic pain resolves over a period of weeks.

Rarely, a large midline disc herniation, usually L4–5, compresses the cauda equina. This is a surgical emergency because neurological results are affected by the time to decompression. The full cauda equina syndrome has a symptom complex that includes LBP, bilateral sciatica, bilateral motor weakness of the lower extremities, loss of sensation in a saddle distribution (over the genitals, anus and inner thighs), with bladder and bowel incontinence. Whenever possible, the cauda equina syndrome should be recognized before incontinence becomes established. The spectrum of symptoms is presented in Box 4.2.

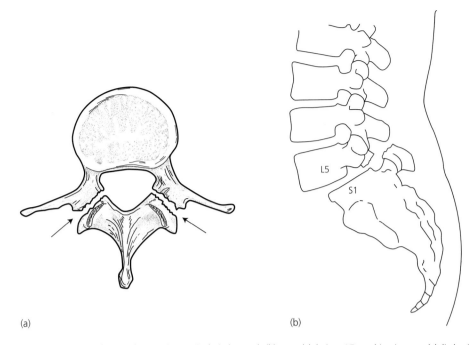

(a)   (b)

Figure 4.3 (a) Spondylolysis with bilateral defects in the pars interarticularis (*arrows*); (b) spondylolysis at L5 resulting in spondylolisthesis at L5–S1

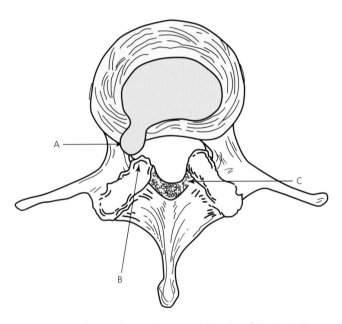

Figure 4.4 Spinal stenosis secondary to a combination of disc herniation (A), facet joint hypertrophy (B) and hypertrophy of the ligamentum flavum (C)

Box 4.3 **Causes of lumbar spinal stenosis**

Congenital
- Idiopathic
- Achondroplastic

Degenerative
- Hypertrophy of facet joints
- Hypertrophy of ligamentum flavum
- Disc herniation
- Spondylolisthesis
- Scoliosis

Iatrogenic
- Post-laminectomy
- Postsurgical fusion

Miscellaneous
- Paget's disease
- Fluorosis
- Diffuse idiopathic skeletal hyperostosis
- Ankylosing spondylitis

Spondylolisthesis

Spondylolisthesis is the anterior displacement of a vertebra on the one beneath it. It is usually secondary to degenerative changes in the disc and facet joints (degenerative spondylolisthesis) but may result from a developmental defect in the pars interarticularis of the vertebral arch (spondylolysis), which produces isthmic spondylolisthesis (Figure 4.3). Patients with minor degrees of spondylolisthesis are usually asymptomatic, although some may have mechanical LBP. Greater degrees of spondylolisthesis occasionally cause sciatica, spinal stenosis or cauda equina syndrome.

Spinal stenosis

Spinal stenosis (ST) is defined as a narrowing of the spinal canal and its lateral recesses and neural foramina, which may result in a compression of lumbosacral nerve roots (20% of adults over age 60 have imaging evidence of ST but are asymptomatic). Degenerative changes (leading to disc herniation, facet joint osteophytes and ligamentum flavum hypertrophy) are the causes of ST in most patients (Figure 4.4, Box 4.3). The prevalence of ST increases with age.

The hallmark of ST is pseudoclaudication (neurogenic claudication). Symptoms are often bilateral with pain, weakness and sometimes paraesthesiae in the buttocks, thighs and legs. Symptoms are induced by standing or walking and relieved by sitting or flexing forward. Forward flexion increases the canal diameter and may lead to the adoption of a simian stance. Unsteadiness of gait is common. The finding of a wide-based gait in a patient with LBP has a 90% specificity for ST. Physical examination is usually unremarkable, and severe neurological deficits are rarely seen. The diagnosis is best confirmed by magnetic resonance imaging (MRI).

Idiopathic (non-specific) low back pain

A definitive pathoanatomical diagnosis with precise identification of the pain generator cannot be made in 80% of patients. Non-specific terms such as lumbago, strain and sprain (which have never been anatomically or histologically characterized) have come into use for this mostly self-limited syndrome of acute LBP.

Neoplasms

Neoplasms are an uncommon, but nevertheless important, cause of LBP. Most cases result from involvement of the spine by metastatic carcinoma (especially prostate, lung, breast, thyroid or kidney) or multiple myeloma. A majority of patients present with persistent and progressive pain that is often worse at night. A history of cancer, unexplained weight loss and older age are associated with a higher likelihood for cancer.

Infection

Vertebral osteomyelitis may be acute (usually pyogenic) or chronic (pyogenic, fungal or granulomatous). It usually results from hematogenous seeding, direct inoculation at the time of surgery or contiguous spread from adjacent soft tissue. *Staphylococcus aureus* and *Escherichia coli* are the most common organisms. A source of infection is detected in about half the cases. Vertebral osteomyelitis may be complicated by an epidural or paravertebral abscess. Persistent back pain, often worse at night, is the initial symptom in most. Fever is present in only half the patients and leucocytosis is seen in two-thirds. However, almost all the patients have increases in ESR and CRP.

Assessment

A major focus of the evaluation is to identify the few patients with an underlying systemic disease (infection, neoplasm or spondyloarthritis) or significant neurological involvement (Box 4.4, Figure 4.5) that may require urgent and/or specific intervention. It is essential to take a full history and perform a comprehensive physical examination.

History

The patient's back pain should be characterized. Severe mechanical LBP with an acute onset in a slender postmenopausal woman is suspicious for a vertebral compression fracture secondary to osteoporosis.

Non-mechanical LBP, especially when accompanied by nocturnal pain, suggests the possibility of underlying infection or neoplasm.

Inflammatory LBP is seen in the spondyloarthritides. It is characterized by morning stiffness of greater than 30 minutes duration, improvement in back pain with exercise but not with rest, awakening because of back pain during the second half of the night, and

Box 4.4 **'Red flags' that indicate need for early diagnostic testing**

Spinal fracture
- Significant trauma
- Prolonged glucocorticoid use
- Age >50 years

Infection or cancer
- History of cancer
- Unexplained weight loss
- Immunosuppression
- Injection drug use
- Nocturnal pain
- Age >50 years

Cauda equina syndrome
- Urinary retention
- Overflow incontinence
- Faecal incontinence
- Bilateral (or unilateral) sciatica
- Motor weakness of lower extremities
- Saddle anaesthesia

Spondyloarthritis
- Morning stiffness >30 minutes
- Back pain improves with exercise but not with rest
- Back pain during the second half of the night
- Alternating buttock pain
- Age <50 years

alternating buttock pain in patients who are usually less than 50 years old.

The radicular pain of sciatica suggests nerve root impingement. It should be differentiated from non-neurogenic sclerotomal pain. Pseudoclaudication is seen with spinal stenosis.

Persistence of disabling LBP has been associated with the presence of maladaptive pain coping behaviour, psychosocial factors, psychiatric co-morbidities, job dissatisfaction, disputed compensation claims, smoking, poor general health status and the presence of non-organic signs.

Physical examination

This rarely leads to a specific diagnosis. Inspection may reveal a structural or functional scoliosis. Structural scoliosis is secondary to structural changes of the vertebral column, generally the result of degenerative changes. Functional scoliosis is usually the result of paravertebral muscle spasm or leg length discrepancy. Functional scoliosis disappears with spinal flexion, whereas structural scoliosis persists.

Paravertebral muscle spasm often leads to loss of the normal lumbar lordosis. Point tenderness on percussion over the spine has sensitivity but not specificity for vertebral osteomyelitis. A palpable step-off between adjacent spinous processes indicates spondylolisthesis.

Limited spinal motion is not associated with any specific diagnosis, because LBP due to any cause may limit motion. Range-of-motion measurements can help in monitoring treatment. Examine the hip for arthritis: this normally causes groin pain and occasionally referred back pain.

A straight leg raise test (Figure 4.6) should be performed on all patients with back pain that radiates into the lower extremities. This test places tension on the sciatic nerve and stretches the sciatic nerve roots (L4, L5, S1, S2 and S3). Patients with existing nerve root irritation, such as impingement from a herniated disc, will experience radicular pain that extends below the knee. This test is very sensitive (95%) but not specific (40%) for clinically significant disc herniation at the L4–5 or L5–S1 level. The straight leg raise test is usually negative in patients with spinal stenosis.

For lower extremities, neurological evaluation should include motor testing, determination of knee and ankle deep tendon reflexes, and dermatomal sensory loss tests (Figure 4.7). This can help identify the specific nerve root involved (Table 4.1), for example a significant left-sided L5–S1 posterolateral disc herniation often impinges upon the left S1 nerve root. Patients will have left-sided sciatica in the distribution of the S1 dermatome and may develop left plantar flexion weakness, diminished light touch and pinprick sensation over the lateral aspect of the left foot, and a diminished or absent left ankle jerk.

Imaging studies

Diagnostic testing is rarely indicated unless symptoms persist beyond 6 weeks, as 90% of patients will have recovered within this time, thus avoiding unnecessary testing. The presence of 'red flags', however, indicates the need for early investigation to detect underlying systemic disease or significant neurological deficit (see Box 4.4).

A major problem with all imaging studies is that many of the anatomical abnormalities (often the result of age-related degenerative changes) are common in asymptomatic people. Abnormalities such as single disc degeneration, facet joint degeneration, Schmorl's nodes, spondylolysis, mild spondylolisthesis, transitional vertebrae (lumbarization of S1 or sacralization of L5), spina bifida occulta and mild scoliosis are equally prevalent in people with and without LBP. Plain radiographs are usually unhelpful in determining the cause of LBP and should be limited to patients with findings suggestive of systemic disease (infection, neoplasm, spondyloarthropathy) or trauma, or those with continued LBP after 6 weeks of conservative care.

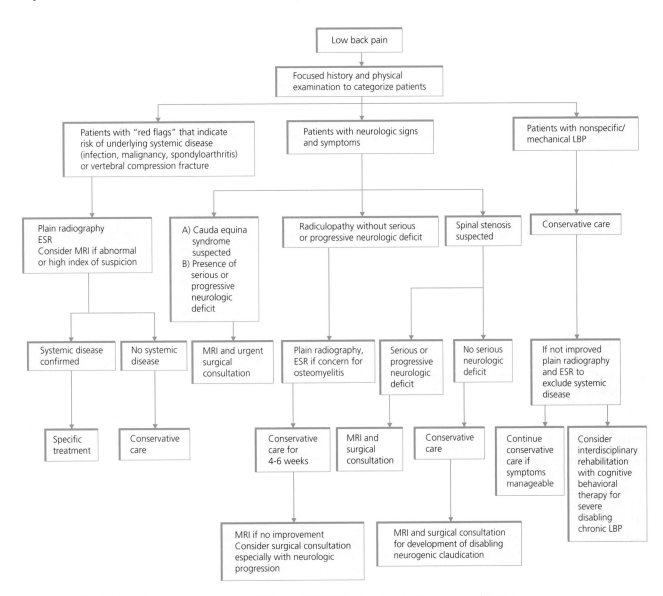

Figure 4.5 Algorithm for the evaluation and treatment of LBP. Source: Dixit (2013). Reproduced with permission of Elsevier

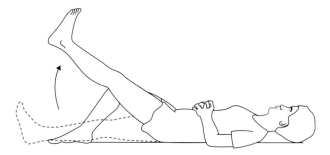

Figure 4.6 Straight leg raise test

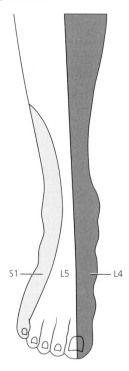

Figure 4.7 Lower extremity dermatomes

Table 4.1 Neurological features of lumbrosacral radiculopathy

Disc herniation	Nerve root	Motor	Sensory (light touch)	Reflex
L3–4	L4	Dorsiflexion of foot	Medial foot	Knee
L4–5	L5	Dorsiflexion of great toe	Dorsal foot	None
L5–S1	S1	Plantar flexion of foot	Lateral foot	Ankle

Computed tomography and MRI (Figure 4.8) should be reserved for patients in whom underlying infection or cancer is suspected, or for patients with significant or progressive neurological deficits. MRI is the preferred modality for the detection of spinal infection, neoplasm, herniated discs and spinal stenosis.

Treatment

Most patients, regardless of the cause, respond to a general programme that includes analgesia, education, back exercises, aerobic conditioning and weight control. Specific treatment is available

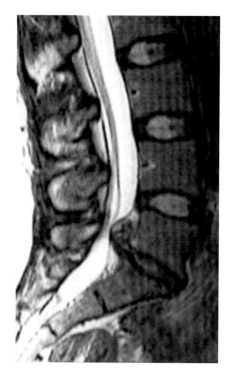

Figure 4.8 MRI showing a disc herniation at the L5–S1 level

only for the small number of patients with major neurological compression or underlying systemic disease. For treatment purposes, patients are considered to have acute LBP (duration <3 months), chronic LBP (duration >3 months) or a nerve root compression syndrome.

Acute low back pain

Patients often seek medical attention for sudden onset of severe mechanical LBP. Examination usually reveals paravertebral muscle spasm and severe decrease in range of motion secondary to pain.

Patients are advised to stay active, and bed rest is discouraged. Acetaminophen/paracetamol and non-steroidal anti-inflammatory drugs (NSAIDs) offer symptomatic relief; some people will need short-term narcotic analgesics, and muscle relaxants used for a few days may help others.

Once the acute episode of pain has subsided, a programme of regular back exercises (including stretching), aerobic conditioning and loss of excess weight is used to prevent recurrences. Back exercises help to stabilize the spine. Flexion exercises strengthen the abdominal muscles and extension exercises the paraspinal muscles. Educational booklets that include back exercises and safe lifting techniques are helpful.

There is no evidence that chiropractic or osteopathic spinal manipulative therapy is superior to standard treatment for acute back pain.

There is limited evidence supporting the use of epidural glucocorticoid injections for short-term relief of radicular pain. However, there is no evidence for the effectiveness of these injections in LBP without radiculopathy. Nerve root blocks and injection of anaesthetic agents or glucocorticoid into trigger points, ligaments, sacroiliac joints and facet joints are of unproven efficacy.

Ultrasound, shortwave diathermy, transcutaneous electrical nerve stimulation and other treatments such as lumbar braces, traction, acupuncture and biofeedback are ineffective.

Chronic low back pain

The clinical spectrum of chronic LBP is wide, with some patients complaining of severe unremitting pain but most having a nagging mechanical LBP, often with periods of acute exacerbation, that may radiate into the buttocks.

Treatment of chronic LBP is focused on relief of pain and restoration of function. Complete relief of pain is an unrealistic goal for most. Acetaminophen/paracetamol and NSAIDs may provide some degree of analgesia. Long-term use of narcotic analgesics should be avoided. Low-dose tricyclic antidepressants and serotonin-norepinephrine reuptake inhibitors may help some patients.

Back exercises, aerobic conditioning, loss of excess weight and patient education are effective in managing chronic LBP. A multidisciplinary approach focusing on functional restoration through an individualized intensive rehabilitation programme based on cognitive behavioural therapy is often helpful in patients with more intractable pain.

The results of back surgery (spinal fusion or artificial discs) for relief of chronic LBP have been disappointing.

Nerve root compression syndromes

Disc herniation – Patients with radicular pain secondary to nerve root compression should be treated conservatively, as described for acute LBP, for the first 6 weeks unless there is severe or progressive neurological deficit: approximately 90% will improve. Elective surgery is considered for the few with persistent and severe sciatica that fails to respond to conservative care. Surgery is indicated for the presence of a severe or progressive neurological deficit. Laminotomy with limited discectomy is generally the procedure of choice.

Spinal stenosis – The symptoms remain stable for years in most patients. Analgesics, NSAIDs, loss of excess weight, and exercises (including those that reduce lumbar lordosis) may provide symptomatic relief. Epidural glucocorticoid injections are ineffective in the treatment of spinal stenosis. Surgical treatment, aimed at decompression of the neural elements, is offered to patients with either disabling, pseudoclaudication or significant neurological deficit.

Spondylolisthesis – The vast majority of patients are treated conservatively. Rarely, a patient may need decompressive surgery with fusion if a significant or progressive neurological deficit develops.

Further reading

Dixit R. Low back pain. In: Firestein G (ed.), *Kelley's Textbook of Rheumatology*, 9th edn. Elsevier, Amsterdam, 2013, pp. 665–682.

Chou R, Qaseem A, Snow V *et al*. Diagnosis and treatment of low back pain: a joint clinical practice guideline from the American College of Physicians and the American Pain Society. *Annals of Internal Medicine* 2007; **147**: 478–491.

CHAPTER 5

Pain in the Hip

Andrew Hamer

Sheffield Teaching Hospitals NHS Foundation Trust, Sheffield, UK

> **OVERVIEW**
>
> - Osteoarthritis of the hip is common in adults, and osteoporotic hip fractures are epidemic in the elderly.
> - Always examine the hip in patients presenting with knee pain, as referred pain from the hip is common.
> - Childhood hip conditions require prompt treatment to reduce the risk of problems in later life.

> Box 5.1 **Important causes of childhood hip pain**
>
> - Developmental dysplasia of the hip
> - Perthes' disease
> - Slipped upper femoral epiphysis
> - Septic arthritis
> - Transient synovitis or 'irritable hip'
> - Other arthritides

Hip pain in children

A child with hip disease often presents to healthcare professionals with an unexplained limp, often in the absence of a history of pain or trauma. Unexplained thigh or knee pain should, however, raise the suspicion of hip abnormalities. See Box 5.1 for a summary of important causes of childhood hip pain.

Developmental dysplasia of the hip (DDH)

This was previously called congenital dislocation of the hip (CDH) and is due to a failure of normal development of the acetabulum leading to failure of normal development of the hip. All babies are screened by physical examination in the neonatal period, although this is unreliable at detecting many cases. Ultrasound screening should detect at risk cases. DDH is associated with a breach presentation, a positive family history and other congenital deformities. Missed cases of DDH may present before 5 years of age as a delay in walking, a limp or discrepancy in leg length. Missed cases may lead to a non-congruent joint and early osteoarthritic degeneration in adulthood (Figure 5.1).

Perthes' disease

Perthes' disease is relatively rare, and is a segmental avascular necrosis of the femoral head. This can lead to subsequent healing and deformity of the hip. This condition occurs in boys usually between the ages of 5 and 10 years. The precise cause is unclear, but the condition is associated with a positive family history, low birth weight and lower socioeconomic groups. A limp, hip pain or knee pain may result. Treatment aims are to contain the femoral head in the acetabulum to reduce the risks of future osteoarthritis.

Slipped upper femoral epiphysis (SUFE)

This condition is typically seen in overweight boys at the time of the adolescent growth spurt, at the ages of 11–15. Girls may also experience the condition but this is more uncommon. The diagnosis may be difficult, but a frog lateral X-ray radiograph will show the deformity (Figure 5.2). Surgical stabilization to fix the slipped epiphysis *in situ* should be carried out urgently. The contralateral hip is at high risk of slippage, and patients and parents should be warned to return if any hip or knee pain occurs on the unoperated side.

Septic arthritis

This is relatively uncommon in children, but should be suspected if a child presents with systemic illness, toxic and inability to walk. Movement of the affected joint is not possible because of pain. Diagnosis is helped by a raised white cell count, erythrocyte sedimentation rate and C-reactive protein. An effusion may be seen on ultrasound, and urgent aspiration will help with diagnosis. Urgent surgical drainage is vital to reduce the risk of late osteoarthritis. *Staphylococcus aureus* is usually the infecting organism, but diagnosis may be particularly difficult in neonates.

Transient synovitis/'irritable hip'

A reactive effusion may occur in the hip joint in association with systemic viral illness. Affected children are not acutely ill and can move the hip, but with some degree of stiffness. An effusion may be seen on ultrasound; the condition is usually self-limiting and responsive to non-steroidal anti-inflammatory drugs. Distinguishing

---

ABC of Rheumatology, Fifth Edition. Edited by Ade Adebajo and Lisa Dunkley.
© 2018 John Wiley & Sons Ltd. Published 2018 by John Wiley & Sons Ltd.

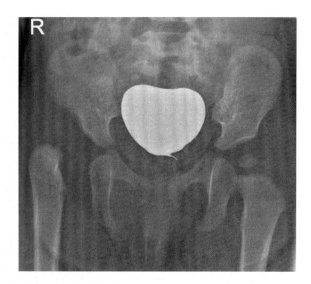

Figure 5.1 Anteroposterior radiograph of child with dislocated right hip. Note the lateral displacement of the femur and poorly developed ossific nucleus of the hip

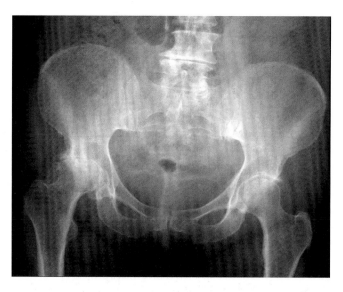

Figure 5.3 Osteoarthritis of the right hip, with joint space loss, subarticular cysts, peripheral osteophytes and subchondral sclerosis

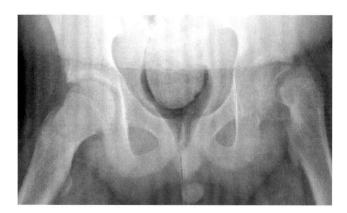

Figure 5.2 X-ray radiograph of a child's left hip. Displacement of the epiphysis relative to the femoral neck is easily seen

Box 5.2 **Causes of hip pain in adults**

- Osteoarthritis
- Other arthritides
  - Rheumatoid arthritis
  - Psoriatic arthritis
  - Ankylosing spondylitis
- Hip fracture
- Paget's disease
- Avascular necrosis
- Malignancy
- Femoro-acetabular impingement
  - Torn acetabular labrum
- Painful soft tissue conditions around the hip
  - Trochanteric bursitis
  - Snapping iliopsoas tendon

this condition from septic arthritis can be difficult, and occasionally these children must undergo aspiration to exclude a septic hip. Perthes' disease in the early stages may present with an effusion without changes visible on X-ray examination.

Other arthritides

Juvenile chronic arthritis may present with hip pain. General management of the arthritic process is important, with physiotherapy to prevent joint contracture. Systemic therapy with disease-modifying agents can be very effective. These therapies have important potential toxicities and must be prescribed knowledgeably.

Hip pain in adults

Pain from the hip is usually felt in the groin or lateral or anterior thigh. Hip pain may also be referred to the knee, and occasionally even down to the front of the ankle; this may confuse the unwary! Although buttock pain may originate from the hip, the lumbar spine is the usual source. Hip disorders often produce a limp, a

reduction in walking distance and associated stiffness. These functional limitations may affect activities of daily living, such as getting in and out of the bath and putting on socks and shoes. Patients with advanced hip disease can become dependent on others, sometimes requiring expensive social services input. See Box 5.2 for a summary of the causes of hip pain in adults.

Osteoarthritis

Osteoarthritis is the most common cause of hip pain in adults, most presenting in their 60s or 70s. Some patients present earlier, their groin pain often being mistaken for pain from an inguinal hernia or a 'groin strain'. An X-ray will confirm the diagnosis, and rest, simple analgesia, range of motion and strengthening exercises may help (Figure 5.3). A walking stick often can relieve the pain. Most cases of osteoarthritis are idiopathic, but may relate to prior hip trauma or congenital abnormalities (see previous section on hip pain in childhood). As the hip abductor muscles weaken, the patient may develop a Trendelenburg gait. In extreme situations, leg length is

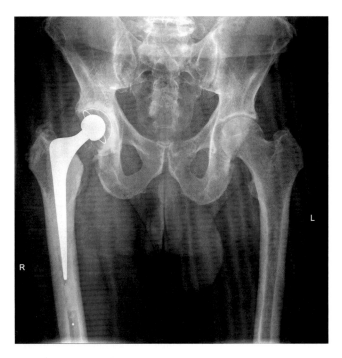

Figure 5.4 Anteroposterior radiograph of a patient following right cemented total hip replacement

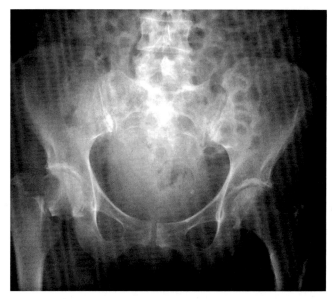

Figure 5.5 Subcapital fracture of the right hip

lost and the hip adopts a fixed flexion and adduction deformity. Total hip replacement (Figure 5.4) is extremely effective at relieving pain and improving functional status in osteoarthritis. Over 80 000 are performed annually in the UK, with expected survival of the implants being approximately 95% at 10 years and 85% at 20 years.

Other arthritides

Rheumatoid arthritis, psoriatic arthritis and ankylosing spondylitis can also produce hip pain and stiffness. The indications for total hip replacement are the same as for osteoarthritis, for the alleviation of intolerable pain, night pain, and the treatment of hip stiffness and associated loss of independence.

Hip fracture

Osteoporotic hip fracture in elderly women is epidemic in the western world. A fall followed by inability to bear weight and a short externally rotated leg are diagnostic (Figure 5.5). An undisplaced fracture may not stop the patient from bearing weight, and it may not be visible on initial X-ray examination. Repeat films are usually required, and in some circumstances magnetic resonance imaging (MRI) may help. Treatment is usually surgical, and includes stabilization with plates/screws, replacement of the femoral head alone (hemiarthroplasty) or total hip replacement in patients with good preinjury activity levels.

Paget's disease

The pelvis is commonly involved in Paget's disease, and can cause hip pain. Paget's disease can co-exist with osteoarthritis, and may lead to diagnostic difficulties in working out which is the source of the pain. Treatment of Paget's disease with bisphosphonates can reduce hip pain, but co-existent osteoarthritis might require hip replacement.

Box 5.3 **Causes of avascular necrosis**

- Most cases are idiopathic
- Associated conditions include:
  - Excess alcohol
  - Prolonged steroid therapy
  - Working in pressurized environments (for example, deep sea divers)

Avascular necrosis

Avascular necrosis of the weight-bearing portion of the femoral head can occur. An accurate history to determine whether predisposing factors are present is important (Box 5.3) but many cases are idiopathic. Plain X-rays may be normal, but an MRI scan will help in diagnosis in the early stages of the disease. Once plain X-ray evidence is apparent, surgical treatment to arrest the disease process is less successful. Hip replacement may be ultimately required. The condition is frequently bilateral, and patients and family should be warned to seek help if pain develops on the contralateral side.

Malignancy

Metastases in the pelvis or proximal femur will produce pain, but often with different characteristics to that of osteoarthritis. Patients may complain of constant deep boring pain, and lesions should be visible on plain X-ray. Treatment with local radiotherapy or bisphosphonates may slow the disease progress. Surgical stabilization of impending fractures may be required. Primary bone tumours as a cause of hip pain are extremely rare.

Femoro-acetabular impingement (FAI)

This is a condition that has become recognized over the past 10–15 years or so. FAI occurs when the normal 'ball and socket' relationship of the femoral head to the acetabulum is abnormal. In 'pincer' type impingement, the rim of the socket is extended, leading to a restriction of movement of the femoral head and

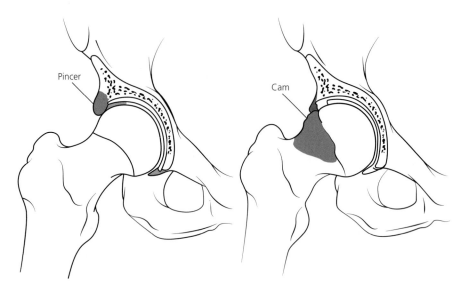

Figure 5.6 Pincer and cam impingement. In 'pincer' type, extra bone extends from the acetabular rim, preventing full movement of the femoral head. In 'cam' type impingement, extra bone around the periphery of the femoral head prevents normal motion inside the acetabulum

neck (Figure 5.6). In 'cam' type impingement, the femoral head is not truly spherical, with extra bone and cartilage causing impingement at the extremes of motion.

Patients with true FAI pain often present if they are involved in sporting activities, particularly those where the hip may be placed in an extreme position (for example, football/gymnastics). The precise aetiology of cam or pincer impingement is not known, although there is speculation that unrecognized SUFE may be responsible for mild cases of cam impingement. Surgical treatment (either open or arthroscopic) to resect the bony prominences of either the acetabulum or femoral head has been shown to improve pain free range of motion in the short term, but whether there is any long-term protective effect against the onset of osteoarthritis is not clear.

Torn acetabular labrum – The acetabular labrum can tear in the presence of FAI and such a tear may be visible on MRI arthrograms. A torn acetabular labrum in the absence of any other previous injury (e.g. hip dislocation) or bony abnormality is most unusual, and is probably an incidental finding at MRI arthrography. The torn labrum can be associated with underlying articular cartilage damage in the superior weight-bearing area of the hip joint. This can be addressed arthroscopically, although the long-term results of debridement or microfracture are unknown.

Painful soft tissue conditions around the hip

Trochanteric bursitis – This is a relatively common self-limiting condition characterized by pain over the tip of the greater trochanter (not in the groin). The name of the condition is somewhat misleading, as inflammation of the trochanteric bursa has never been demonstrated in histological specimens, and the pain may indeed be referred from the lumbar spine. Local physiotherapy, anti-inflammatories, rest and occasional local anaesthetic and steroid injections can help.

Iliopsoas bursitis – The iliopsoas bursa is deep to the psoas muscle and anterior to the hip joint. Pain occurs in the groin and anterior thigh and can be exacerbated by resisted hip flexion and passive hip

extension. The syndrome occasionally has an infectious aetiology. Thus, when the presentation is acute, especially painful and accompanied by systemic features, the work-up should be aggressive and include image-guided aspiration.

Snapping iliopsoas tendon – This causes a painful clunk in the groin when the hip goes from flexion to extension. The hip is otherwise normal. The psoas tendon impinges on the capsule of the hip anteriorly to produce discomfort. Diagnosis is made if movement of fluoroscopic X-ray contrast agent injected into the psoas tendon is abnormal. Surgical release may be needed, although the results are somewhat unpredictable.

Ischial bursitis – The ischial bursa separates the gluteus maximus from the ischial tuberosity. Bursitis can arise from prolonged sitting or trauma to the bursa (hence the name 'weaver's bottom'). Use of a cushion and local corticosteroid injection may be useful.

Meralgia paresthetica – This refers to local compression of the lateral cutaneous nerve of the thigh (L2–3 distribution) at the inguinal ligament. Patients experience numbness and burning pain in the anterior and lateral thigh. Symptoms are felt to arise from direct compression of the nerve as a result of obesity, pregnancy and tight-fitting belts. Hip extension (as can occur with high heels) and diabetes are risk factors. The syndrome generally improves with conservative measures such as weight loss and changes in clothing and shoes.

Management of hip pain

The most important step in management of the painful hip is to establish the underlying pathology and treat it as specifically as possible. Thus, infection in the hip should be diagnosed expeditiously and treated with surgical drainage and prolonged parenteral antibiotics. Fractures should be diagnosed and stabilized. Inflammatory arthritis can be treated with systemic therapy.

Conservative treatment such as a walking stick can be helpful in unloading the painful hip and relieving pain. Patients must be shown the proper use of the stick in the contralateral hand. The hip can become stiff with disuse and develop flexion contractures. These can be avoided with gentle range-of-motion exercises.

Simple analgesia and NSAIDs can help in early osteoarthritis, but referral to an orthopaedic surgeon for consideration of total hip replacement is indicated if conservative treatment fails or pain interferes with the patient's ability to function on a daily basis.

Acknowledgement

With thanks to Jeffry N. Katz for contributing to this chapter in a previous edition of the book.

Further reading

McRae R. *Clinical Orthopaedic Examination*. Churchill Livingstone, Edinburgh, 1997.

Miller MD (ed.). *Review of Orthopaedics*. WB Saunders, Philadelphia, 2000.

Solomon L, Nayagam D, Warwick D. *Apley's System of Orthopaedics and Fractures.*, 8th edn. Arnold, London, 2001.

CHAPTER 6

Pain in the Knee

Adrian Dunbar[1] and Mark Wilkinson[2,3]

[1] Skipton, North Yorkshire, UK
[2] University of Sheffield, Sheffield, UK
[3] Sheffield Teaching Hospitals NHS Foundation Trust, President British Orthopaedic Research Society, UK

OVERVIEW

- Knee pain is a frequent presenting complaint in primary care.
- Knee pain may arise from overuse injuries, trauma, degenerative change and inflammatory conditions.
- Osteoarthritis and rheumatoid arthritis affect the knee commonly.
- In most cases, knee pain responds to simple measures such as lifestyle modification, simple analgesia and physiotherapy.
- Pain poorly controlled by simple measures, mechanical symptoms such as instability and locking, and progressive disability are indications for referral to secondary care.
- Where infection or tumour are suspected as a cause of knee pain, urgent referral to secondary care is required.

The knee is the largest joint in the body. It is a complex hinge that is made up of two separate articulations: the tibiofemoral joint and the patellofemoral joint. Knee motion occurs in a complex manner involving three planes, although the vast majority of its motion occurs in the sagittal plane (from full extension through to 140° of flexion).

Pain in the knee joint is one of the most common musculoskeletal complaints that presents to primary care physicians, and may arise from a broad range of pathologies. In the younger patient, pain most commonly arises from sporting or overuse injuries, which may affect the intra-articular or extra-articular structures of the knee. The knee is also a common site for inflammatory and infective pathologies. In the older patient, the most common cause is degenerative disease. Knee pain arising from osteoarthritis is a major cause of disability in the older patient, the prevalence and healthcare costs of which continue to rise as the population ages.

The evaluation of knee pain centres on a thorough history and physical examination supplemented, where necessary, with appropriate imaging and laboratory tests (Figure 6.1).

Traumatic causes of knee pain

Injuries are a common cause of knee pain. Most knee injuries in sport occur as a result of indirect trauma, such as a twisting moment to the knee. The structures most commonly injured by this mechanism are the menisci, the collateral ligaments and the cruciate ligaments. These structures may be damaged in isolation, or damage may occur in combination (for example, the anterior cruciate ligament, medial collateral ligament and medial meniscus may be injured in O'Donoghue's triad). Direct trauma to the knee (such as during contact sport, an industrial accident or a motor vehicle collision) most commonly causes bone contusions, fracture or dislocation that may affect the patellofemoral or tibiofemoral joint. Dislocation of the tibiofemoral joint indicates high-energy trauma, and is often associated with neurovascular damage.

Meniscus injury

Meniscus injury in young people can present as an acute injury or as a chronic condition with an insidious onset. The majority of meniscus tears in young people occur after mild to moderate energy twisting injuries and are typically isolated injuries or associated with a collateral ligament strain. The medial meniscus is damaged three times more commonly than the lateral meniscus (Figure 6.2). Higher energy twisting injuries are commonly associated with an anterior cruciate ligament injury, an acute haemarthrosis and inability to bear weight. Patients with meniscus tears have focal tenderness over the joint line and may experience mechanical catching and locking symptoms in the knee in addition to joint effusion and pain.

Ege's test and the Thessaly test, performed with the patient in standing, have much higher sensitivity and specificity for meniscal tears than McMurray's test and are easy to perform (Figures 6.3, 6.4). Magnetic resonance imaging (MRI) can aid in establishing the diagnosis and in identifying associated conditions, such as

ABC of Rheumatology, Fifth Edition. Edited by Ade Adebajo and Lisa Dunkley.
© 2018 John Wiley & Sons Ltd. Published 2018 by John Wiley & Sons Ltd.

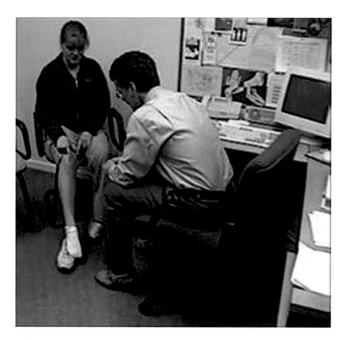

Figure 6.1 A detailed history and examination are required to make an accurate clinical diagnosis in the patient presenting with knee pain

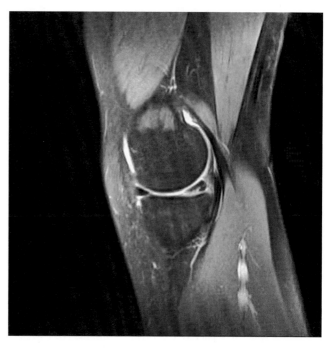

Figure 6.2 MRI of meniscus injury (sagittal view). The anterior part of the medial meniscus can be seen as a black triangle on the left side of the joint line; the black triangle of the posterior part of the meniscus has a white line running through it, representing an oblique tear

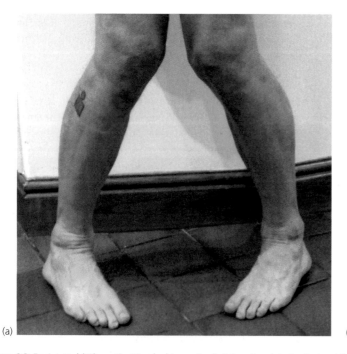

(a)

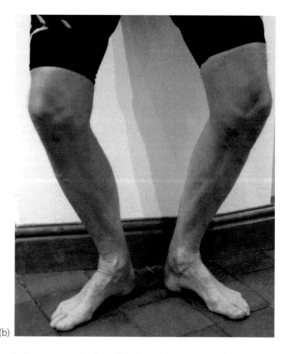

(b)

Figure 6.3 Ege's test. (a) The patient is asked to maximally internally rotate the feet and flex the knees. A meniscal tear is indicated if the patient's knee pain is reproduced. (b) The patient is asked to maximally externally rotate the feet and flex the knees. A meniscal tear is indicated if the patient's knee pain is reproduced

degenerate disease affecting the articular cartilage. Acute tears that occur in the well-vascularized peripheral portion of the meniscus are amenable to arthroscopic repair, which preserves meniscal function. Where an anterior cruciate ligament injury is also present, this is commonly reconstructed concurrently. Chronic meniscal tears are typically avascular with degenerative characteristics and will not heal if repaired.

Arthroscopic resection is confined to the torn and degenerate portions of meniscus, as early-onset osteoarthritis of the knee commonly follows complete meniscal resection.

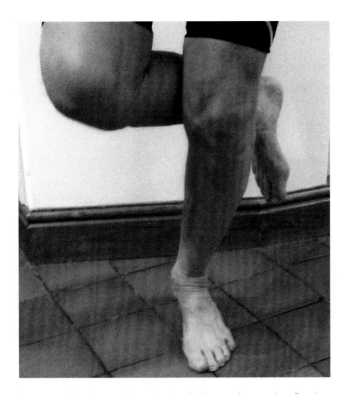

Figure 6.4 Thessaly test. The patient is asked to stand on one leg, flex the knee to approximately 20°, then rotate on the knee, medially then laterally. A meniscal tear is present if the patient's knee pain is reproduced by rotation on the flexed knee

Articular cartilage injury

Articular cartilage injury is often the result of a traumatic episode that involves an impact injury to the cartilage surface. Articular cartilage injuries can result in focal pain, joint effusion and mechanical catching symptoms. Treatment comprises graduated physiotherapy for undisplaced injuries and arthroscopic repair or removal for displaced osteochondral fragments. Occult episodes of trauma to the knee may result in separation of cartilage from the subchondral bone, termed osteochondritis dissecans. Patients complain of poorly localized pain. The diagnosis is made from plain radiographs or MRI scans, and treatment commonly involves arthroscopic resection of loose cartilage.

Differentiation of cause

A detailed history of the mechanism of injury and physical examination provide valuable information to differentiate between the various traumatic causes of knee pain. Knee pain from injury has a sudden onset at the time of the injury episode and is often accompanied by local soft tissue swelling and an effusion. Certain fractures and dislocations may exhibit gross deformity but the majority of knee and patellar dislocations spontaneously reduce before presentation. A haemarthrosis develops quickly (over a period of minutes to a few hours) and indicates significant intra-articular injury, such as an anterior cruciate ligament tear, intra-articular fracture or osteochondral injury, or patellar dislocation. Effusions develop more slowly (over several hours) and tend to be associated with meniscal injuries (Table 6.1).

Table 6.1 Post-traumatic knee swelling and the most common associated diagnoses

Immediate haemarthrosis	Delayed effusion	Minimal effusion
Anterior cruciate ligament tear	Meniscus tear	Collateral ligament tear
Osteochondral fracture	Posterior cruciate ligament tear	
Patellar dislocation		

Table 6.2 Symptoms associated with overuse injuries

Symptom	Likely diagnosis
Pain adjacent to patella Pain ascending/descending stairs Pain when sitting for prolonged periods ('movie theatre sign')	Anterior knee pain syndrome
Pain in patellar tendon Pain with jumping	Patellar tendonopathy
Lateral knee pain with repetitive activity	Iliotibial band friction syndrome
Medial knee pain distal to joint line	Pes anserine bursitis

Radiographs should be obtained when evaluating any knee injury to exclude a fracture, dislocation or other significant abnormality. After obtaining radiographs, additional diagnostic tests may be indicated, including a computed tomography scan in the case of intra-articular fractures or MRI when a soft tissue or osteochondral injury is suspected. In the absence of neurovascular compromise or gross deformity, initial treatment of traumatic knee pain should consist of restricted weight bearing, ice and elevation. Severe injuries require immediate referral for orthopaedic surgical evaluation.

Knee pain in younger people and athletes

Knee pain in younger people and athletes can be caused by overuse syndromes, meniscus injury or articular cartilage abnormality. Common overuse syndromes include patellar tendonopathy, anterior knee pain syndrome, pes anserine bursitis and iliotibial band friction syndrome (Table 6.2).

Patellar tendonopathy

Patellar tendonopathy is caused by repetitive activity, particularly 'explosive' athletics such as jumping. Patients complain of pain and soft tissue swelling about the patellar tendon, usually at its proximal attachment to the patella. Treatment consists of ice, pain-relieving medication, activity modification, to reduce inappropriate stress on the tissue as healing takes place, and strengthening exercises, focusing on eccentric loading of the tendon.

Anterior knee pain syndrome

Anterior knee pain syndrome occurs in patients who engage in repetitive athletic activity, in those with abnormalities in extensor mechanism alignment and in those who are overweight. Patients with anterior knee pain syndrome complain of pain in the front of the knee, which is accentuated by ascending and descending stairs, squatting, kneeling and sitting for long periods of time. The pain may be located directly behind the patella or in the medial or lateral retinaculum. Treatment should include activity modification, weight control if necessary, physiotherapy to strengthen the quadriceps muscles (particularly vastus medialis) and core musculature, and appropriate pain-relieving medication.

Pes anserine bursitis

Pes anserine bursitis is an inflammation of the bursa overlying the insertion site of the semitendinosus, gracilis and sartorius tendons in the anteromedial aspect of the proximal tibia. Patients complain of medial knee pain distal to the medial joint line. Treatment can include activity modification, strengthening exercises and anti-inflammatory medication. Chronic symptoms may respond to local corticosteroid injection.

Iliotibial band friction syndrome

Iliotibial band friction syndrome is an inflammation of the iliotibial band, the distal portion of the tensor fascia lata muscle that inserts into the anterolateral aspect of the proximal tibia. Patients are usually runners or cyclists who complain of activity-related lateral knee pain. This condition responds well to activity modification, stretching and strengthening exercises, ice and anti-inflammatory medication.

Knee pain in older people

Twenty five percent of people over the age of 50 years report chronic knee pain, and degenerative arthritis of the knee is common in this age group (Box 6.1). However, clinical symptoms and radiological severity of arthritis are poorly correlated. Many older people with knee pain have minor radiological evidence of arthritic change. Conversely, many people with advanced radiological changes have little pain. Arthritis of the knee is often associated with periarticular soft tissue problems, and indeed, these can often be a major source of knee pain. Pes anserine bursitis is a common example. Plain radiographic imaging is not always helpful in the assessment of patients with knee pain, and the diagnosis of osteoarthritis is often a clinical one.

Anterior knee pain due to patella maltracking can occur in the degenerative knee and will respond to weight loss and knee strengthening exercise. This should always be done before more risk-laden, invasive or expensive interventions. An MRI scan may assist in the diagnosis of an occult degenerate meniscal tear, but may not change the management plan.

Box 6.1 **Diagnosis of osteoarthritis**

Osteoarthritis is diagnosed clinically by the presence of:

- Chronic knee pain
- Morning stiffness lasting less than 30 minutes
- Joint crepitus
- Range of movement restricted by pain or degenerative change
- Presence of palpable osteophytes or visible joint deformity

---

Box 6.2 **Non-pharmacological treatments**

Non-pharmacological treatments with an evidence base include:

- Weight loss
- Aerobic exercise
- Specific knee-strengthening exercise
- Patellar taping
- Acupuncture
- Knee bracing

The management of osteoarthritis is, for most people, the management of their knee pain and lifestyle modification (Box 6.2). The high prevalence of knee pain in the community means that such treatments should be simple, safe, cost-effective and, ideally, self-administered. Initial treatments consist of simple analgesia. The place of oral glucosamine and similar nutraceuticals is still debated in the presence of conflicting reports from different studies, and no treatment interventions have yet been convincingly shown to alter the course of osteoarthritis. Oral non-steroidal anti-inflammatory drugs (NSAIDs) are prescribed commonly; however, there is little evidence of benefit over simple analgesia, and they are associated with significant risk of serious adverse effects in the older patient. Their use should be considered only after failure of simple measures such as weight loss, exercise regimes and use of simple analgesics.

Local treatments, such as topical non-steroidal anti-inflammatory gels, are effective in the short term, particularly in the setting of acute symptomatic flares. Injected treatments include corticosteroids and hyaluronans. Intra-articular steroids can be very effective in relieving knee pain for several weeks or months. Use of hyaluronans is controversial; they are more expensive and require a series of injections over time, and are recommended not to be used for knee osteoarthritis by the National Institute for Health and Care Excellence (NICE). Certain hyaluronans can cause pseudoseptic joint inflammation and effusion.

Arthroscopic surgical treatment for arthritis of the knee is reserved for the treatment of mechanical symptoms such as joint catching, locking or instability due to a loose body or meniscal tear. In the absence of mechanical symptoms, arthroscopic interventions are no more effective than placebo.

In up to 40% of patients, disease does not progress significantly after initial presentation, or does so very slowly. In these patients use of simple, safe, cost-effective treatments is essential for effective and economic management.

Joint replacement surgery is indicated in those patients whose disease progresses such that their symptoms, such as pain, stiffness, loss of function or progressive deformity, become poorly controlled despite the treatment measures outlined above. The main indication for referral for joint replacement surgery is poor joint pain control and loss of function. In most patients, joint replacement surgery entails total knee replacement (Figure 6.5).

In a small proportion of patients, the arthritis is limited to one compartment of knee, in which case a unicompartmental joint replacement may be considered as an alternative to total knee

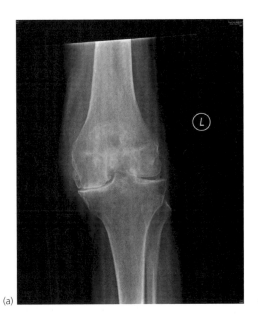
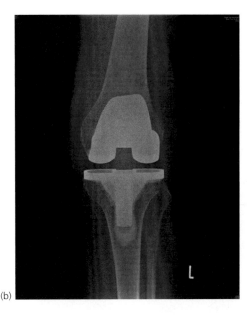

(a) (b)

Figure 6.5 Radiograph showing the typical features of knee osteoarthritis, joint space narrowing, subchondral sclerosis and osteophyte formation (a), and following treatment with total knee replacement (b)

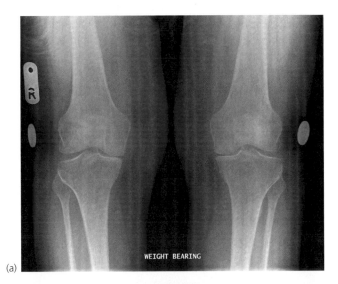

(a)

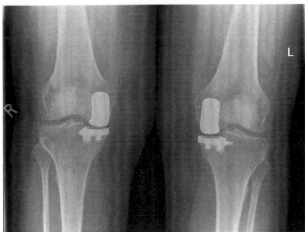

(b)

Figure 6.6 Radiographs showing bilateral isolated osteoarthritis of the medial compartment of the knee (a), and following treatment with bilateral unicompartmental knee replacement (b)

replacement (Figure 6.6). Unicompartmental joint replacement is associated with good functional outcomes in suitable patients, but progression of arthritis in the non-replaced parts of the knee and higher prosthesis failure rates mean that the long-term survival of these prosthesis types is lower than total knee replacement. The results of joint replacement surgery are excellent in over 90% of patients in terms of improvement in health-related quality of life.

Knee pain in systemic disease

Pain and swelling in the knee may be a feature of systemic illness. Patients should be asked about pain in other joints, previously painful, swollen joints and a family history of joint disease. Systemic symptoms such as malaise, pyrexia, anorexia and weight loss may provide clues to the origin of the knee pain. Symptoms affecting other organs, such as the skin, bowel, eyes or genitourinary tract, may also be of diagnostic relevance.

The knee is the most commonly affected large joint in rheumatoid arthritis. The knees are usually affected bilaterally and symptom onset usually occurs early in the course of the disease. The knee is also commonly affected in the other chronic inflammatory arthritides, including psoriatic arthritis and ankylosing spondylitis. The treatment of the knee pain in these conditions is considered along with the management of the systemic disease and includes lifestyle modification, physiotherapy, NSAIDs, disease-modifying agents, biological agents (genetically engineered drugs that target specific disease pathways or cell types) and total joint replacement surgery.

The knee is also the most commonly infected joint. Joint infection presents with a red, swollen, hot knee, difficulty in weight bearing and a limitation in the range of passive motion. Occasionally, the infection may originate in the metaphyseal region of the tibia or femur, rather than the knee joint itself (Figure 6.7). A suspected infection of the knee requires immediate referral to secondary care

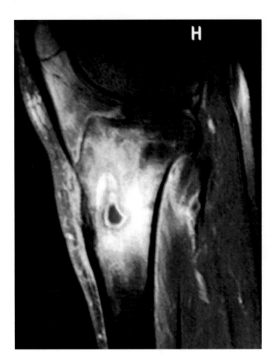

Figure 6.7 MRI scan of the knee (sagittal view) in a patient presenting with an acute, red knee. In this case, the diagnosis was acute staphylococcal osteomyelitis of the proximal tibial metaphysis

for assessment and treatment. The most common infecting organism is *Staphylococcus aureus*. Less common infections include *Streptococcus*, *Gonococcus*, *Brucella* and, rarely, tuberculosis. Infective arthritis should always be considered in the immunocompromised and other patients with increased infective risk, such as intravenous drug users and the immunosuppressed patient.

Aspiration of the joint for microbiological culture is the most important investigation for the accurate diagnosis of infection. This must be carried out at initial assessment, and before the administration of antibiotics. Aspiration of the knee after antibiotic administration usually results in a false-negative microbiological culture result and a missed diagnosis. Other useful diagnostic tests include concurrent aspirate microscopy for crystals and serological measurement of white cell count, erythrocyte sedimentation rate and C-reactive protein.

The treatment of the infected knee includes initiation of systemic antibiotics immediately after knee aspiration, typically using an agent with broad Gram-positive antimicrobial activity, and serial joint aspiration or arthroscopic-assisted washout. The choice of antibiotic is adjusted as indicated by the aspirate microbiological culture sensitivities, and may be continued for up to 6 weeks orally, although specialist microbiological advice should be taken where infection is confirmed from aspirate culture.

The differential diagnosis of the hot, swollen, painful knee includes systemic inflammatory conditions such as calcium pyrophosphate arthropathy, gout, reactive arthritis and prepatellar bursitis. Aspiration of joint fluid for crystal microscopy and culture,

and appropriate serological investigations, are both important in confirming the correct diagnosis and excluding joint infection. Rarely, infections of the genitourinary tract and viral infections may present with bilateral swollen, tender knees with a large effusion of sympathetic origin. Radiographs are frequently of limited diagnostic utility in such cases.

Other causes of knee pain

Hip pain may occasionally refer to the anterior distal thigh or the knee. A complete examination of the patient with knee pain includes an examination of the hip to exclude this cause of knee pain. Knee pain may also present as part of a chronic widespread pain syndrome. An adequate general musculoskeletal assessment is essential if appropriate treatment of the knee pain is to be effected. In the presence of polyarthralgia or symptoms suggestive of a fibromyalgia syndrome, the knee pain is unlikely to be adequately managed by focusing on the knee alone. Attention should be paid to management of the global pain problem.

'Red flags'

Although primary bone tumours are rare, the knee is one of the most commonly affected sites for both benign tumours, including osteoid osteoma, enchondroma and chondroblastoma, and malignant tumours, including osteosarcoma and chondrosarcoma. Ewing's sarcomas also commonly affect the knee. In children and young adults who are very active, knee pain may be related to recent activity. Unexplained pain, pain that is worse at night, unexplained swelling and systemic symptoms are all 'red flag' features that may indicate a bone tumour. Patients in whom a bone tumour is suspected should be referred early to a centre specializing in their management.

Further reading

Akseki D, Özcan Ö, Boya H, Pınar H. A new weight-bearing meniscal test and a comparison with McMurray's test and joint line tenderness. *Arthroscopy* 2004: **20**: 951–958.

Brukner P, Khan K. Lateral, medial and posterior knee pain. In: Brukner P, Khan K (eds), *Clinical Sports Medicine*, 3rd edn. McGraw Hill, London, 2007.

Brukner P, Khan K, Cooper R, Morris H, Arendt L. Acute knee injuries. In: Brukner P, Khan K (eds), *Clinical Sports Medicine*, 3rd edn. McGraw Hill, London, 2007.

Brukner P, Khan K, Crossley K, Cook J, Cowan S, McConnell J. Anterior knee pain. In: Brukner P, Khan K (eds), *Clinical Sports Medicine*, 3rd edn. McGraw Hill, London, 2007.

Karachalios T, Hantes M, Zibis A *et al.* Diagnostic accuracy of a new clinical test (the Thessaly test) for early detection of meniscal tears. *Journal of Bone and Joint Surgery American Volume* 2005; **87**(5): 955–962.

Panayi G, Dickson DJ. *Clinical Practice Series: Arthritis.* Churchill Livingstone, London, 2004.

Underwood M. *Chronic Knee Pain in the Elderly.* Reports on the Rheumatic Diseases Series 5, no. 5. Arthritis Research Campaign, York, 2005.

CHAPTER 7

Pain in the Foot

Philip S. Helliwell[1] and Heidi J. Siddle[1,2]

[1] Leeds Institute of Rheumatic and Musculoskeletal Medicine, University of Leeds, Leeds, UK
[2] Foot Health Department, Leeds Teaching Hospitals NHS Trust, Leeds, UK

OVERVIEW

- Foot pain is common and can be associated with a number of local or generalized conditions.
- Clinical examination and simple investigations can usually identify the cause of the pain.
- Foot pain is a common feature in most rheumatic diseases, including rheumatoid arthritis and osteoarthritis.
- Podiatrists, general practitioners, rheumatologists and orthopaedic surgeons are involved in the management of foot pain.

Foot pain is common; 8% of primary care consultations are related to foot and ankle problems. It may be caused by local disease, be associated with systemic disease, or be a reflection of chronic widespread pain. In general, a multidisciplinary approach to treatment is preferable. This is reflected in increasingly close liaison between podiatry, rheumatology and orthopaedic departments. Chiropodists and podiatrists registered with the Health and Care Professions Council (HCPC) offer a range of treatments from skin lesion care to orthoses and, more recently, ambulatory foot surgery and local steroid injections.

To understand dysfunction, clinicians should be familiar with the normal development and anatomical variants of the foot (Boxes 7.1 and 7.2, Figures 7.1 and 7.2). This information can be found in *Neale's Disorders of the Foot* (Frowen *et al.*, 2010) and in the following paragraphs.

Foot pain in children

Pain may be associated with congenital abnormalities such as equinovarus deformity. Such structural abnormalities may reflect underlying neurological diseases, such as cerebral palsy. A rigid pronated foot in the early teens may be the first symptom of a tarsal coalition (Figure 7.3). Gait abnormalities, such as in-toeing, may be of concern to parents, but they are seldom treated actively. Juvenile idiopathic arthritis is the most common rheumatic disease in children and a primary cause of paediatric disability in the UK.

Juvenile idiopathic arthritis

The foot and ankle joints are most often affected in all subtypes of juvenile idiopathic arthritis. Children may present with a limp or reluctance to walk. In the hindfoot, pain and inflammation can lead

to valgus deformity (in two-thirds of cases) or varus deformity (in one-third of cases). In some patients, this may progress to bony ankylosis. The child may be reluctant to push off with the forefoot

---

Box 7.1 **Characteristics of the adult foot**

Three main types of foot

- Normal
- Pronated (flat) (Figure 7.1)
- Supinated (high arch) (Figure 7.2)

Examination

- Examine the foot when weight bearing and when non-weight bearing and be sure to look at the plantar surface of the foot for callus formation (often associated with high pressure)
- Inspect patient's shoes for abnormal or uneven wear
- Consult a podiatrist if a structural or mechanical abnormality is suspected – many can be treated with orthoses

---

Box 7.2 **Characteristics of children's feet**

Normal foot

- Flexible foot structure (may look flat with a valgus heel)
- Medial longitudinal arch forms when child stands on tiptoe
- Heel to toe walking
- Forefoot in line with rear foot
- Mobile joints with painless motion and no swelling
- Adopts adult morphology by about eight years of age

Abnormal foot

- Inflexible
- Lesser toe deformities
- Rigid valgus (pronated) foot with everted heel position (arch doesn't form when standing on tiptoe)
- High arch foot with toe retraction and tight extensor tendons
- Toe walking
- Delay or difficulty in walking or running
- Abducted or adducted forefoot relative to heel
- Pain, swelling, or stiffness of joints
- Hallux deformity

ABC of Rheumatology, Fifth Edition. Edited by Ade Adebajo and Lisa Dunkley.
© 2018 John Wiley & Sons Ltd. Published 2018 by John Wiley & Sons Ltd.

during walking, and pressure studies show poor contact of the foot to the floor. Lack of use can lead to delayed maturation of bone or soft tissue, and routine examination should include an assessment of leg length discrepancy.

Pain in the forefoot (metatarsalgia)

Morton's neuroma (interdigital neuroma)

This normally affects the proximal part of the plantar digital nerve and accompanying plantar digital artery. Trauma to these structures leads to histological changes, including inflammatory oedema, microscopic changes in the neurolemma, fibrosis and, later, degeneration of the nerve. Morton's neuroma is the result of irritation or compression of the interdigital nerve.

Clinical features – Clinical features include a gradual onset, with sudden attacks of neuralgic pain (burning) or paraesthesia during walking, often in the third and fourth toes. Examination may show lesser toe deformities, slight splaying of the forefoot, abnormal pronation and hallux valgus. These often occur in people who wear footwear with a narrow toe box or those who undertake sporting activities with increased movement in the forefoot. Compression of

the cleft or laterally across the metatarsal heads may produce acute pain and the characteristic 'Mulder's click'.

Treatment – An ultrasound scan is the most useful diagnostic tool. Patients should be given advice about suitable footwear and the provision of orthoses to address abnormal foot function. Treatment is with injections of local anaesthetic and hydrocortisone into the interdigital space, or surgical excision if this fails.

Stress fracture (march fracture)

Stress fractures are associated with increased activity, and lesions can affect any of the metatarsal shafts (Figure 7.4), often along the line of the surgical neck. They can occasionally be seen in patients with osteoporosis as a pathological fracture. Other common sites of stress fractures in the foot include the navicular and the calcaneus.

Clinical features – Patients will often report an increase in the frequency, duration or intensity of activity or exercise they undertake, which may coincide with a change in occupation or footwear. The symptom is a dull ache along the affected metatarsal shaft, which changes to a sharp ache just behind the metatarsal head. The pain is

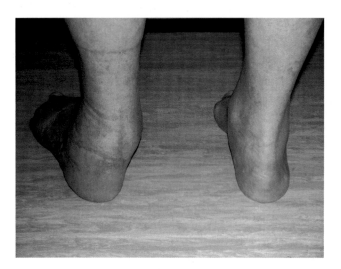

Figure 7.1 Abnormally pronated left foot demonstrating a significantly everted heel position

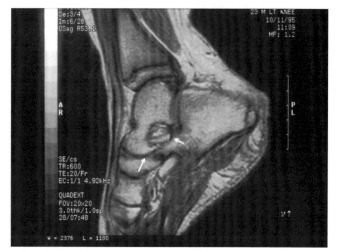

Figure 7.3 Tarsal coalition. Magnetic resonance image in a patient with calcaneonavicular coalition. Note synostosis between the calcaneus and navicular bones (*arrows*)

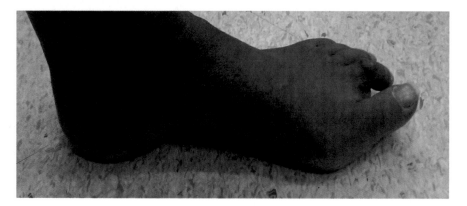

Figure 7.2 Abnormally supinated foot with a high arch profile and non-weight-bearing toes

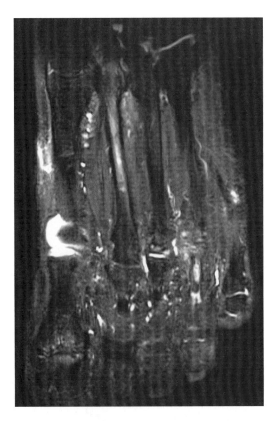

Figure 7.4 MR image demonstrating high signal in the shaft of the second metatarsal indicating a stress fracture

exacerbated by exercise and is more acute at 'toe off'. Tenderness and swelling are felt over the dorsal surface of the shaft. Pain is produced by compression of the metatarsal head or traction of the toe. X-ray examination may not show the fracture for up to 6 weeks, but if it is important to confirm the diagnosis, for example, for an athlete who needs advice on whether to continue playing sport, a bone scan or MRI can reveal it earlier.

Treatment – Rest and local immobilization are usually enough; the use of an Aircast boot allows mobilization during this period and is usually required for 6 weeks. These fractures rarely require casting or surgical fixation.

Acute synovitis

This condition is normally associated with acute trauma, which leads to inflammation of the synovial membrane and effusion. Freiberg's disease (avascular necrosis of the second metatarsal head) may also contribute. Systemic causes of acute synovitis, such as rheumatoid arthritis (Figure 7.5) or infection, should be excluded when making a diagnosis.

Clinical features – It is rare in children but often affects young adults in puberty. Patients complain of a sudden onset of painful throbbing that is made worse by movement. The patient may have experienced trauma or infection or have a systemic inflammatory disorder. Any movement of the joint produces pain. Fusiform swelling is present around the distended joint, and crepitus may be felt.

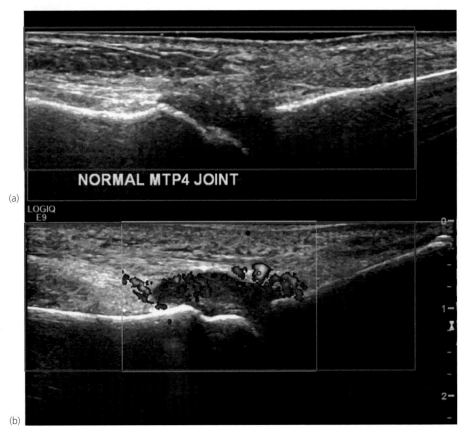

(a)

(b)

Figure 7.5 Ultrasound images of (a) normal MTP joint and (b) MTP joint demonstrating synovial hypertrophy and power Doppler signal indicating acute synovitis

Treatment – Rest, immobilization and ultrasound treatment may help if trauma is the cause. Anti-inflammatory drugs sometimes help. Previously unsuspected systemic arthritis, such as psoriatic arthritis, should be investigated.

Differential diagnosis: inflammation of anterior metatarsal soft tissue pad

This common condition is generally found in middle-aged women. It affects the soft tissues of the plantar aspect of the forefoot and is associated with increased shear forces, such as occur when wearing 'slip-on' and high-heeled court shoes.

Clinical features – Patients present with a burning or throbbing pain localized to the soft tissues anterior to the metatarsal heads. The pain usually develops over a few weeks, is often associated with walking in a particular pair of shoes, and is usually relieved by rest. The tissues are inflamed, warm and congested. Direct palpation, rotation and simulation of shear forces on the foot exacerbate the pain. Examination of patients' shoes may reveal a worn insole, with a depression under the metatarsal heads.

Management – Advice on footwear, with adequate support or cushioning, should be given. Associated abnormal pronation or lesser toe deformities should be corrected with orthoses.

Plantar metatarsal bursitis

This condition may affect the deep anatomical or superficial adventitious bursae. In the acute form, such as in dancers, squash players or skiers, the first metatarsal is usually affected, while the second to fourth metatarsals are predominantly affected in chronic inflammatory arthritis.

Clinical features – Patients present with a throbbing pain under a metatarsal head that usually persists at rest and is exacerbated when the area is first loaded. The acute condition affects men and women equally, usually in younger adults. If a superficial bursa is affected there will be signs of acute inflammation, with fluctuant swelling and warmth. With deep bursitis, the tissues are tight and congested. Direct pressure or compression produces pain, as does dorsiflexion of the associated digit.

Treatment – Anti-inflammatory drugs are useful; in practice, local gels and systemic oral drugs help. Injections of corticosteroid may be indicated in severe cases. Patients must rest the affected part; this may be achieved by immobilization of the forefoot (rocker-soled shoe or Aircast). Any underlying deformity or foot type with abnormal function should be assessed and treated.

A summary of causes of pain in the forefoot is presented in Box 7.3.

Pain along the medial longitudinal arch

Pain along the medial longitudinal arch is quite common. Most affected patients have abnormal foot mechanics, such as abnormal pronation, valgus heel or a flat foot. Mechanical dysfunction and

---

Box 7.3 **Causes of pain in the forefoot**

Primary
- Functional and structural forefoot pathologies

Secondary
- Inflammatory arthritis
- Stress lesions
- Post-traumatic syndromes
- Diabetes
- Gout
- Neurological conditions
- Sesamoid pathology
- Osteoarthritis

Unrelated to weight distribution
- Nerve root pathology
- Tarsal tunnel nerve compression syndrome

Box 7.4 **Common causes of painful heel**

Pain within heel
- Disease of calcaneus – osteomyelitis, tumours, Paget's disease
- Arthritis of subtalar joint complex

Pain behind heel
- Haglund's deformity ('pump bumps', 'heel bumps')
- Rupture of Achilles tendon
- Achilles paratendinitis
- Posterior tibial paratendinitis or tenosynovitis
- Peroneal paratendinitis or tenosynovitis
- Retrocalcaneal bursitis
- Subcutaneous calcaneal bursitis
- Calcaneal apophysitis

Pain beneath heel
- Tender heel pad
- Plantar fasciitis (Figure 7.6)
- Plantar calcaneal bursitis

---

change in medial arch posture can place strain on soft tissues, which results in localized or more diffuse pain – the foot's equivalent to 'low back pain' syndrome. Other conditions include true plantar fasciitis, which is characterized by a thickened plantar fascia, and plantar fibromatosis, which is characterized by fibrous nodules and contracture of the fascia.

Treatment of true plantar fascial strain requires rest and control of abnormal function with orthoses, and stretching exercises. Ultrasound treatment seems helpful and injections of corticosteroid into a thickened plantar fascia appear beneficial, but controlled trials are lacking.

Painful heel (Box 7.4)

Sever's disease (calcaneal apophysitis)

This was thought to be an avascular necrosis of growing bone but is now interpreted as a chronic strain at the attachment of the

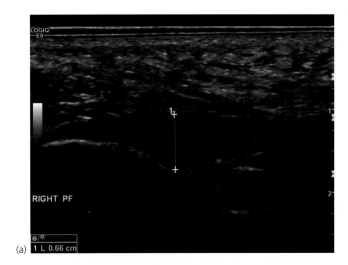 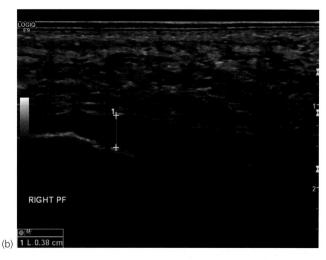

Figure 7.6 Ultrasound images of (a) normal plantar fascia (<0.45 cm) and (b) thickened plantar fascia (0.66 cm) indicating plantar fasciitis

posterior apophysis of the calcaneus to the main body of the bone, possibly from pull of the Achilles tendon. It therefore is analogous to Osgood–Schlatter disease of the tibial tuberosity.

Clinical features – The condition usually affects boys aged 8–13 years, who complain of a dull ache behind the heel of gradual onset that is exacerbated by jumping or occurs just before heel lift. A limp is usually seen with early heel lift. Rest normally relieves the pain. Tenderness is seen over the lower posterior part of the tuberosity of the calcaneus. Radiographs are usually normal.

Treatment – In most cases, reassurance and advice about reducing activities will suffice: the condition usually subsides spontaneously. In some cases, heel lifts help; occasionally, if the pain is severe, an Aircast walker boot is needed.

Plantar calcaneal bursitis

This is inflammation of the adventitious bursa beneath the plantar aspect of the calcaneal tuberosities. It is associated with shearing stress caused by an altered angle of heel strike.

Clinical features – The condition is characterized by an increasingly severe burning, aching and throbbing pain on the plantar surface of the heel. A history of increased activity or weight gain is usual. The heel seems normal but may feel warm. Direct pressure or sideways compression causes pain. The tissues may feel tight and congested.

Treatment – Rest and anti-inflammatory drugs may be useful. Heel cushions and medial arch supports are also used. Stretching exercises such as rolling a bottle under the foot and calf stretches can help. Little evidence supports ultrasound treatment, local steroid injections or shortwave diathermy.

Chronic inflammation of the heel pad

This is a distinct clinical condition that usually results from trauma (jumping) or heavy heel strike. It sometimes is seen in elderly people as their fat pads atrophy or in those who suddenly become more active.

Clinical features – A generalized warm dull throbbing pain is felt over the weight-bearing area of the heel; this develops over a few months. The pain is most intense typically on first rising. Tenderness is experienced over the heel, which feels tight and distended.

Treatment – Normally, this condition improves with time and rest. Footwear should be addressed: a suitably tight heel cap to hold the heel pad in place under the heel, and with shock-absorbing soles. If the condition does not improve then an ultrasound and X-ray assessment are recommended to exclude other acute pathologies.

Achilles tendon affections

Inflammation of the Achilles tendon and surrounding soft tissue may be associated with overuse or systemic inflammatory disorders (Box 7.5). Inflammation of the tendon, peritendon tissues and bursae give slightly different clinical pictures. Conditions such as xanthoma can also affect the Achilles tendon and produce fusiform swelling in the tendon. In such cases, cholesterol concentrations should be checked and treated if raised.

Rheumatoid nodules, and occasionally gouty tophi, can also be found within the substance of the Achilles tendon

Treatment depends on the primary cause. Partial or complete ruptures of the tendon need immobilization and surgical repair. For inflammatory conditions, non-steroidal anti-inflammatory drugs may help, as may ultrasound treatment, friction, rest and shock-absorbing heel lifts. Inflammation may be triggered by overuse through poor foot mechanics; in such cases, orthoses may control pronation, if present. Hydrocortisone injections may be useful if the bursa or peritendons are affected, but they are contraindicated for the tendon itself. Dry needling, platelet-rich plasma (PRP) and saline injections are also used. Ultrasound imaging may be useful both as a diagnostic tool and to aid intervention.

Osteochondritis

Osteochondritis is an aseptic necrosis or epiphyseal infraction associated with trauma and localized minute thrombosis of the epiphysis.

This quite common condition generally affects the second metatarsal head, calcaneus (both discussed above), the dorsal aspect of the talus (talar dome) and the navicular (Kohler's disease).

Clinical features – Osteochondritis affects teenagers and is associated with increased sporting activity. The presenting complaint is often a limp, with dull pain associated with movement of the affected area. The long-term result is destruction of the bone, which can progress to arthritis. The affected joint may be slightly swollen, with the potential for a change in the biomechanical function of the foot. Traction causes pain. Restricted movement may be due to muscle spasm in the early stages and later to arthritis. Radiographs show distortion of the involved bone.

Treatment – In the early stages, rest and immobilization are enough; foot orthoses will be required to improve the function of any resulting deformation. Unfortunately, sometimes patients eventually need corrective surgery.

Arthropathies that affect the foot

Osteoarthritis

Osteoarthritis in the foot may be asymptomatic, but it can lead to pain, joint stiffness, functional loss and disability. The most common sites are the first metatarsophalangeal joint (hallux rigidus),the midfoot joints and ankle, but foot osteoarthritis rarely occurs alone. Biomechanical factors are often involved in the development of degenerative joint changes. Trauma, recurrent inflammation and the demands of fashion footwear such as high heels and pointed toes may play a part.

Rheumatoid arthritis

Rheumatoid arthritis often starts in the foot, particularly at the metatarsophalangeal (MTP) joints. The forefoot is painful and stiff, and direct transverse pressure to the forefoot or squeezing a single metatarsophalangeal joint is often painful. Non-specific metatarsalgia is frequently diagnosed. In the early stages of the disease, the hindfoot, particularly the subtalar joint, may also be painful. Synovitis of tendon sheaths around the ankle may also occur. In chronic rheumatoid disease, severe pain in the forefoot may continue, with a sensation of walking on pebbles. Gross deformity causes dysfunction and disability (Figure 7.8).

Spondyloarthritis

This group includes ankylosing spondylitis, psoriatic arthritis, the arthropathy of inflammatory bowel disease, undifferentiated spondyloarthropathy and reactive arthritis. Inflammation at the insertion of the Achilles tendon, and retrocalcaneal bursitis can be seen. In radiographs, inflammatory spurs (bony spurs with irregular new bone formation and erosion) may be seen on the calcaneum at the insertion points of the Achilles tendon and plantar fascia. Asymmetrical heel pain may result from a plantar calcaneal enthesopathy.

The pattern of articular involvement in the foot may vary from a single 'sausage toe' (dactylitis) (Figure 7.9) to a very destructive arthritis. Painful stiff interphalangeal and metatarsophalangeal joints, often in an asymmetrical pattern, are common. Claw toe and hallux valgus deformity are more obvious. Nail dystrophy may be seen, with typical psoriatic pitting, onycholysis, subungual hyperkeratosis, discoloration and transverse ridging.

Pustular psoriasis and keratoderma blennorrhagica on the plantar aspect of the foot may contribute to pain when walking.

Neuropathic joint disease

Charcot neuropathic joint disease is a rare and disabling joint disease affecting people with diabetes and other sensory neuropathy disorders such as alcoholism. The acute progressive Charcot-like arthropathy primarily affects the midfoot and ankle. Patients complain of (paradoxically) pain and swelling in the foot, often after minor trauma. Untreated, this will rapidly deteriorate, leaving a disorganized and dysfunctional foot. Treatment must be immediate and intensive with immobilization of the foot and possibly intravenous bisphosphonates. Early referral is recommended.

Complex regional pain syndrome, type 1

A similar condition can develop in the non-diabetic foot following trauma. Complex regional pain syndrome type 1 (formerly known as reflex sympathetic dystrophy or Sudek's atrophy) is a painful condition of the foot and ankle associated with regional bone loss, tissue

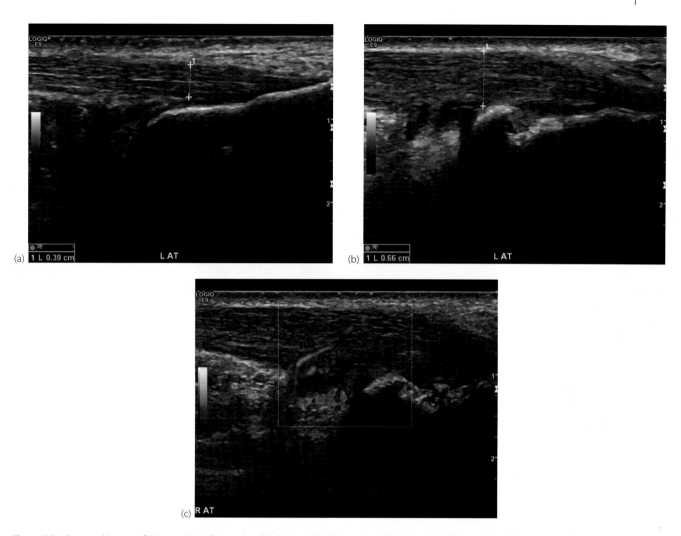

Figure 7.7 Ultrasound images of (a) normal Achilles tendon, (b) thickened Achilles tendon, (c) thickened Achilles tendon with power Doppler indicating tendonitis

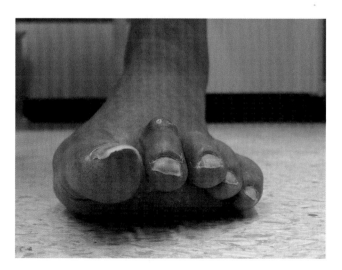

Figure 7.8 Extensive forefoot deformity in a patient with rheumatoid arthritis; hallux valgus with subluxation of the lesser MTP joints and retracted, non-weight-bearing toes

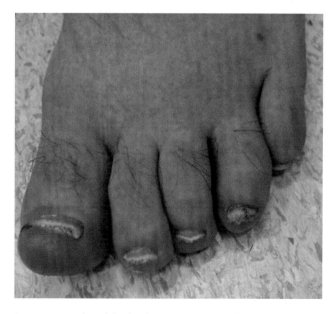

Figure 7.9 Dactylitis of the fourth toe and nail dystrophy in a patient with psoriatic arthritis

inflammation and vascular abnormalities. This may be mediated by abnormalities of the autonomic nervous system. The foot may look blue and swollen and is painful at rest and exercise. Plain X-ray may show widespread osteoporosis in the affected area. Treatment is effective pain control and physical therapies. Sympathetic blockade and intravenous bisphosphonates are treatments used.

Gout

Chapter 10 discusses the manifestations of acute gout in the foot. In the chronic state, tophi in the foot may ulcerate if they act as pressure points. Permanent destructive joint damage and deformity may result and lead to painful dysfunction in the foot. A single leaking tophus over an interphalangeal joint may be mistaken for chronic infection and underlying osteomyelitis. Instead of a swab sent for microbiology, the discharge should be examined for uric acid crystals.

Management of rheumatic foot conditions

Patients with rheumatic diseases (Box 7.6) affecting the feet are best managed by a team that includes a physician, a surgeon and allied health professionals. Podiatrists have a defined role in several aspects of foot health management.

Tissue viability

Joint deformity causes pressure lesions such as callosities, corns or ulceration and may be compounded by other factors such as ingrowing toe nails, peripheral neuropathy, reduced circulation or the effects of systemic drug therapies. Podiatrists undertake procedures such as scalpel reduction, design and manufacture of insoles and orthoses, and surgery under local anaesthesia to relieve pain and reduce deformity or restore function to maintain tissue viability.

Box 7.6 **Common abnormalities in the foot in rheumatoid arthritis**

- Hallux valgus
- Lesser toe deformities, for example, hammer toes and claw toes
- Prominent metatarsal heads with overlying painful callosities, bursae or ulceration
- Pronation of foot with valgus heel deformity and collapse of midtarsal joint, giving a flat-footed appearance
- Tenosynovitis, especially of tibialis posterior and peroneal tendons, plantar heel bursitis, calcaneal spur and tendo Achilles bursitis
- Tarsal tunnel nerve compression syndrome

Foot function and joint protection

Foot dysfunction due to arthritis can be improved with orthoses, which can be prefabricated or individually designed from casts. Orthoses may be used to control deformities such as the valgus heel seen in rheumatoid arthritis, but they also have a major role in maintaining tissue viability and relieving pain (be it joint, soft tissue or skin lesion in origin). Training towards gait modification may be necessary, and pressure-relieving orthoses of a total contact design may serve to reduce pressures at painful joint sites. Improvement in foot function may be aided by the injection of local corticosteroids.

Foot health promotion

Patients will often need advice on daily care of feet. Family members may be involved when patients cannot reach their feet or are unable to perform tasks on the feet because of other disability. Advice may be needed on splints, walking aids, footwear, insoles, foot hygiene and exercise.

Foot surgery

Foot surgery may be effective for relieving pain and improving deformity when conservative measures have failed. Many patients with rheumatic diseases have conditions of the toenails that need surgery under local anaesthetic; they are best dealt with by an experienced clinician such as a podiatrist.

Further reading

Frowen P, O'Donnell M, Burrow JG, Lorimer DL (eds). *Neale's Disorders of the Foot*, 8th rev edn. Elsevier Health Sciences/Churchill Livingstone, Edinburgh, 2010.

Helliwell P, Woodburn J, Redmond A, Turner D, Davys H. *The Foot and Ankle in Rheumatoid Arthritis. A Comprehensive Guide.* Churchill Livingstone/Elsevier, Edinburgh, 2007.

Podiatry Rheumatic Care Association. *Standards of Care for People with Musculoskeletal Foot Health Problems.* PRCA, London, 2008.

Redmond A. Foot and ankle. In: Watts RA, Conaghan PG, Denton C, Foster H, Isaacs J, Müller-Ladner U (eds), *Oxford Textbook of Rheumatology*, 4th edn. Oxford University Press, Oxford, 2013, p.156.

Redmond A, Helliwell PS. Musculoskeletal disorders. In: Frowen P, O'Donnell M, Burrow JG, Lorimer DL (eds). *Neale's Disorders of the Foot*, 8th rev edn. Elsevier Health Sciences/Churchill Livingstone, Edinburgh, 2010, pp. 199–230.

Redmond A, Helliwell PS, Robinson P. Investigating foot and ankle problems. In: Conaghan PG, O'Connor PJ, Isenberg DA (eds), *Oxford Specialist Handbook in Radiology: Musculoskeletal Imaging.* Oxford University Press, Oxford, 2010.

CHAPTER 8

Fibromyalgia Syndrome and Chronic Widespread Pain

Sarah Ryan[1] and Andrew Hassell[2]

[1] Staffordshire and Stoke on Trent Partnership NHS Trust, Haywood Hospital, Stoke on Trent, UK
[2] Staffordshire and Stoke on Trent Partnership NHS Trust; Keele University School of Medicine, Keele, UK

OVERVIEW

- Fibromyalgia is common and characterized by widespread musculoskeletal pain, muscle stiffness, fatigue and non-restorative sleep.
- There are physical, psychological and cognitive associations.
- Diagnosis is made on the presence of clinical symptoms.
- Simple investigations will exclude other causes of musculoskeletal pain.
- Management includes education, graded exercise, pacing activities, psychotherapeutic interventions and limited drug therapy.

Chronic widespread pain is very common in the general population, with an estimated point prevalence of 11% in the United Kingdom. Living with pain has a significant impact on the individual and society, in terms of reduced physical functioning, depressive symptoms, increased use of healthcare resources and work productivity loss. The focus of this chapter will be fibromyalgia as the prototype condition that manifests with chronic widespread pain and fatigue

Fibromyalgia or fibromyalgia syndrome (FMS), a heterogeneous pain syndrome of unknown aetiology, affects 0.5–5% of the population and is much more common in women. As the treatment effects of single interventions are modest at best, the European League against Rheumatism (EULAR) recommends a multidisciplinary approach to the management of fibromyalgia tailored according to symptom intensity, patient function and associated features. The aim of management is to optimize physical, psychological and social functioning.

Diagnosis

As there are currently no diagnostic tests for FMS, the diagnosis is exclusively clinical. Most patients will have had symptoms for 2–3 years before a diagnosis is made. The main symptoms are chronic widespread musculoskeletal pain, muscle stiffness, non-restorative sleep and fatigue, in the absence of an alternative explanation such as active inflammatory arthritis, endocrine or metabolic disorder. Commonly associated physical, psychological and cognitive symptoms are identified in Box 8.1.

The original American College of Rheumatology (ACR) criteria for fibromyalgia have been considered the gold standard for diagnosis for research studies since their introduction in 1990. The criteria include the presence of widespread pain of at least 3 months' duration and pain at 11 of 18 designated tender points when finger pressure (just enough to blanch the clinician's fingertips) is applied (Figure 8.1). These criteria have not been widely used in clinical practice, perhaps owing to the reliance on tender spots and the lack of consideration of other symptoms. In 2010, the ACR proposed an additional/alternative set of diagnostic criteria for use in primary care, recognizing perhaps that fibromyalgia is a common spectrum disorder rather than a discrete one. The new criteria do not require tender point examination. They include a widespread pain index (number of defined areas, between 0 and 19, in which a patient has had pain in the previous week) and a symptom severity score (0–9) which includes fatigue, waking unrefreshed and cognitive symptoms identified in Box 8.1.

Box 8.1 **Physical, psychological and cognitive associations with fibromyalgia**

Physical	Psychological	Cognitive
Urinary frequency and urgency	Panic attacks	Memory lapses
Irritable bowel syndrome	Anxiety	Word mix-ups
Migraine	Depression	Reduced concentration
Muscle spasm	Irritability	
Dizziness		
Perception of swelling (typically of limb extremities)		
Paraesthesia		
Temperature changes		

ABC of Rheumatology, Fifth Edition. Edited by Ade Adebajo and Lisa Dunkley.
© 2018 John Wiley & Sons Ltd. Published 2018 by John Wiley & Sons Ltd.

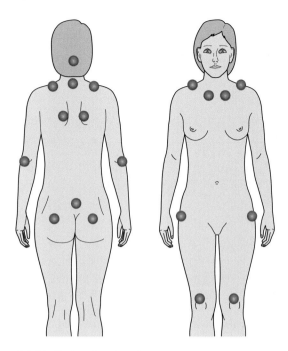

Figure 8.1 Distribution of tender points

Aetiology and symptoms

The aetiology of fibromyalgia is unknown and has been the subject of some controversy with, at the two ends of a spectrum, some believing that there is an entirely physical explanation, for example a viral infection, and others proposing that it represents a somatization syndrome. Our current understanding is that the primary abnormality is in pain processing within the central nervous system resulting in maladaptive pain responses. Patients can experience pain from sensory stimuli including heat, touch and auditory tones. This dysfunctional pain processing results from a number of factors including central sensitization, blunting of inhibitory pain pathways, altered neurotransmitters and psychological stressors.

Predisposing factors may include anxiety, depression, viral infection or exposure to physical and/or emotional trauma. Psychological factors have been identified as contributing to the symptoms of fibromyalgia including previous pain conditions, anxiety and stressful life events. Fibromyalgia is not solely a pain syndrome and patients often experience stiffness, fatigue and sleep disturbance among other physical, psychological and cognitive symptoms (see Box 8.1).

A typical patient will tend to be female aged 30–50 years with long-standing diffuse pain. She will describe pain in the muscles and joints. Fatigue will be pronounced (there is considerable overlap with chronic fatigue syndrome and 55% of chronic fatigue syndrome patients fulfil the diagnostic criteria for fibromyalgia). She will often have a history of previous physical or psychological trauma. She will describe a disturbed sleep pattern and difficulties in concentration and short-term memory recall. Her symptoms are always present and are exacerbated when she encounters a period of stress. She is anxious and low in mood as her symptoms are affecting her work and social activities. Often, she will have tried a number of analgesics and non-steroidal anti-inflammatory tablets without any improvement.

Investigations

There are no confirmatory investigations to arrive at a diagnosis of fibromyalgia but it is important that investigations are carried out to exclude other causes of musculoskeletal pain (Box 8.2). It is helpful to explain to the patient why these investigations are required and the expectation that they will be normal. Patients often feel that normal investigation results reduce the validity of their condition and the clinician can help by validating that their symptoms are genuine and recognized, irrespective of the investigation results. Useful investigations to exclude other disorders are listed in Box 8.3.

Management

The management of patients with fibromyalgia involves education about the condition and the treatments available, including graded exercise, pacing activities, psychotherapeutic interventions, sleep hygiene and drug therapy. The goal of treatment is to minimize symptoms and optimize physical, psychological and social function. All interventions must be tailored to the individual needs of the patient.

Education

It is important to be able to explain the concept of fibromyalgia to the patient. The clinician can explain that the pain system has

---

Box 8.2 Other causes of diffuse or widespread musculoskeletal pain

- Inflammatory arthritis
- SLE/Sjogren's syndrome
- Hypermobility syndromes
- Polymyalgia rheumatica
- Polymyositis/dermatomyositis
- Vasculitides
- Hypo- and hyperthyroidism
- Multiple sclerosis
- Neuropathies
- Osteomalacia
- Chronic fatigue syndrome
- Treatment with statins

Box 8.3 Suggested investigations

- Full blood count
- Tests of inflammation (erythrocyte sedimentation rate and C-reactive protein)
- Muscle enzymes (creatinine kinase)
- Bone profile (calcium, alkaline phosphatase, phosphate; perhaps vitamin D)
- Blood glucose
- Thyroid-stimulating hormone
- A simple autoantibody screen: rheumatoid factor and antinuclear antibody (weakly positive ANA generally insignificant)
- Urinalysis for protein, blood and glucose

become more sensitive by demonstrating the patient's response to light touch which will manifest as pain. Patients appear more satisfied by explanations of fibromyalgia that make sense to them, remove blame, integrate psychological and biological factors and include practical ideas for management.

The patient will often need guidance, support and motivation from a health professional before feeling able to take an active role in the management of their symptoms. Coping with symptoms includes the acceptance of symptoms and of some limitations as well as continuous self-management. Patient-centred goals need to be realistic to prevent failure and increased feelings of helplessness.

Some areas may run pain management programmes to help patients cope with their symptoms. It can be useful to signpost patients to the Arthritis Research UK website which contains patient-specific information on the condition.

Graded exercise

Patients experiencing pain and fatigue can understandably find it difficult to engage in exercise due to the bothersome nature of these symptoms. There can often be a fear of increasing symptoms and patients will very commonly have reduced or even stopped any form of exercise. Swimming, walking and/or cycling are forms of exercise that are good for maintaining muscle health and there is evidence to support the use of aerobic exercise in patients with fibromyalgia. One of the most successful ways to help the patient re-engage in exercise is to use a graded approach.

The principle of graded exercise is to start with a small, achievable and maintained amount of exercise, for example a 10-minute walk three times a week, to allow the muscles to become accustomed to a regular demand. It is helpful if such exercise is linked to a functional goal such as walking the children to school for it to be meaningful to the person and for it to be carried out. Breaking down exercise into small manageable times throughout the week may help avoid the situation where the person exercises less frequently and then experiences several days of heightened pain and fatigue following a burst of exercise.

Pacing activities

Pacing involves breaking down everyday activities into small realistic goals to accommodate the pain and fatigue and to maintain function. Many patients wait for a day when their symptoms are less bothersome and then overexert themselves, leading to increased symptoms and several days when they are unable to do anything. It is important to support the patient to break this 'boom-and-bust' cycle. By encouraging patients to plan and prioritize their activities, they can remain functionally active. For example, by cleaning one room in the house a day instead of doing all the rooms in one go, the desired outcome is still achieved and the symptoms of pain and fatigue are less intense.

Psychotherapeutic interventions

Psychological therapies including cognitive behavioural therapy, mindfulness-based treatments, relaxation and biofeedback are used to treat fibromyalgia. Cognitive behavioural therapy focuses on thoughts and behaviour to modify emotional responses to pain and improve personal control and function. For example, patients can become fearful about engaging in exercise as they think this will increase their pain. By explaining the purpose of exercise and supporting the patient to engage in small, realistic amounts of exercise, the patient's confidence and willingness to try exercise can improve as they adjust their thoughts as to what exercise involves and the benefits it can have.

Mindfulness-based techniques including relaxation, meditation and stress management are focused on acceptance of the condition and an awareness of how emotions may affect coping. For example, dwelling on the pain may lead to a reduction in daily functioning. Once acceptance and awareness have been gained, it will be easier to support the patient in setting meaningful goals (e,g. walking to the shops) which will increase their sense of control over the condition

Sleep

Patients with fibromyalgia often report a poor quality of sleep. Behavioural measures (Box 8.4) can help here and may be complemented by medications such as amitriptyline and duloxetine.

Complementary/alternative medicine

Patients often ask about the use of complementary and alternative therapies but there is a lack of available evidence to inform patients in this area. Tai chi, yoga and meditation have been shown to improve muscle stiffness, stress, depression, anxiety and self-esteem. The use of acupuncture has been associated with a small reduction in pain in patients with FMS.

Drug therapy

Patients with fibromyalgia often exhibit multiple symptoms in addition to pain and may be prescribed a combination of medications. If a trial of a specific medication is ineffective after a sufficient period of use, it should be discontinued as it is common to see patients on a number of different medications which are not being effective. Analgesics such as paracetamol or co-codamol may be prescribed. There is little evidence to support the use of stronger opioids. Other medications that have been shown to be of benefit in randomized controlled trials are shown in Box 8.5. The choice of which drug to start is an individual, tailored one, depending on the patient's main symptoms, co-morbidities and preferences.

Box 8.4 **Behavioural measures to assist sleep**

- Develop a sleep routine that involves going to bed and getting up at a set time
- Avoid daytime sleeping
- Reduce intake of stimulants such as coffee and alcohol
- Exercise early in the day and not in the evening
- Increase the amount of exercise taken during the day
- Avoid watching television in the bedroom
- Ensure the bedroom is well ventilated
- Have a hot bath as part of a sleep routine

Conclusion

Chronic widespread pain conditions, including fibromyalgia, are characterized by pain, fatigue, unrefreshing sleep and other somatic symptoms. The diagnosis is made from the clinical history and physical examination with investigations to eliminate other causes of the symptoms. A multidisciplinary approach to management is required to help patients cope with their symptoms and to optimize physical, psychological and social function.

Further reading

Choy E. (2015) *Fibromyalgia Syndrome*, Oxford Rheumatology Library. Oxford University Press

Kuttikat A, Shenker N. Fibromyalgia and chronic widespread pain syndromes – adult onset. In: Watts R, Conaghan P, Denton C *et al.* (eds), *The Oxford Textbook of Rheumatology*, 4th edn. Oxford University Press, Oxford, 2013, pp. 1373–1379.

Sosa-Reina MD, Nunez-Nagys S, Gallego-Izquierdo T *et al.* (2017) Effectiveness of Therapeutic Exercise in Fibromyalgia Syndrome. *BioMed Research International*. doi 1155/2017/2356346.Epub 2017.

CHAPTER 9

Osteoarthritis

Michael Doherty and A. Abhishek

Academic Rheumatology, University of Nottingham; Nottingham University Hospitals Trust, Nottingham, UK

OVERVIEW

- Osteoarthritis (OA) presents with usage-related joint pain in middle-aged and older people.
- Typically affects the knees, hips, thumb bases and finger interphalangeal joints.
- Risk factors for OA include age, female sex, obesity and joint injury.
- OA can be diagnosed confidently on clinical grounds alone as there is only a modest correlation between radiographic changes and symptoms.
- Management of OA should be individualized with emphasis on patient education, exercise, analgesia, functional optimization, and managing adverse biomechanical factors.

Osteoarthritis (OA) is the most common condition to affect synovial joints. It is also the most important cause of locomotor disability and a major challenge for healthcare providers. OA was previously regarded as a degenerative disease due to trauma and ageing (Figure 9.1). However, it is now regarded as a dynamic process characterized by joint tissue injury and attempted joint repair. This may result from either abnormal biomechanical stress on a normal joint or normal stress applied to an inherently compromised joint (Figure 9.2). Frequently, both factors contribute. Therefore, OA is a consequence of a number of interacting processes and risk factors. Risk factors for OA may vary in importance from joint to joint, and risk factors for development of OA may differ from risk factors for its progression (Box 9.1). Often inherent joint repair compensates for the triggering insults, resulting in asymptomatic structural OA. In other cases, however, repair cannot compensate, leading to symptoms and disability.

Presentation

Osteoarthritis is traditionally separated into primary and secondary OA. Primary OA typically involves joints in characteristic locations (Figure 9.3) and is likely to result mainly from genetic and other constitutional predisposition. Multiple Heberden's nodes

(bony enlargement of distal interphalangeal joints (DIPJs) of the hand) (Figure 9.4) appear in middle age and are a strong marker for subsequent development of knee OA, and OA at other common target sites (nodal generalized OA). However, OA can occur in any synovial joint. When OA occurs in atypical joints, such as the ankle, the presentation alone should trigger consideration of secondary OA. Typical aetiologies of secondary OA include previous joint trauma, fracture and inflammatory arthritis like gout. Joint injury is the most common of these, and can lead to OA 15–20 years after the joint insult. It is a common cause of young-onset mono- or pauciarticular OA. When abnormal joint stress occurs in those with abnormal joint physiology, the outcome is even more severe. For example, severe knee meniscal damage is more likely to cause eventual knee OA in patients with hand OA (suggesting genetic predisposition to OA) compared to patients without hand OA (Englund and Lohmander, 2004).

Symptoms

The main symptoms of OA include pain, stiffness and reduced range of movement. Hyaline cartilage is not innervated, and pain in OA arises from nociceptive fibres and mechanoreceptors in the synovium, capsule, subchondral bone and periarticular tissues (e.g. ligaments, bursae). Pain in OA has insidious onset and slow progression, and affects just one or a few joints at a time. It is use related. However, night pain does occur in severe OA. Although not universal, pain in OA frequently progresses through three sometimes overlapping stages (Hawker *et al.*, 2008).

- Stage 1: sharp, predictable pain often brought on by a mechanical insult that limits high-impact activities with modest effect on function.
- Stage 2: constant pain which affects daily activities.
- Stage 3: constant dull/aching pain with short-lived, often unpredictable exacerbations resulting in severe functional limitations.

Early-morning stiffness in OA is short-lived (<30 minutes), and brief periods of inactivity-related stiffness ('gelling') is common.

ABC of Rheumatology, Fifth Edition. Edited by Ade Adebajo and Lisa Dunkley.
© 2018 John Wiley & Sons Ltd. Published 2018 by John Wiley & Sons Ltd.

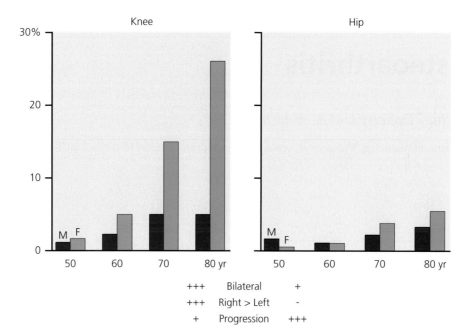

Figure 9.1 Differences between knee and hip OA in terms of age and sex prevalence, symmetry and likelihood for clinical progression, supporting consideration of OA at each site as discrete conditions. Source: van Sasse *et al.* (1989), reproduced with permission of BMJ Publishing Group Ltd

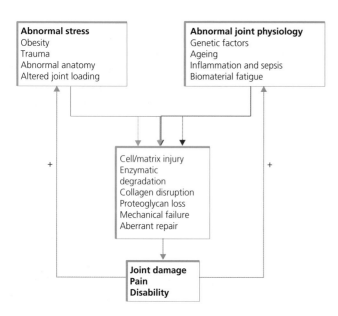

Figure 9.2 Pathways to osteoarthritis. Source: Modified from Poole *et al.* (2007), with permission of Dr Farshid Guilak and Lippincot Williams and Wilkins

Both these quickly improve with joint use. Joint stiffness arises at least in part from the accumulation of hyaluronan (joint lubricant and the most abundant constituent of synovial fluid) and hyaluronan fragments in the deep layers of arthritic synovium during rest, thereby excluding water from within the synovial tissue. Joint movement mobilizes hyaluronan to the lymphatics and blood with attendant hydration of synovial tissue and improvement in joint stiffness (Engstrom-Laurent and Hallgren, 1987). Other symptoms of OA such as locomotor restriction, functional impairment and

Box 9.1 Risk factors of OA

Age	Not a direct consequence of ageing. This association reflects cumulative effects of joint insults and failure of repair mechanisms
Sex	More common in women. More likely to be severe and symptomatic (except hip OA)
Race	Lateral compartment knee OA and hip OA are more common in Chinese and African-American men respectively compared to Caucasians
Obesity	Important risk factor for knee and hand OA
Genetics	40–65% of OA is heritable. Heritability is stronger for hand and hip OA. Polymorphisms in GDF 5, 7q22 and MCF$_2$L associate with OA with genome-wide association significance
Joint injury and use	Major joint injury can cause OA at any site. Recognized occupational hazards include farming, lifting (hip OA); kneeling or squatting, professional soccer (knee OA); heavy manual jobs and frequent pincer movement (hand and thumb base OA)
Joint shape and alignment	Varus or valgus knee alignment (knee OA); excessive medially or laterally placed patella, high-riding patella (patellofemoral OA); acetabular dysplasia, pistol grip femoral deformity and femoro-acetabular impingment (hip OA); ≥1 cm lower limb length inequality (lower limb OA)
Bone mineral density (BMD)	High BMD associates with OA but not its progression. Paradoxically, low BMD associates with OA progression

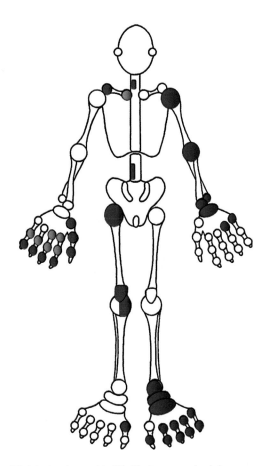

Figure 9.3 Joint involvement in OA. Most common (*red*), less common (*yellow*), least common (*blue*). OA may still be the most common arthritis to affect joints coloured blue

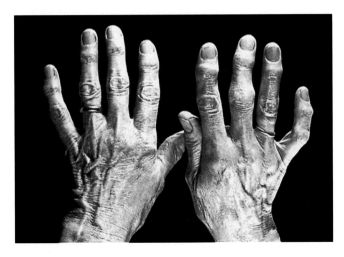

Figure 9.4 Hands with Heberden's nodes (bony enlargement of distal interphalangeal joints) and Bouchard's nodes (bony enlargement of proximal interphalangeal joints)

disability depend on the site and severity of OA, and on the individual's activities. Cartilage matrix changes in OA promote calcium pyrophosphate, basic calcium phosphate and monosodium urate crystal deposition, and this may result in superimposed attacks of acute crystal synovitis.

Examination

Common signs include bony swelling, tenderness, crepitus, reduced range of motion, deformity and instability. Bony swelling results from marginal osteophytosis and bone remodelling. Joint line tenderness suggests articular pathology, while tenderness away from the joint line suggests secondary periarticular lesions due to altered joint biomechanics. Crepitus, a coarse crunching sensation or sound due to friction between damaged articular cartilage and/or bone, occurs during both active and passive movement. Reduced active and passive movement is typical of OA, and predominantly results from marginal osteophytosis, capsular thickening and synovial hyperplasia +/− effusion. Muscle weakness and wasting, when present, suggest moderate to severe OA. Deformity and instability suggest severe joint damage. Marked inflammation is not a feature, and any erythema or acute painful effusion and warmth suggest co-existent crystal synovitis.

In contrast to the distribution of joint involvement in OA (see Figure 9.3), RA simultaneously involves multiple small and large joints in a symmetrical fashion. As co-morbidities like fibromyalgia, sleep deprivation, anxiety, depression and adverse social factors affect symptoms and response to treatment in OA, the evaluation of patients should include focused assessment to establish their presence.

Investigations

Osteoarthritis is a clinical diagnosis and may be reached without radiographic or laboratory investigations in the presence of typical symptoms and signs in the at-risk age group. This is supported by the fact that there is only a poor correlation between structural changes and symptoms in OA (Figures 9.5, Figures 9.6). Effusion, synovial hypertrophy and low-grade power Doppler signal have been observed on ultrasound evaluation of joints with OA but this is much less than in inflammatory arthropathies. Synovial fluid examination is indicated only if co-existent crystal deposition or sepsis is suspected.

Management

The goals of OA management (Figure 9.7) are to provide patient education and information, relieve pain, optimize function and minimize disease progression. Treatment should be individualized according to patient preference, location and risk factors for OA, severity of structural changes, level of pain and restriction of daily activities (Fernandes *et al.*, 2013). Symptoms are often episodic. It is therefore advisable to provide the patient with an armamentarium of treatment options to choose from during periods of relative quiescence and exacerbations.

Patient education and information access

This is a professional responsibility but education also improves outcome and is a treatment in its own right. The myth that OA is a progressive wearing out of joints due to old age still persists and leads to inappropriate reduction in activity. Education on weight loss should be incorporated (Fernandes *et al.*, 2013). Good evidence

Pain and radiographic OA

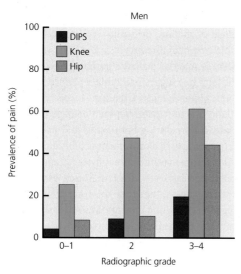
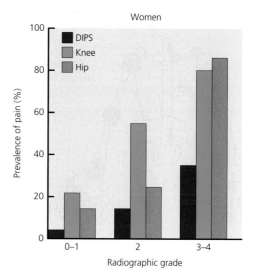

Figure 9.5 The discordance between radiographic OA and symptoms in hands, knees and hips. Source: Reproduced from Arden and Nevitt (2006), with permission of Elsevier

supports the use of educational programmes to help patients understand OA and develop self-management strategies.

Exercise

People with OA should be taught a regular individualized daily exercise regime that includes sustained isometric exercise, aerobic activity and adjunctive range of movement/stretching exercises (Fernandes *et al.*, 2013). Aerobic activity reduces pain and disability from OA, improves well-being and sleep quality and is beneficial for common co-morbidities. Increased activity and exercise can be accomplished in a variety of ways, including home exercise or group classes. Pool exercise, during which patients weigh one-eighth of their land weight, can mitigate the negative effects of excessive joint loading due to obesity and allow freedom of joint movement and aerobic training for individuals with lower extremity OA.

Reducing adverse biomechanical factors

Spreading physically demanding jobs (e.g. housework, mowing the lawn) throughout the day with breaks in between ('pacing') reduces sustained mechanical loading. Weight reduction improves function, reduces pain in obese and overweight patients and slows progression of knee OA. Appropriate footwear (thick soft sole, no raised heel, broad forefoot and deep soft uppers) can reduce the impact of loading in people with knee and hip OA. A walking stick used by the contralateral hand and other walking aids reduce loading across OA joints. Wedged insoles and thumb-base splints are effective for knee and trapeziometacarpal OA respectively. Other modifications such as raising seat height, stair hand rails, walk-in shower and appropriate car modifications help with symptoms (Fernandes *et al.*, 2013).

Pharmacological treatments

Cardiovascular, gastrointestinal, renal and other co-morbidities often co-exist with OA, and may influence choice of adjunctive drug management. Pain is the main reason for patients seeking

help. Paracetamol or topical non-steroidal anti-inflammatory drugs (NSAIDs) should be the first choice. Topical NSAIDs may be preferred over paracetamol in knee or hand OA as they have minimal systemic side effects, and are more analgesic (Cibere *et al.*, 2010; Zhang *et al.*, 2007).

Oral NSAIDs, selective COX-2 inhibitors and weak opioids (e.g. codeine, tramadol) may be considered for patients who obtain insufficient relief from topical NSAIDs and/or paracetamol. The risk of upper gastrointestinal bleeding and ulceration from NSAIDs can be decreased by co-prescription of proton pump inhibitors. Selective COX-2 inhibitors, although safer for the gut, increase the risk of cardiovascular events just like some traditional NSAIDs. Traditional NSAIDs can also adversely affect renal function, especially in the elderly. NSAIDs and selective COX-2 inhibitors should therefore be given at lowest effective dose on an as-required basis. Weak opioids provide good analgesia but side effects such as headache, confusion and constipation often limit their usefulness. Several studies have shown slowing of progressive joint space narrowing in OA patients on glucosamine and chondroitin sulphates. However, there are also negative trials and they are not recommended by NICE (2008) and other OA guidelines (Hochberg *et al.*, 2012).

Intra-articular corticosteroid injection is a valuable treatment that often gives quick effective analgesia that may last from a few weeks to several months. It is particularly useful to tide a patient over an important personal event and to improve pain during initiation of other events such as an exercise programme. A variety of hyaluronan preparations are also available, given as a single injection or a course of one per week for 3–5 weeks. However, there is again trial heterogeneity, the cost and logistics of the treatment are limiting, and they are not recommended by NICE (2008).

Surgery

The success of total joint replacement (TJR) has advanced the management of end-stage knee or hip OA. Surgery is also used for the management of end-stage shoulder, elbow and thumb base OA.

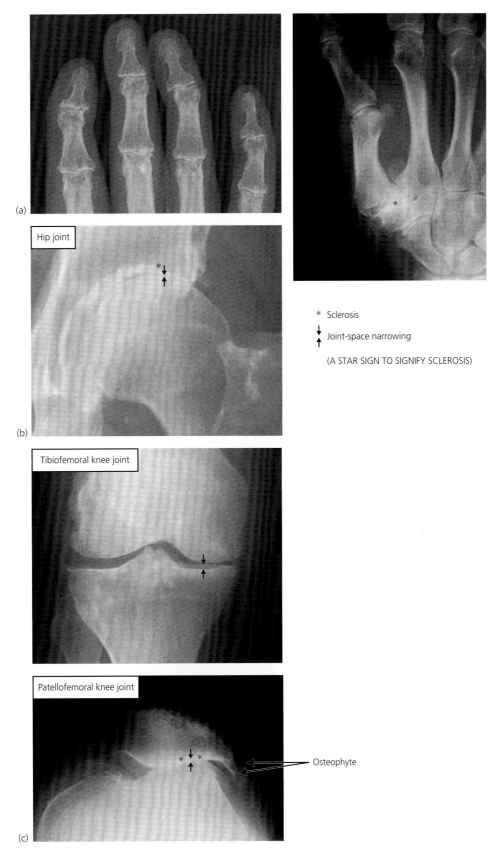

* Sclerosis

↓
↑ Joint-space narrowing

(A STAR SIGN TO SIGNIFY SCLEROSIS)

Figure 9.6 Radiographic OA: representative images of a hand (a), a hip (b) and a knee (c) with radiographic OA

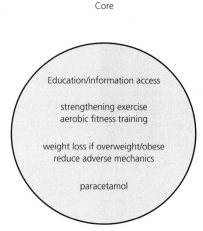

Core	Options
	Topical NSAID
	topical capsaicin
	oral NSAID
	opioids
Education/information access	nutripharmaceuticals
	ia steroid
strengthening exercise	ia hyaluronan
aerobic fitness training	walking aid
	mechanical supports
	assistive devices
weight loss if overweight/obese	acupuncture
reduce adverse mechanics	thermotherapy
	electrotherapy
	telephone contact
paracetamol	coping strategies
	washout
	surgery

Figure 9.7 Summary of the medical management of OA, illustrating the need for holistic approach. i.a., intra-articular

The criteria for referral for consideration of TJR are not universally agreed upon but include uncontrolled pain and severe impairment of function despite conservative treatment. Age itself is not a contraindication. Surgical correction of anatomical predisposition to knee and hip OA (e.g. tibial osteotomy, hip labral repair) may prevent disease progression.

Conclusion

In summary, OA is a condition of increasing prevalence which, although often asymptomatic, may cause a range of symptom severity and disability. An individualized and holistic approach to management is essential as the best means for relieving pain, minimizing disability and improving quality of life. The core management is non-pharmacological.

References

Arden N, Nevitt M. Osteoarthritis: epidemiology. *Best Practice and Research in Clinical Rheumatology* 2006; **20**: 3–25.

Cibere J, Zhang H, Thorne A *et al*. Association of clinical findings with pre-radiographic and radiographic knee osteoarthritis in a population-based study. *Arthritis Care and Research* 2010; **62**: 1691–1698.

Englund M, Lohmander LS. Risk factors for symptomatic knee osteoarthritis fifteen to twenty-two years after meniscectomy. *Arthritis and Rheumatism* 2004; **50**: 2811–2819.

Engstrom-Laurent A, Hallgren R. Circulating hyaluronic acid levels vary with physical activity in healthy subjects and in rheumatoid arthritis patients. Relationship to synovitis mass and morning stiffness. *Arthritis and Rheumatism* 1987; **30**: 1333–1338.

Fernandes L, Hagen KB, Bijlsma JW *et al*. EULAR recommendations for the non-pharmacological core management of hip and knee osteoarthritis. *Annals of the Rheumatic Diseases* 2013; **72**: 1125–1135.

Hawker GA, Stewart L, French MR *et al*. Understanding the pain experience in hip and knee osteoarthritis – an OARSI/OMERACT initiative. *Osteoarthritis and Cartilage* 2008; **16**: 415–422.

Hochberg MC, Altman RD, April KT *et al*. American College of Rheumatology 2012 recommendations for the use of nonpharmacologic and pharmacologic therapies in osteoarthritis of the hand, hip, and knee. *Arthritis Care and Research* 2012; **64**: 465–474.

National Institute for Health and Care Excellence. *Osteoarthritis: The Care and Management of Osteoarthritis in Adults*. Clinical Guideline 59. NICE, London, 2008.

Poole AR, Guilak F, Abramson SB. Etiopathogenesis of osteoarthritis. In: Moskowitz RW, Altman RD, Hochberg MC, Buckwalter JA, Goldberg VM (eds), *Osteoarthritis: Diagnosis and Medical/Surgical Management*, 4th edn. Lippincott Williams and Wilkins, Philadelphia, 2007, pp. 27–49.

van Saase JL, van Romunde LK, Cats A, Vandenbroucke JP, Valkenburg HA. Epidemiology of osteoarthritis: Zoetermeer survey. Comparison of radiological osteoarthritis in a Dutch population with that in 10 other populations. *Annals of the Rheumatic Diseases* 1989; **48**: 271–280.

Zhang W, Doherty M, Leeb BF *et al*. EULAR evidence based recommendations for the management of hand osteoarthritis: report of a Task Force of the EULAR Standing Committee for International Clinical Studies Including Therapeutics (ESCISIT). *Annals of the Rheumatic Diseases* 2007; **66**: 377–388.

CHAPTER 10

Gout, Hyperuricaemia and Crystal Arthritis

Martin Underwood

Warwick Clinical Trials Unit, Warwick Medical School, The University of Warwick Coventry, UK;
Department of Epidemiology and Preventive Medicine Monash University, Clayton, Australia

---

OVERVIEW

- Asymptomatic hyperuricaemia does not need treating.
- Steroids, NSAIDs or colchicine can be used to treat acute gout.
- Patients with recurrent gout ≥ twice a year should be offered urate lowering medication.
- Target serum urate for patients on urate-lowering drugs is <0.36 mmol/L (or <0.30 if tophi present).
- Dose of urate-lowering medication should be titrated according to response; many patients with recurrent gout get inadequate doses of urate-lowering drugs.

Gout and hyperuricaemia

Gout is a common metabolic disorder, typically presenting as an acute monoarthritis, most commonly of the first metatarsal phalangeal joint. The term 'gout' includes an acute attack, the propensity for repeated episodes and also for chronic gouty arthritis. The underlying problem is a build-up of urate, a purine breakdown product. Humans, and some primates, lack uricase, which in other mammals oxidizes urate to allantoin, which is readily soluble. Both an increased dietary purine intake and an increased breakdown of endogenous proteins (e.g. cancer treatment or haematological malignancy) can increase urate levels.

Urate excretion is mainly renal. The rate of renal excretion is affected by urine flow, pH and competition for renal tubular exchange (e.g. diuretics). People whose problems are primarily due to increased purine turnover will have a high urinary urate and those whose problems are primarily renal will have a low urinary urate. This distinction is rarely of clinical importance. For uric acid crystals to form, the serum needs to be saturated with urate, i.e. >0.42 mmol/L (>7.0 g/dL). This is coincidentally the upper limit of the reference range in men and postmenopausal women in many laboratories. For premenopausal women, the upper limit of the reference range for serum urate is commonly 0.36 mmol/L (6.0 mg/dL).

Epidemiology

Globally, the age-standardized prevalence of gout is 0.076% (95% uncertainty interval (UI) 0.072–0.082). This overall figure, from the Global Burden of Disease, conceals striking differences in prevalence between regions and within regions according to age and sex. Population prevalences range from 0.39% (95% UI 0.35–0.43) in Australasia to 0.03% (95% UI 0.02–0.05) in parts of sub-Saharan Africa. For men living in Australasia, southern Latin America, North America (high income) and western Europe, prevalences all exceed 1% by the age of 60, peaking at over 2.5% in elderly Australasian men (Figure 10.1). Even in high-prevalence regions, only around 0.5% of elderly women are affected. See http://vizhub.healthdata.org/gbd-compare/ for detailed breakdown.

There is no pattern of change of age-standardized prevalence of gout over time. Nevertheless, with an ageing population, the absolute number of people affected and the disease burden are increasing. However, there are few reliable data on how many people are affected each year or how many people are taking prophylactic drugs. Some non-white populations are more prone to gout/hyperuricaemia; there is generally a higher prevalence of gout in indigenous ethnic groups around the Pacific Rim. Environmental factors also have a part to play; for example, increasing age and obesity have resulted in a >50% increase in disease burden from gout in high-income Asian Pacific countries in the 20 years to 2010.

Risk factors for gout/hyperuricaemia

Age and sex – Gout becomes more common with increasing age. The diagnosis is rare in premenopausal women. It is more common in older women but still much less prevalent than in men (see Figure 10.1). The later age of onset in women may relate to the uricosuric effects of oestrogens.

Obesity – Relative risk of gout increases with increasing body mass index (BMI). Compared to people with a BMI of 21–25, those with BMI of >35 are four times as likely to develop gout (Figure 10.2).

ABC of Rheumatology, Fifth Edition. Edited by Ade Adebajo and Lisa Dunkley.
© 2018 John Wiley & Sons Ltd. Published 2018 by John Wiley & Sons Ltd.

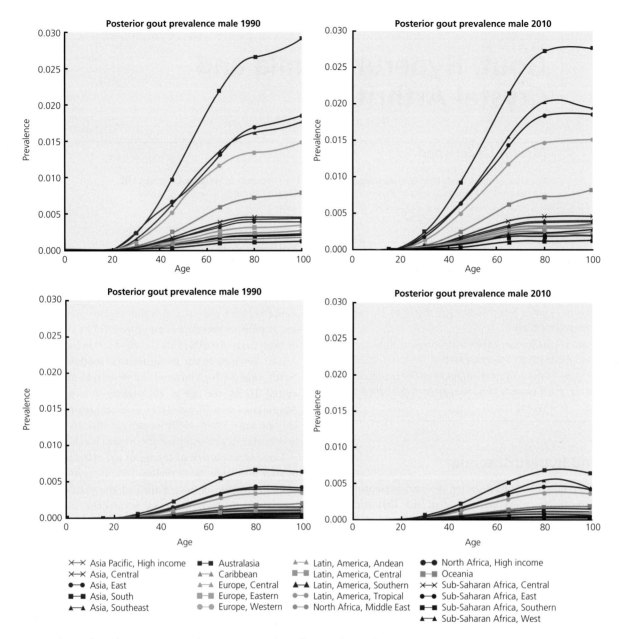

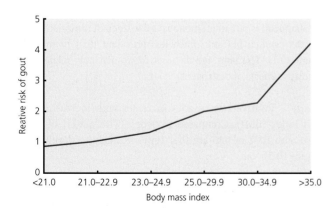

Figure 10.1 Prevalence of gout by region, 1990 and 2010. Source: Redrawn from Smith *et al.* (2014)

Figure 10.2 Obesity and the incidence of a first attack of gout in men. Source: Data from Choi *et al.* (2005)

Diet – Each additional portion of meat per day increases the risk of gout by 20%. Purine-rich vegetables do not appear to increase the risk, whilst consuming more dairy products reduces the risk of developing gout (Table 10.1). Dietary fructose may also increase the risk of developing gout. This occurs naturally and is also present in high fructose corn syrup (HFCS) which is commonly used as a sweetener for soft drinks and other foods in the USA. Its use in the European Union, where it is known as isoglucose, is set to increase with planned lifting of production quotas in 2017.

Drugs – A number of drugs can increase serum urate; diuretics are common culprits. Aspirin and salicylates at low doses decrease urate excretion but at high doses (4–6 g/day) they have a uricosuric effect.

Table 10.1 Effect of diet and alcohol on incidence of a first attack of gout in men*.

Portion	Relative risk (95% CI)
Alcohol	
Beer 335 ml	1.49 (1.32 to 1.70)
Sprits 44 ml	1.15 (1.04 to 1.28)
Wine 118 ml	1.04 (1.88 to 1.22)
Food:	
Meat	1.21 (1.04 to 1.41)
Seafood (fish)*	1.07 (1.01 to 1.12)
Purine rich vegetables	0.97 (0.79 to 1.19)
Total dairy products	0.82 (0.75 to 0.90)
Low fat dairy products	0.79 (0.71 to 0.87)
High fat dairy products	0.99 (0.89 to 1.10)

Data from the professionals follow-up-study.
*Additional weekly serving.
Source: Data from Choi et al. (2014a & b)

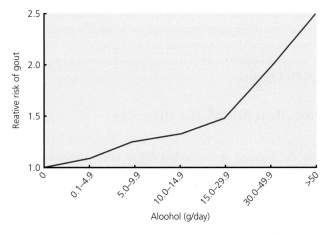

Figure 10.3 Effect of total alcohol intake on the relative risk of a first attack of gout. Source: Data from Choi *et al*. (2005)

Alcohol – Compared to non-drinkers, people consuming >50 g alcohol per day are 2.5 times as likely to develop gout. Whilst there is a strong relationship between beer intake and gout, there is only a weak relationship between intake of spirits and gout. There does not appear to be a relationship between wine intake and gout. Alcohol is catabolized to ketones that compete with urate for excretion by the renal tubule. Beer typically contains substantial amounts of purines, from yeast, that are catabolized to urate by gut bacteria. Alcohol may also increase the dose of allopurinol needed by decreasing the conversion of allopurinol to its effective metabolite, oxipurinol (Figure 10.3).

Relationship between gout and hyperuricaemia

Hyperuricaemia is necessary for the development of gout. Crystal deposition can only occur when the serum is saturated with urate: ≥0.42 mmol/L. This may be different from some laboratories' reference ranges which are based on population norms. Only a minority of people with hyperuricaemia develop gout. For example, the annual incidence of gout is only 6% in people with a urate of 0.60 mmol/L (Figure 10.4). Serum urate can fall during an acute attack, and patients

Box 10.1 Investigation of patients with gout

Diagnosis	*Serum urate*
	May fall during an attack
	Joint aspiration
	Consider if diagnosis uncertain. Will enable the alternative diagnosis of pseudogout to be made if pyrophosphate crystals present. Note, however, that both types of crystals can co-exist
Causes	*Full blood count*
	To exclude myelo- and lymphoproliferative disorders, secondary polycythaemia, haemolytic anaemia, haemoglobinopathies. White count may be slightly raised; if very high, consider septic arthritis
	Liver enzymes
	Possible alcohol abuse
	Renal function
	Drug doses might need adjusting if renal function is poor
	Review medication
	Diuretics and some other drugs increase urate
	Investigations if pseudogout suspected
	Calcium, magnesium, ferritin, thyroid function
Co-morbidities	*Blood pressure*
	Cholesterol
	Blood sugar
	Thyroid function
	15% of patients with gout have hypothyroidism
	Uric acid excretion
	Consider if strong family history of gout, if onset under age 25 or if renal stones present

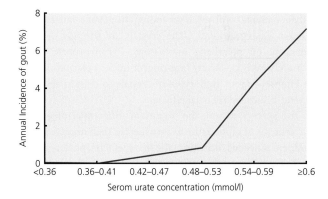

Figure 10.4 Relationship between serum urate and the annual incidence of gout. Source: data from Campion *et al*. (1987)

on urate-lowering medication can still be affected until crystal deposits have cleared from the joints. Thus, demonstrating a raised serum urate is not an essential prerequisite for diagnosing gout.

Hyperuricaemia and cardiovascular disease

There is a well-recognized association between hyperuricaemia and cardiovascular disease. A meta-analysis of prospective studies suggested that people with the highest urate levels have a 37%

(95% confidence interval (CI) 19–57%) greater risk of cardiovascular death when compared to the lowest urate levels. It is not known if reducing urate will reduce cardiovascular risk. However, assessing cardiovascular risk in people presenting with gout is worthwhile.

Clinical features

Acute gout

Typically, gout presents as rapid onset of a monoarthritis associated with severe pain and inflammation, classically affecting the first metatarsophalangeal joint (podagra). Low-grade fever, general malaise and anorexia may accompany the joint symptoms. Onset may follow a drinking bout or local trauma. Untreated, acute gout usually resolves spontaneously within 7–10 days but can on occasion last several weeks. The other most commonly affected areas are the other joints in the foot, ankle, knee, wrist, finger and elbow. The affected joint is warm, tender and swollen and in most cases, the overlying skin is erythematous. The predilection for peripheral joints is probably because crystals are more likely to form in cooler joints. Typically, the attack occurs during the night. After the acute attack, patients may be symptom free for months or years.

Diagnosis – The diagnosis of acute gout is usually clinical. The European League Against Rheumatism (EULAR) recommendations for gout suggest that: 'the rapid development of severe pain, swelling and tenderness that reaches its maximum within just 6–12 hours, especially with overlying erythema, is highly suggestive of crystal inflammation though not specific for gout' and that: 'for typical presentations of gout (such as podagra with hyperuricaemia) a clinical diagnosis alone is reasonably accurate but not definitive without crystal confirmation'. The gold standard is demonstrating urate crystals in synovial fluid. However, few generalists (or their patients) will relish aspirating an acutely inflamed first metatarsophalangeal joint. Urate crystals are strongly negatively birefringent on polarizing microscopy. Pyrophosphate crystals which are weakly positively birefringent under polarized light are found in pseudogout. Both types of crystals co-exist in about 10% of crystal-associated synovial effusions.

In the acute situation, the important differential diagnosis is septic arthritis. If septic arthritis is suspected then urgent specialist assessment is needed. Bursitis of the first metatarsophalangeal joint can mimic podagra and is often mislabelled and mistreated as gout, especially in young women.

Investigations – All patients with a suspected first episode of gout should be investigated to obtain some confirmatory evidence to support the diagnosis, to look for underlying causes and to identify associated co-morbidities (see Box 10.1). X-rays are not helpful in the diagnosis of acute gout.

Chronic gout

Chronic, poly- or oligoarticular gout can cause inflammatory arthritis in older people, especially those on diuretics. No diagnostic pattern exists, although lower limb joint involvement is common. Crystal deposits (tophi) can develop around hands, feet, elbow and ears; they are particularly common in older women with secondary, diuretic-induced gout, in whom they may develop without a history of acute gout. Tophi are chalky deposits of urate embedded in a matrix of lipid, protein and calcific debris. They are usually subcutaneous, but may occur in bone and other organs, including heart valves and the eye. Tophi can contribute to a destructive arthropathy and secondary osteoarthritis. This picture can also develop in patients with recurrent acute gout.

Diagnosis – Urate crystals can be demonstrated in aspirates from tophi. These can be seen radiographically as soft tissue swellings (occasionally with associated calcification) and there may be characteristic gouty X-ray changes of subcortical cysts without erosions and/or geodes (punched-out type erosions with sclerotic margins and overhanging edges).

Urate stones

One in five patients with gout overexcrete urate and may develop urate stones. Around 5% of renal stones are pure urate. However, urinary urate may co-precipitate in calcium oxalate or phosphate stones. Serum urate should be measured in patients with a history of renal colic. Uricosuric drugs should be avoided in patients with a history of urate-containing renal stones. Patients with ileostomies are prone to urate stones as a consequence of producing concentrated acidic urine.

Inherited metabolic disorders

Gout in childhood may be a manifestation of one of the several rare inherited disorders of metabolism such as Lesch–Nyhan syndrome and G6PD deficiency and should be investigated in detail. Adults with new-onset gout may be heterozygous for one of these conditions but investigations should be restricted to those with indicative family histories.

Treatment

There are few robust data to inform the management of gout. Recommendations for treatment are largely based on clinical experience rather than randomized controlled trial evidence.

Acute gout

The choice of drug treatment for acute gout is dependent on the balance of risks and benefits. It is likely that oral treatment with colchicine, corticosteroids or NSAIDS will be similarly effective for treating acute gout. The choice of preparation should be based on an assessment of relative risks of each drug for an individual patient and patient preference. If the initial response to treatment is poor, or an attack is particularly severe, then combination treatment with colchicine and an NSAID or corticosteroid may be appropriate.

NSAIDs – There is one small randomized controlled trial of NSAIDs compared to placebo for acute gout. Decades of clinical experience and guideline recommendations attest to their efficacy for acute gout. The only firm conclusion from comparative studies of NSAIDs is that pain reduction from indomethacin, etoricoxib or celecoxib is similarly effective. There is probably little to choose in terms of efficacy between different NSAIDs/COX-2 inhibitors. If they are used, a co-prescription of a proton pump inhibitor is usually indicated.

Colchicine – There are two controlled trials of colchicine compared to placebo for acute gout. These show that colchicine is effective and that low-dose colchicine appears to be as effective as high-dose colchicine. Since colchicine can have unpleasant side effects, including severe diarrhoea, bone marrow and neuromuscular dysfunction, using a lower dose of 0.5 mg three times a day is advisable.

Corticosteroids/ACTH – There are no controlled trials comparing steroids/ACTH with placebo for acute gout. A systematic review of identified six comparative studies comparing corticosteroids with NSAIDs for acute gout. They did not find any differences in response to treatment between the two treatments. However, people taking NSAIDs had more gastrointestinal side effects. Clinical experience supports the use of intra-articular steroids but septic arthritis must be positively excluded. Intra-articular injections in acute gout can be difficult and very painful, particularly in smaller joints Billy CA *et al.* (2018).

Analgesics – Gout is painful. Patients may need potent analgesic in addition to specific treatments. For some frail patients, just using analgesics may be appropriate.

Other treatments – Experience and some controlled trial evidence suggest that some non-drug pain relief modalities such as the use of ice packs may give additional pain relief. The monoclonal antibody canakinumab is licensed for the treatment of acute gout, if conventional treatment is ineffective, but its cost is prohibitive.

Intercritical and chronic gout

The mainstay of treatment for prevention of recurrent acute gout and chronic gout is reducing serum urate enough to allow crystals to clear. Different authorities suggest <0.30 mmol/L or <0.36 mmol/L as the therapeutic target; <0.30 mmol/L is appropriate if tophi are present. Asymptomatic hyperuricaemia does not require treatment.

Patients with two or more attacks of gout per year should be offered urate-lowering medication. Usual advice is not to start urate-lowering drugs during an attack as this may delay resolution and should be avoided as lowering serum urate can trigger acute gout. There is, however, one RCT that did not find a difference in recurrent attacks if allopurinol was started during an attack or 10 days later. An NSAID, probably with a proton pump inhibitor, or colchicine should be co-prescribed for the first 3 months.

Medication review – Consider stopping diuretics or any other drugs known to increase serum urate.

Lifestyle interventions – Patients should be advised to:

- Lose weight (if appropriate)
- Reduce meat and fish eaten
- Reduce alcohol intake and avoid beer
- Increase intake of low-fat dairy products.

Xanthine oxidase inhibitors – These prevent the purine breakdown products xanthine and hypoxanthine being converted into urate. Allopurinol has been available for nearly 50 years; more recently, a second xanthine oxidase inhibitor, febuxostat, has become available (see below).

Allopurinol – Allopurinol reduces serum urate, but its effect on recurrent gout is unclear. Only a minority of patients taking the typical dose of 300 mg/day achieve a target urate of 0.36 mmol/L. Its dose should be titrated according to response up to 900 mg/day. Allopurinol hypersensitivity may occur in up to 2% of patients; this can be severe or even fatal. Desensitizing regimens of allopurinol can be tried in milder cases of hypersensitivity.

Febuxostat – Febuxostat 80 mg is superior to allopurinol 300 mg at achieving a serum urate of <0.36 mmol/L. However, febuxostat does not appear to be more effective at reducing recurrent gout over 1 year. It may have a role in patients who cannot take allopurinol either because of intolerance or because it is contraindicated.

Uricosuric drugs – Uricosuric drugs lower serum urate by inhibiting its tubular reabsorption. There is no RCT evidence supporting their use for prevention of recurrent gout. Only sulfinpyrazone is generally available for the treatment of gout. Benzbromarone can also be used, but it is not universally available and there are concerns about it causing liver problems. Historically, probenecid has also been used. New selective uric acid reabsorption inhibitors are being tested and may become available. One should consider measuring urinary urate before starting uricosurics.

NSAIDs and colchicine – Both regular NSAIDs and colchicine can be used to prevent recurrent gouty attacks but have no effect on serum urate.

Uricase drugs – Uricase drugs that work by oxidizing uric acid to the more soluble allantoin are available in some jurisdictions.

Other drugs – Several other drugs have, coincidentally, been found to have urate-lowering effects. These include losartan, fenofibrate, atorvastatin and amlodipine. Although they are not licensed for the treatment of gout, they may have a role if other drugs cannot be tolerated or if they are otherwise indicated for patients with multiple pathology.

Pseudogout

Pseudogout, which can be easily confused with gout, is caused by deposition of calcium pyrophosphate crystals. It most commonly affects knees, wrists, shoulders, ankles, elbows or hands. Typically, it produces an episodic monoarthritis but it can also have a clinical picture similar to osteoarthritis or rheumatoid arthritis. Its prevalence increases from 3% in people in their 60s to half of those in their 90s. It can be associated with hypothyroidism, hypercalcaemia, haemochromatosis or hypomagnesaemia.

Diagnosis is based on identifying pyrophosphate crystals or chondrocalcinosis seen on X-ray. Acute episodes can be treated with NSAIDs or intra-articular steroids. Long-term NSAIDs or colchicine can be used to try and prevent recurrence.

Other crystal diseases

A number of other crystals can produce acute musculoskeletal inflammation. Most common are hydroxyapatite crystals which typically deposit in tendons, periarticular soft tissue and synovium. Hydroxyapatite deposition may be asymptomatic but can on occasion lead to significant joint destruction. Involvement of the shoulder is sometimes called Milwaukee shoulder, but virtually any joint may be affected. Identifying and correcting an underlying cause of hypophosphataemia or hypercalcaemia may reduce the risk of future attacks. Calcium oxalate may also cause acute arthritis. Its identification in joint fluid requires special staining with alizarin red dye. Treatments for acute attacks include NSAIDs and intra-articular steroids.

References

Campion EW, Glynn RJ, DeLabry LO. Asymptomatic hyperuricemia. Risks and consequences in the Normative Aging Study. *American Journal of Medicine* 1987; **82**: 421–426.

Choi HK, Atkinson K, Karlson EW, Willett W and Curhan G. Purine-rich foods, dairy and protein intake, and the risk of gout in men. *The New England Journal of Medicine* 2004a; **350**: 1093–103.

Choi HK, Atkinson K, Karlson EW, Willett W and Curhan G. Alcohol intake and risk of incident gout in men: a prospective study. *Lancet* 2004b; **363**: 1277–81.

Christy Amanda Billy, Ricky Tanujaya Lim, Marinella Ruospo, Suetonia C. Palmer and Giovanni F.M. Strippoli: corticosteroid or nonsteroidal antiinflammatory drugs for the treatment of acute gout: a systematic review of randomized controlled trials. *The Journal of Rheumatology* 2018; **45**(1): 128–136; DOI: https://doi.org/10.3899/jrheum.170137

Smith E, Hoy D, Cross M et al. The global burden of gout: estimates from the Global Burden of Disease 2010 study. *Annals of the Rheumatic Diseases* 2014; **73**: 1470-6.2012

Further reading

Khanna D, Fitzgerald JD, Khanna PP et al. American College of Rheumatology guidelines for management of gout. Part 1: systematic nonpharmacologic and pharmacologic therapeutic approaches to hyperuricemia. *Arthritis Care and Research* 2012; **64**(10): 1431–1446.

Khanna D, Khanna PP, Fitzgerald JD et al. American College of Rheumatology guidelines for management of gout. Part 2: therapy and antiinflammatory prophylaxis of acute gouty arthritis. *Arthritis Care and Research* 2012; **64**: 1447–1461.

Sivera F, Andrés M, Carmona L et al. Multinational evidence-based recommendations for the diagnosis and management of gout: integrating systematic literature review and expert opinion of a broad panel of rheumatologists in the 3e initiative. *Annals of the Rheumatic Diseases* 2014; **73**: 328–335.

Underwood M. Gout. *BMJ Clinical Evidence*. Available at: http://clinicalevidence.bmj.com/x/systematic-review/1120/overview.html

Zhao G, Huang L, Song M, Song Y. Baseline serum uric acid level as a predictor of cardiovascular disease related mortality and all-cause mortality: a meta-analysis of prospective studies. *Atherosclerosis* 2013; **231**: 61–68.

CHAPTER 11

Osteoporosis and Metabolic Bone Disease

Eugene McCloskey[1], Nicola Peel[2], Jennifer Walsh[1] and Richard Eastell[1]

[1] Northern General Hospital; Academic Unit of Bone Metabolism, Mellanby Centre for bone research, Department of Oncology & Metabolism, University of Sheffield, Sheffield, UK
[2] Metabolic Bone Centre, Northern General Hospital (Sheffield Teaching Hospitals Foundation Trust), Sheffield, UK

OVERVIEW

- Osteoporotic fractures cause substantial morbidity and place a significant burden on healthcare resources.
- An individual's risk of fracture in the next 10 years can be readily estimated by the FRAX tool and incorporated into clinical management.
- The measurement of bone mineral density plays an important role in the diagnosis of osteoporosis and contributes to fracture risk assessment as part of the FRAX tool.
- Effective treatments include the bisphosphonates, selective oestrogen receptor modulators, denosumab and parathyroid hormone peptides.
- Falls risk assessment and prevention is an important consideration in patient management.

Normal physiology of bone

Bone undergoes a continual process of remodelling through the processes of osteoclastic resorption and osteoblastic formation in discrete remodelling units (Figure 11.1). About 10% of the adult skeleton remodels each year; remodelling maintains skeletal strength and plays a role in calcium homeostasis. The process is coupled so that resorption is followed by formation. Many systemic hormones and inflammatory mediators regulate osteoclastic resorption, and thus bone remodelling, through the generation of proresorptive RANK-ligand (RANKL) and antiresorptive osteoprotegerin by osteocytes and osteoblasts. Regulatory pathways for osteoblast function are being elucidated; the Wnt pathway and its inhibitors (e.g. sclerostin) are of prime importance and provide novel targets for potential therapies.

Osteoporosis

Osteoporosis is a systemic skeletal disease characterized by low bone mass and microarchitectural deterioration of bone tissue that results in a high risk of fragility fracture. With increasing age and in some disease states (Table 11.1), irreversible bone loss results from increased remodelling rates combined with an imbalance between the rates of resorption and formation; formation rates are particularly lowered during prolonged glucocorticoid therapy. Thinning and perforation of the trabecular plates, primarily in the early post-menopausal years, are followed by age-related increases in cortical porosity in both women and men (Figure 11.2). Bone mineral density (BMD) measured by dual X-ray absorptiometry (DXA) at the femoral neck, total hip or lumbar spine is used to diagnose osteoporosis; a T-score ≤ -2.5 (i.e. 2.5 or more standard deviations below the young adult mean) is the WHO threshold for osteoporosis in postmenopausal women and men aged 50 years and older. BMD results in children and young adults who have not yet completed skeletal development are more appropriately interpreted by comparison to the mean value of the same age and gender (the Z-score).

One in two women and one in five men will sustain a fracture related to osteoporosis by the age of 90 years; all fragility fractures in the elderly (e.g. women aged 75 years and older) should be regarded as osteoporotic once pathological fracture (e.g. metastatic disease) has been excluded. Recent estimates suggest that the cost of managing incident fractures in the UK is approximately £3.2 billion a year, rising to around £10 billion when loss of quality of life is included.

Assessment of osteoporosis

While most fragility fractures are age related, an underlying cause (secondary osteoporosis) can be identified in up to 40% of cases of osteoporosis in women and 60% of cases in men (Table 11.1); appropriate investigations should be undertaken, especially if there is clinical suspicion. Individuals with a low-trauma vertebral fracture or low BMD for age should certainly be investigated. In addition to a good clinical history, a small number of investigations can exclude the most common causes or alternative diagnoses, such as myeloma (Box 11.1).

A history of prior low-trauma fracture in adult life is a very important risk factor; it is important to remember that prior vertebral fractures may be asymptomatic and may not be identified without spinal imaging. Low radiation imaging of the thoracolumbar spine using DXA machines (vertebral morphometry) can now be undertaken in high-risk groups as part of their routine assessment.

ABC of Rheumatology, Fifth Edition. Edited by Ade Adebajo and Lisa Dunkley.
© 2018 John Wiley & Sons Ltd. Published 2018 by John Wiley & Sons Ltd.

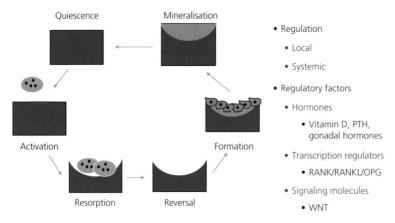

Figure 11.1 A schematic representation of the bone remodelling cycle in which osteoclastic bone resorption is followed by osteoblastic bone formation. Bone loss can occur as a result of increased resorption or decreased formation, relative to each other. Source: Courtesy of Richard Eastell

Table 11.1 Relatively common causes of secondary osteoporosis

Endocrine	Gastrointestinal	Rheumatological	Malignancy	Drugs
Thyrotoxicosis	Malabsorption syndrome, e.g. coeliac disease, partial gastrectomy	Rheumatoid arthritis	Multiple myeloma	Glucocorticoids
Primary hyperparathyroidism	Inflammatory colitis	Ankylosing spondylitis	Cancer treatment-induced bone loss (see drugs)	Anticonvulsants
Cushing's syndrome	Liver disease, e.g. primary biliary cirrhosis			Heparin
Hypogonadism including anorexia nervosa				Aromatase inhibitors
Diabetes (types 1 and 2)				Androgen deprivation therapy

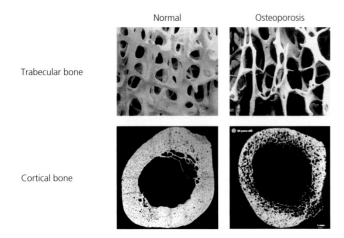

Figure 11.2 The impact of osteoporosis on trabecular and cortical bone. Loss of bone mass is associated with structural deterioration in both bone envelopes, contributing to an even greater decrease in bone strength. Source: Zebaze et al. (2010). Reproduced with permission of Elsevier

Box 11.1 **Investigations to exclude underlying causes of osteoporosis**

- Serum calcium, phosphate, alkaline phosphatase, parathyroid hormone and creatinine
- 24-hour urinary calcium and creatinine excretion
- Serum protein electrophoresis and urinary Bence Jones protein
- Thyroid-stimulating hormone
- Full blood count and erythrocyte sedimentation rate
- Serum testosterone (in males)
- Coeliac screen, if clinically indicated (endomysial and/or tissue transglutaminase antibodies)

DXA measurements of BMD are usually accurate and precise, though those reporting the scans should be aware of potential technical artefacts and limitations. Other measurement techniques, such as quantitative ultrasound, can predict osteoporotic fractures but appropriate intervention thresholds remain uncertain, as does their role in monitoring responses to treatment.

The decision to undertake a DXA scan or to treat an individual is increasingly based on an assessment of absolute fracture risk, as recommended by NICE. Two fracture risk tools are available for use in the UK, QFracture and FRAX, with the latter having the advantage of taking BMD into account. The FRAX tool (www.shef.ac.uk/FRAX) estimates the probability of a major osteoporotic fracture (clinical vertebral, hip, wrist or proximal humerus) or a hip fracture in the next 10 years from a small number of clinical risk factors, with or without femoral neck BMD (Figure 11.3). For risk assessment, BMD measurements are best targeted to individuals whose risk of fracture lies at or near an intervention threshold, an approach endorsed by NICE, and implemented for FRAX by guidance from the National Osteoporosis Guideline Group (www.shef.ac.uk/NOGG) (Figure 11.4).

Reducing fracture risk
The ultimate goal of osteoporosis management is to reduce the future risk of fracture through patient education, falls prevention, lifestyle modification and pharmacological approaches. If access to DXA is

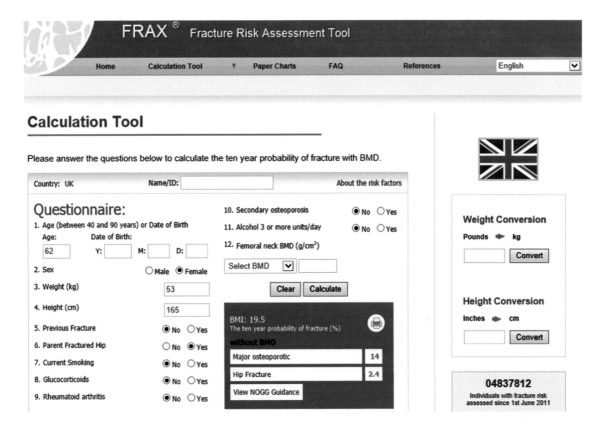

Figure 11.3 A screenshot of the FRAX UK calculation page. The tool provides estimates of 10-year probability of major fractures and hip fractures. The UK tool contains a link to transfer the result to the guidance page provided by the National Osteoporosis Guideline Group (see Figure 11.4). Source: Courtsey of Eugene McCloskey

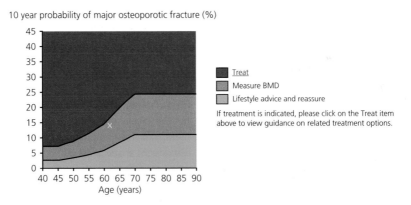

Figure 11.4 A screenshot of the NOGG guidance page. In the absence of a BMD result, the major fracture probability is plotted on a 'traffic light' graph as shown to recommend reassurance, BMD assessment or intervention if high risk. Source: Courtsey of Eugene McCloskey

limited, it may be appropriate to treat high-risk individuals without DXA, such as elderly people with typical osteoporotic fractures or those who need high-dose glucocorticoid therapy. It is important to remember that in secondary osteoporosis, treating the underlying cause often leads to at least partial recovery of bone mass. Groups such as the National Osteoporosis Society (www.nos.org.uk) provide excellent education and support for the patient and their carers.

Pharmacological agents

Two broad classes of treatments exist, namely antiresorptive and anabolic agents, and new agents in both classes are likely to be available in the next few years. Current treatments reduce the risk of vertebral fracture by 40–70%, hip fractures by 40% and other non-vertebral fractures by 20–30%. Lifestyle advice with or without calcium and/or vitamin D supplementation should be regarded largely as adjuncts to osteoporosis treatments (Box 11.2). Vitamin D supplementation, alone or combined with calcium, may be of particular importance in frail elderly patients who are housebound or in residential care. Hypocalcaemia should be corrected by adequate intake of calcium and vitamin D before initiating other therapies, particularly intravenous bisphosphonates or subcutaneous denosumab. Poor adherence remains an issue with some therapies, so patient choice and ease of administration should be taken into account when making treatment choices.

Antiresorptive treatments

Hormone replacement therapy – This plays a useful role in women under 50 who have undergone an early menopause and in the early postmenopausal years to prevent bone loss and relieve climacteric symptoms. The safety profile of oestrogen-only therapy appears somewhat better than combined oestrogen-progestogen therapy, but is limited to use in hysterectomized women. *Selective oestrogen receptor modulators (SERMs)* act as oestrogen agonists on bone and lipids but without stimulation of breast and endometrial tissues. Used alone, they may exacerbate menopausal vasomotor symptoms, but combined preparations of SERMs and oestrogens are being developed for the treatment of vasomotor symptoms, vaginal atrophy and prevention of postmenopausal osteoporosis. All oral oestrogen-like treatments may be associated with small increases in the risk of thromboembolic events. SERMs are associated with a significant reduction in breast cancer.

Bisphosphonates – These agents remain the most widely used class of treatments in the management of osteoporosis, with several generic bisphosphonates now available. Administration can range from daily, once weekly or monthly oral preparations to 3-monthly and annual intravenous preparations. NICE recommends the use of generic bisphosphonates, particularly alendronate, as first-line therapy but these may not be suitable for or tolerated by all. GI intolerance is quite common and can be addressed by using intravenous bisphosphonates or alternative therapies. Poor absorption of the oral preparations means they must be taken on an empty stomach 30–60 minutes before breakfast and washed down with tap water only. All bisphosphonates should be avoided in patients with renal impairment (CKD 4/5).

Denosumab – This is a fully humanized monoclonal antibody against receptor activator of nuclear factor kappa B ligand (RANKL), a major regulator of osteoclast development and activity. It is approved for the treatment of osteoporosis in postmenopausal women and men at increased risk of fractures and is given as a subcutaneous injection every 6 months. No dose adjustment is required in patients with renal impairment.

Two potential but rare adverse events of bisphosphonates and denosumab have garnered recent attention though it is important to remember that in the vast majority of patients, the benefits of treatment far outweigh the risks. Osteonecrosis of the jaw occurs rarely in patients receiving these agents for osteoporosis. A dental examination with appropriate preventive dentistry should be considered prior to treatment in patients with concomitant risk factors, for example poor oral hygiene, dental disease or glucocorticoid therapy. Treatment should not be regarded as a contraindication to necessary dental treatment. Atypical fractures, mainly of the subtrochanteric and diaphyseal regions of the femoral shaft, have also been reported. These fractures are often bilateral, associated with prodromal pain and tend to heal poorly. During treatment, patients should be advised to report any unexplained thigh, groin or hip pain and if such symptoms develop, imaging of the whole femur should be performed. If an atypical fracture is present, the contralateral femur should also be imaged, treatment discontinued and alternative treatment options considered where appropriate. Surgical treatment with intramedullary nailing may be recommended to protect against progression of incomplete fractures.

Anabolic treatments

Parathyroid hormone peptide (teriparatide, PTH 1-34) initially increase bone formation, with a later increase in bone resorption. It improves bone mass and structure, particularly in trabecular sites such as the vertebrae. Expense limits its use to patients with severe, progressive osteoporosis despite exposure to antiresorptive therapy. Treatment is limited to 24 months duration and patients require treatment with antiresorptive agents after discontinuation to maintain the improvements in bone mass. Teriparatide is also licensed for use in men and patients with glucocorticoid-induced osteoporosis (GIO).

In development

Other therapies, for example analogs of parathyroid hormone-related peptide (abaloparatide) and inhibitors or sclerostin (e.g. romosozumab), are being developed for the treatment of osteoporosis.

Pain relief and falls prevention

In addition to analgesia and/or physical measures, such as hydrotherapy or transcutaneous nerve stimulators, some patients require assessment at specialist pain clinics. Fracture pain usually resolves within 6 months, but patients with vertebral fractures may need long-term analgesia because of secondary degenerative disease. Techniques such as vertebroplasty (Figure 11.5) and kyphoplasty can be useful in selected patients with persisting or severe pain resulting from recent vertebral fractures.

Predisposing factors for falls, such as postural hypotension or drowsiness due to drugs, should be eliminated where possible. Patients may benefit from physiotherapy to improve their balance and saving reflexes. Appropriate walking aids, vision assessments and removal of environmental hazards should be considered. Referral to a specialized falls clinics may be appropriate.

Monitoring of treatment

A proportion of patients fail to respond to treatment, commonly due to non-persistence with therapy or poor dosing compliance

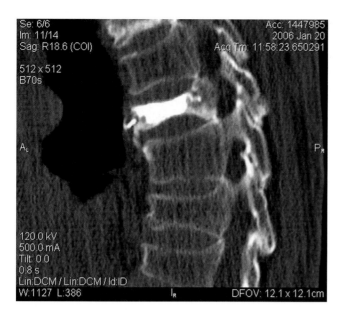

Figure 11.5 A CT scan showing the results of vertebroplasty with filling of cement (*white*) within a collapsed thoracic vertebra. There are other fractures lower down but only symptomatic fractures need treating.

with oral therapies or, less commonly, due to underlying disease. Baseline DXA prior to treatment is useful in individuals in whom it is anticipated that a review of the need for continuing therapy after 5 years is likely. Repeat spine DXA after 18–24 months of treatment is frequently used to monitor response, but doesn't detect early loss of adherence. Biochemical markers of bone turnover can assess response within 3–6 months.

Osteomalacia

Osteomalacia ('soft bones') is characterized by undermineralization of bone and may cause bone pain, muscle weakness and occasionally fractures in adults. In children, bone deformity can also occur (rickets). Vitamin D deficiency is by far the most common cause of osteomalacia (Box **11.3**), though not all patients with apparent vitamin D deficiency develop osteomalacia. The people most at risk of vitamin D deficiency are those with limited exposure to sunlight, for example the frail elderly or individuals wearing clothing that covers almost all of the skin. In these higher risk groups, the diagnosis should be suspected in the presence of symptoms or on finding hypocalcaemia, hypophosphataemia, secondary hyperparathyroidism and/or increased alkaline phosphatase levels on biochemical testing.

In deficiency, high-dose oral colecalciferol over 3 months (up to 300 000 IU in divided doses, e.g. 20 000 IU once weekly for 12 weeks) restores most individuals safely to the replete state. Longer term maintenance therapy should be given using either combined calcium/vitamin D supplements or low-dose cholecalciferol alone if the combined preparation is not tolerated. Active metabolites may be required in the presence of renal failure.

Recent advances in our knowledge of phosphate regulation, for example the role of FGF-23 in tumour-induced osteomalacia, may

Box 11.3 **Causes of osteomalacia**

Vitamin D deficiency

- Inadequate sunlight exposure or synthesis in skin
- Inadequate dietary intake
- Malabsorption including cholestatic liver disease
- Impaired renal hydroxylation, e.g. CKD, type 1 VDDR
- Renal wasting, e.g. nephrotic syndrome
- Abnormal vitamin D receptor function, e.g. type II VDDR

Renal phosphate wasting

- X-linked hypophosphataemic rickets
- Renal tubular acidosis
- Fanconi' syndrome
- Tumour-induced osteomalacia

Other

- Hypophosphatasia

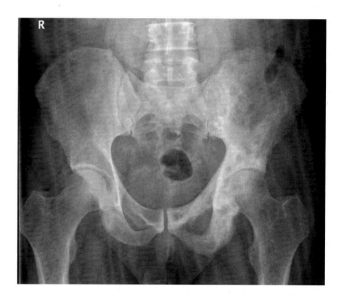

Figure 11.6 Paget's disease of bone in the hemipelvis of an elderly man. Note the bone expansion and sclerosis in the left periacetabular bone compared to the opposite side. Source: Courtsey of Eugene McCloskey

open new therapeutic pathways in diseases of phosphate retention such as CKD.

Paget's disease of bone

Paget's disease of bone (PDB) affects 1–2% of Caucasians aged 55 and over and is characterized by focal increases in bone remodelling, predominantly in the axial skeleton, resulting in disorganized bone. The pelvis is the most commonly involved site (70% of cases) (Figure 11.6), followed by the proximal femur, the lumbar spine, skull and tibia. Complications include bone pain, pathological fracture, deafness, nerve compression and, rarely, osteosarcoma. There is increasing evidence that it is an inherited disease caused by a number of alleles; mutations of SQSTM1, a gene encoding p62, an adaptor protein in the NF-kappa-B signalling pathway that also plays a role in autophagy, occur in about 10% of patients. Seven other loci that predispose to PDB have recently been identified by genome-wide association studies. It is estimated that the combined effects of these genes account for about 86% of the population-attributable risk of PDB in SQSTM1-negative patients.

The activity of PDB is well suppressed by treatment with bisphosphonates, particularly intravenous zoledronic acid, and the disease may only require treatment every few years.

Reference

Zebaze RM, Ghasem Zadeh A, Bohte A *et al.* Intracortical remodelling and porosity in the distal radius and post-mortem femurs of women: a cross-sectional study. *Lancet* 2010; **375**: 1729–1736.

Further reading

Compston J, Bowring C, Cooper A *et al.* Diagnosis and management of osteoporosis in postmenopausal women and older men in the UK: National Osteoporosis Guideline Group (NOGG) update 2013. *Maturitas* 2013; **75**(4): 392–396.

Hosking D, Lyles K, Brown JP *et al.* Long-term control of bone turnover in Paget's disease with zoledronic acid and risedronate. *Journal of Bone and Mineral Research* 2007; **22**(1): 142–148.

National Institute for Health and Care Excellence. *Osteoporosis: Assessing the Risk of Fragility Fracture.* Clinical Guideline No. 146. NICE, London, 2012.

National Institute for Health and Care Excellence. *TA161 (amended) Alendronate, Etidronate, Risedronate, Raloxifene, Strontium Ranelate and Teriparatide for the Secondary Prevention of Osteoporotic Fragility Fractures in Postmenopausal Women.* NICE, London, 2010.

National Osteoporosis Society. *Vitamin D and Bone Health: A Practical Clinical Guideline for Patient Management.* Available at: https://nos.org.uk/media/2073/vitamin-d-and-bone-health-adults.pdf

CHAPTER 12

Rheumatoid Arthritis: Clinical Features and Diagnosis

Mohammed Akil[1] and Robert Moots[2]

[1] Sheffield Teaching Hospitals NHS Foundation Trust, Sheffield, UK
[2] University of Liverpool; Aintree University Hospital, Liverpool, UK

OVERVIEW

- Rheumatoid arthritis (RA) is a chronic systemic inflammatory disease, associated with significant morbidity and increased mortality.

- It has a wide spectrum of disease manifestations, both articular and non-articular. Progressive joint destruction and extra-articular manifestations account for the disability and increased mortality. Early recognition and intervention with disease-modifying therapy are key to preventing the progressive disability.

- It is vital that clinicians develop expertise in identifying early disease and recognizing the spectrum of its manifestations. Geographical variations in disease pattern have been reported and attributed to lifestyle differences in populations; however, genetic differences have also been implicated in the severity of the disease.

- RA occurs with varying prevalence in different parts of the world; the highest incidence is reported in some Native American tribes (5%), but it is far less common in Chinese and Japanese people (0.3%).

- It is three times more common in women than men.

Pathogenesis

Whilst the cause of rheumatoid arthritis (RA) is not fully established, it is clear that there is a complex dysregulated inflammatory process that, in the presence of a yet undefined environmental trigger, develops in genetically predisposed individuals. This leads to the development of an autoimmune synovitis with subsequent hypertrophy that, if inadequately treated, leads to cartilage and bone destruction, progressive joint damage and disability. The inflammatory process also potentially affects many other tissues, including the lungs and cardiovascular system.

Many cells and molecules appear to play central roles in the pathogenesis of RA. T-cells, which orchestrate the immune response, appear to be important, and biologic drugs that selectively target them are effective, but not in all patients. Similarly, drugs targeting other cells, such as B-cells, have also proven highly

effective. Small soluble immune system messengers, cytokines, also play a crucial role. These include tumour necrosis factor-alpha (TNF-α) and interleukin-6 (IL-6), both of which are targeted successfully by highly effective biologic drugs. The majority of the genetic predisposition lies in the class II MHC (the 'shared epitope' on the hypervariable region of DRB1), the presence of which may also correlate with disease severity.

A possible environmental trigger is smoking. It is thought that this might lead to citrillination of proteins that in turn can act as antigens and trigger the development of an autoimmune response. Indeed, anticitrillinated peptide antibodies, anti-CCP (also referred to as ACPA), can be used in the diagnosis of RA and may precede onset of symptoms by many years.

Clinical features

The objectives of clinical assessment for RA are to:

- establish the diagnosis
- evaluate the disease activity (is the disease active or quiescent?)
- assess the disease severity (amount of damage and disability)
- examine for extra-articular manifestations.

The disease may be insidious in nature, rarely occurring in men younger than 30 years, with gradually rising incidence with advancing age. In women, the incidence steadily increases from the mid-20s to peak incidence between 45 and 75 years. In the typical presentation, the most common variant, the small joints of the hands and feet are affected in a symmetrical pattern. The joints predominantly involved are the metacarpophalangeal joints, proximal interphalangeal joints and wrists (Figure 12.1); in the feet, the metatarsophalangeal joints and the forefoot joints are typically affected.

Less common forms of presentation are acute monoarticular, palindromic rheumatism and asymmetrical large joint arthritis. Theoretically, any synovial joint can be affected but spine joints other than the cervical spine are very rarely involved.

Extra-articular manifestations (Figure 12.2) are also varied and may differ in different populations. They can affect almost any

ABC of Rheumatology, Fifth Edition. Edited by Ade Adebajo and Lisa Dunkley.
© 2018 John Wiley & Sons Ltd. Published 2018 by John Wiley & Sons Ltd.

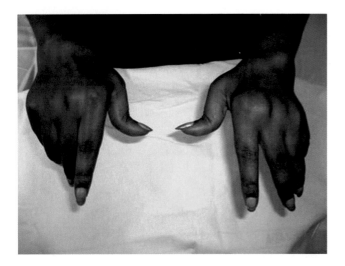

Figure 12.1 Typical changes in the hands in rheumatoid arthritis

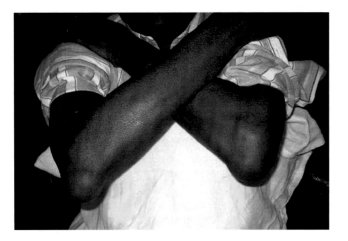

Figure 12.2 Large rheumatoid nodules over the elbows

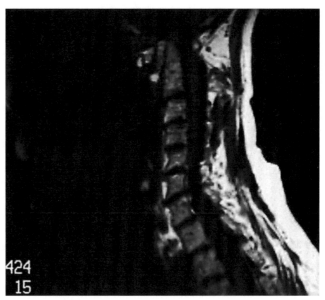

Figure 12.3 Magnetic resonance image of the cervical spine showing atlantoaxial involvement in rheumatoid arthritis

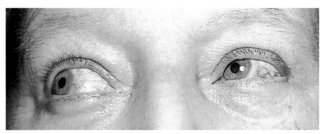

Figure 12.4 Scleritis in rheumatoid arthritis

system of the body and are mediated by various inflammatory mechanisms, which include immune complex deposition, cytokine production and direct endothelial injury, all of which can mediate distant and local effects. Also, mechanical insults such as synovial hypertrophy and subluxation of joints may cause entrapment of nerves or vessels. The abnormal mechanics and disuse lead to degenerative changes and osteoporosis, compounding disability.

'Red flags'

As many complications of RA or its treatment can occur, vigilance on the part of clinicians is required to pick them up early and intervene, preventing severe morbidity and even mortality in certain cases; some of these are detailed below.

Atlantoaxial subluxation – This results from involvement of the atlantoaxial joint, which may be clinically asymptomatic until the subluxation develops. Development of pain around the occiput, radiating arm pain, numbness or weakness of the limbs and vertigo on neck movement are warning signs; if not detected, this may lead to sudden death, especially if patients undergo neck manipulation

for endotracheal intubation during surgery. It is essential to actively look for this during presurgical evaluation by performing lateral views of the cervical spine in flexion (Figure 12.3) and extension, measuring the distance between the posterior margin of the atlas ring and the anterior surface of the odontoid process.

Pericarditis – Onset of central chest pain worsened by lying flat, accompanied by a pericardial rub, merits urgent echocardiogram to confirm and urgent initiation of steroid therapy. Infective causes such as tuberculosis need to be ruled out by aspiration and analysis when suspected.

Monoarticular flare – A single joint worsening should always be viewed with suspicion in RA, and septic arthritis excluded by aspiration. It is prudent to initiate treatment for possible septic arthritis as soon as possible after aspiration, until the results of the joint aspirate rule it out.

Eye involvement – Sudden onset of eye pain and increased lacrimation should alert the clinician to the possibility of scleritis (Figure 12.4); if left untreated, this may lead to full-thickness involvement of the sclera, with thinning and risk of perforation. Called scleromalacia perforans, this sinister condition is thankfully rare but needs to be looked out for.

Other manifestations of RA are given in Box 12.1.

Box 12.1 **Other manifestations of rheumatoid arthritis**

Haematological
Anaemia, thrombocytosis, Felty's syndrome

Neurological
Entrapment neuropathies such as carpal tunnel syndrome
Mononeurits multiplex, peripheral neuropathy

Pulmonary
Pleural effusions, interstitial lung disease, bronchiolitis obliterans

Cardiac
Pericarditis, coronary vasculitis (rare)

Cutaneous
Rheumatoid nodules, cutaneous vasculitis, leg ulcers

Ocular
Xerophthalmia, scleritis, episcleritis, corneal melt

Others
Dry mouth, osteoporosis

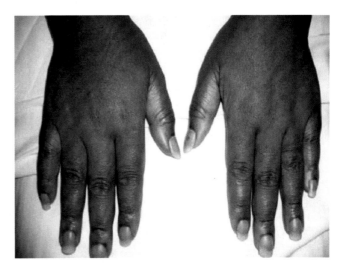

Figure 12.5 Subtle features of synovitis in early rheumatoid arthritis

Table 12.1 Specificity and sensitivity of RF and anti-CCP

	RF	**Anti-CCP**
Specificity	Fair (80%)	Excellent (95%)
Sensitivity	Fair (78%)	Fair (78%)
Frequency in healthy individuals	10–15%	1–2%
Effect of age	Increased levels	None
Presence in other diseases	Infection, other autoimmune diseases, e.g. Sjogren's syndrome, cryoglobulinaemia, lymphoproliferative disorders	Very rare
Association with X-ray damage	Positive	Positive

Diagnosis

The diagnosis of RA is predominantly a clinical one; no diagnostic test has been shown to be foolproof and both false-positive and false-negative results occur with varying frequency. The 2010 ACR/EULAR classification criteria are listed in box 12.2.

History

A detailed history of the problem, its onset and progression with time, relieving and aggravating factors and the distribution of the symptoms are all important elements in the history. A progressive pattern of joint involvement, stiffness and increased pain after a period of inactivity and a history of joint swellings is indicative of inflammatory joint disorders. A family history of autoimmune disease can raise the suspicion further. The distribution of joint involvement helps in distinguishing other forms of arthritis such as spondyloarthritis.

Clinical examination

The objective of the clinical assessment is to identify signs of inflammatory arthritis, such as swelling, tenderness and restriction of movement of the joints. A symmetrical involvement of the hands, especially the metacarpophalangeal and proximal interphalangeal joints, with relative sparing of the axial skeleton, are some key elements that support the diagnosis of RA. Clinical evaluation may also pick up extra-articular findings that can support the diagnosis or refute it – for example, the presence of rheumatoid nodules and psoriatic skin patches, respectively. In early disease, the classic signs of structural changes are usually missing and subtle synovitis (Figure 12.5) may escape notice; however, tenderness and restriction without history of trauma should arouse suspicion.

Laboratory tests

Active RA is associated with a variety of haematological responses. Acute-phase responses such as a high erythrocyte sedimentation rate and C-reactive protein, a high platelet count and high serum ferritin can be seen in some patients with widespread synovitis. Anaemia of chronic disease may also be present. A very high leucocyte response is uncommon and usually indicative of an infection, which should be excluded in such situations. Acute-phase response may sometimes not be seen in early RA patients, if disease is confined to small joints.

The traditional test of rheumatoid factor that detects immunoglobulin M (IgM) antibodies directed against IgG can be used as supporting evidence in establishing the diagnosis, but is neither conclusive nor universal in patients with RA.

Anticyclic citrullinated peptide antibodies (anti-CCP) are more specific and sensitive for the diagnosis of RA. It is also a marker of erosive disease and can predict eventual development of RA in undifferentiated arthritis. The specificity and sensitivity of RF and anti-CCP are given in Table 12.1.

Imaging

Radiological features of periarticular erosions (Figure 12.6) are characteristic and may appear within the first 3 years of disease in the majority of the patients; more subtle changes, such as juxta-articular osteopenia and early joint space narrowing, are less specific and can be misleading. Conventional radiology can still be useful in monitoring progression of the disease in established diagnosis and to plan corrective surgeries when there is significant disability. Magnetic resonance imaging detects soft tissue changes, including synovitis, as well as bone oedema and early erosive changes. The high cost limits

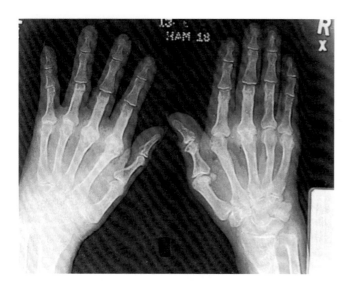

Figure 12.6 Radiograph of the hands, showing erosions at the metacarpophalangeal and proximal interphalangeal joints

its use in everyday practice. Ultrasound of small joints, relatively cheap, quick and sensitive in the detection of synovitis and joint erosions, is increasingly used by rheumatologists to confirm the diagnosis and monitor disease progress. Ultrasound and MRI are superior to clinical examination in the detection of joint inflammation and should be considered for more accurate assessment of inflammation, especially when there is diagnostic doubt.

High-resolution computed tomography is the modality of choice to detect interstitial lung disease and pulmonary fibrosis and should be performed in patients with abnormal lung function.

Synovial fluid analysis

This test is rarely required to establish diagnosis in a typical presentation; however, in atypical presentations with large joint involvement, especially monoarticular, it is vital to rule out infective aetiology and crystal arthropathy. The fluid would typically show a high protein and leucocyte count and the absence of crystals and organisms on Gram stain.

Differential diagnosis

Other arthritides can be distinguished on the basis of joint involvement pattern; however, atypical presentations may prove challenging to rule out. A careful search for evidence of nail pitting or skin

lesions may clinch the diagnosis in psoriatic disease, but joint aspiration for crystals may be needed to exclude polyarticular gout. Nodal osteoarthritis, chronic pyrophosphate arthropathy and connective tissue diseases (i.e. SLE) can have similar presentation to RA. In areas of high incidence, conditions such as hepatitis B and C and HIV need to be borne in mind.

Box 12.2 2010 ACR/EULAR classification criteria for RA

Target population: Patients who (i) have at least one joint with clinical synovitis, and (ii) with the synovitis not better explained by another disease
Add score of categories A–D; score of 6/10 or more is needed to classify patient as having definite RA

A. Joint involvement (tender/swollen)

1 large joint	0
2–10 large joints	1
1–3 small joints (with or without involvement of large joints)	2
4–10 small joints (with or without involvement of large joints)	3
>10 joints (at least 1 small joint)	5

B. Serology

Negative RF and anti-CCP	0
Low positive RF/low positive anti-CCP	2
High positive RF/high positive anti-CCP	3

C. Acute-phase reactants

Normal CRP and ESR	0
Abnormal CRP and ESR	1

D. Duration of symptoms

Less than 6 weeks	0
6 weeks or more	1

Further reading

Firestein GS, Panayi G, Wollheim F (eds). *Rheumatoid Arthritis*, 2nd edn. Oxford University Press, Oxford, 2006.

Isaacs J, Moreland LW. *Fast Facts: Rheumatoid Arthritis*. Health Press, Oxford, 2002.

Isenberg D, Maddison P, Woo P, Glass D, Breedveld F (eds). *Oxford Textbook of Rheumatology*. Oxford University Press, Oxford, 2004.

Taylor P. *Rheumatoid Arthritis in Practice*. Royal Society of Medicine Press, London, 2006.

CHAPTER 13

Treatment of Rheumatoid Arthritis

Edwin S. L. Chan[1], Anthony G. Wilson[2] and Bruce N. Cronstein[1]

[1] Department of Medicine, New York University, New York, NY, USA
[2] EULAR Centre of Excellence/UCD Centre for Arthritis Research, Conway Institute of Biomolecular & Biomedical Research, University College Dublin, Dublin, Ireland

---

> ## OVERVIEW
>
> - Rheumatoid arthritis is a disease requiring life-long treatment.
> - Treatment should begin early since radiological damage can occur much earlier than previously thought.
> - Disease-modifying antirheumatic drugs (DMARDs) and biological response modifiers have been proven to retard disease progression.
> - Combination therapy is often more efficacious than monotherapy.
> - Inadequately treated rheumatoid arthritis is associated with increased mortality.

Remarkable strides have been made in recent years in controlling clinical and radiological progression of RA. However, the usefulness of small molecules such as methotrexate remains and has not been overshadowed by the current interest in biological response modification. Our understanding of the molecular mechanisms responsible for the pathogenesis of RA has heralded a shift from empiricism to selective molecular targeting in immunomodulatory pharmacotherapeutics. While symptomatic control and reduction of the clinical signs of synovitis have been the foremost considerations in the past, modern pharmacotherapy has emphasized the need to slow down if not halt disease progression as well as prevention of the development of potential complications.

It is now recognized that significant radiological damage can occur in this disease much earlier than previously thought, certainly within the first 2 years of disease onset. Disease-modifying therapy is therefore introduced early following confirmation of diagnosis, particularly in those with poor prognostic indicators such as severe disease activity, radiological damage or anticyclic citrullinated peptide positivity. The old 'pyramidal' treatment approach has been called into question and new advances have dramatically improved the disease outlook for the RA patient.

Non-steroidal anti-inflammatory drugs

Non-steroidal anti-inflammatory drugs are inhibitors of cyclo-oxygenase, an enzyme that catalyses the conversion of arachidonic acid to prostanoids. The enzyme exists in two isoforms.

Cyclooxygenase-1 is constitutively expressed in many tissues, including platelets, blood vessels and the upper gastrointestinal mucosa where production of prostaglandin E_2 mediates a protective mucosal effect that includes mucus secretion and diminution of acid production. Expression of cyclooxygenase-2 is induced at sites of inflammation, particularly on polymorphonuclear cells and macrophages. Thus, non-selective inhibition of both isoforms by traditional NSAIDs may affect the desirable gastroprotective effects mediated by cyclooxygenase-1, and reported hospitalization of RA patients as a result of upper gastrointestinal complications may exceed 1% of patients treated per year. Selective inhibition of cyclooxygenase-2, on the other hand, has met with concerns over potential cardiovascular risks. Despite these concerns, NSAIDs continue to be used for symptomatic control in RA, but it must be emphasized that they have little effect in limiting joint damage or radiological progression.

Corticosteroids

The demonstration of the anti-inflammatory efficacy of corticosteroids in RA resulted in the first Nobel prize awarded for a clinical observation, and 70 years hence, these potent anti-inflammatory agents continue to have an important place in the management of RA. Furthermore, multiple routes of administration, including depot injections (methylprednisolone and triamcinolone acetonide) and local intra-articular injections, offer a variety of therapeutic options. Given orally, the onset of action is quick and these agents are therefore useful in relieving symptoms while awaiting the onset of DMARD activity. Lower oral doses have been favoured (prednisolone up to 10 mg/day) owing to fear of suppressing the hypothalamus-pituitary-adrenal axis, and prevention of corticosteroid-induced osteoporosis must be considered in patients receiving these medications long term.

Conventional disease-modifying antirheumatic drugs (DMARDs)

Gold

Originally intended for the treatment of infectious diseases, gold is one of the oldest of DMARDs and has been in use for almost a

---

ABC of Rheumatology, Fifth Edition. Edited by Ade Adebajo and Lisa Dunkley.
© 2018 John Wiley & Sons Ltd. Published 2018 by John Wiley & Sons Ltd.

century for the treatment of RA. An intramuscular drug of proven efficacy, radiological improvement with decrease in radiological damage gave evidence of its disease-modifying capacity. However, weekly injections may be cumbersome, and an oral form proved inefficacious. This, together with the fact that over half of drug discontinuations were reported to be the result of toxicity, heralded a decline in its popularity over the years.

Methotrexate

A dihydrofolate reductase inhibitor originally used for its antiproliferative effects in the treatment of cancer, methotrexate is now an anchor drug amongst DMARDs and a gold standard against which all emerging therapies are compared. An oral drug administered on a weekly basis, its anti-inflammatory mechanisms of action are thought to differ from its antimalignant effects, and are largely related to its induction of adenosine release to the inflammatory environment (Box 13.1).

Sulfasalazine

Sulfasalazine, the first drug developed specifically for the treatment of RA, was first synthesized in the 1940s. It is composed of sulfapyridine and 5-aminosalicylic acid moieties and should be avoided in patients allergic to sulfa medications. Plasma half-life is greatly influenced by acetylation status, and slow acetylators are more likely to develop serious toxicities. While minor upper gastrointestinal side effects and rashes are common, drug-induced hepatitis, cytopenias and Stevens–Johnson syndrome may also occur.

Hydroxychloroquine

Hydroxychloroquine is an antimalarial with proven efficacy in the treatment of RA, particularly in early and mild disease. Unlike its sister drug, chloroquine, occurrence of retinopathy is extremely rare. However, evidence for radiological protection has been unconvincing, and this benign medication in most often used in conjunction with other DMARDs in combination therapy rather than alone.

Leflunomide

The newest member amongst the DMARDs, leflunomide inhibits the *de novo* synthesis of pyrimidines by inhibiting dihydro-orotate

dehydrogenase, and this action principally affects lymphocytes which lack salvage pathways for pyrimidine synthesis. It may be useful in patients who have failed to respond to methotrexate, but can also be administered together with methotrexate to improve response. It has a long half-life, requiring a loading dose for 1–3 days. Since a long washout period of up to 2 years is suggested prior to conception, careful planning is needed in premenopausal women.

Other DMARDs in use include:

- penicillamine
- azathioprine
- cyclophosphamide
- ciclosporin
- tacrolimus
- mycophenylate mofetil
- minocycline.

Combination therapy

Although DMARDs represent a marked improvement over previous symptom-oriented therapies, response to monotherapy is often partial at best and discontinuation, whether due to toxicity or lack of response, is commonplace. It has been suggested that using these medications with different but complementary mechanisms of action in combination not only allows for greater efficacy, but also limits effective required dosage and hence toxicity. Various combinations, including step-up and step-down regimens, have been tried, often with the inclusion of methotrexate.

Biological response modifiers

A major development in the treatment of RA in the last decade was the emergence of biological response-modifying therapy. Previous attempts at drug development have largely been empirical efforts. Understanding of the molecular and cellular mechanisms that contribute to the generation and maintenance of the inflammatory processes that culminate in synovial inflammation and joint destruction has escalated astronomically in recent decades. These fundamental elements of the inflammatory cascade, whether it be a cytokine or an inflammatory cell subset, have become the targets of new treatment modalities. These drugs are much larger than conventional DMARDS in molecular weight (150 000 compared with 500 daltons), are produced using recombinant DNA technology and complex purification techniques and are administered parenterally, but the onset of action, unlike DMARDs, is rapid (Table 13.1).

Tumour antagonists

Tumour necrosis factor (TNF) is a pivotal cytokine released in excess in RA, and is a major contributor to synovial inflammation and cartilage destruction. Blockade of its actions by the human TNF receptor 2-immunoglobulin constant region fusion protein, etanercept, resulted in the first success of biological response-modifying therapy in RA. Since then, monoclonal antibodies to human TNF have come into use, whether chimeric (infliximab) or fully humanized (adalimumab, certolizumab and golimumab) (Table 13.2). These agents

---

Box 13.1 **Side effects of methotrexate**

Mucosal ulceration
  Alopecia
  Gastrointestinal – nausea and vomiting, oesophagitis, anorexia, diarrhea, gingivitis, GI bleeding, GI perforation, pancreatitis, elevated transaminases, cirrhosis
  Bone marrow suppression – anaemia, leucopenia, thrombocytopenia, aplastic anaemia
  Malignancy – lymphoproliferative disorders
  Infections
  Interstitial pneumonitis
  Renal impairment
  Teratogenesis

Table 13.1 Biological properties

	Infliximab	Etanercept	Adalimumab	Certolizumab	Golimumab	Rituximab	Tocilizumab	Abatacept
Structure	Monoclonal antibody	P75TNFR/Fc fusion	Monoclonal antibody	Pegylated monoclonal antibody	Monoclonal antibody	Monoclonal antibody	Monoclonal antibody	CFLA-4/Fc
Dosing method	IV	SC	SC	SC	SC	IV	IV or SC	IV or SC
Dosing frequency	8 weeks	Weekly	2 weeks	2 weeks	Monthly	Dependent on response	4 weeks (IV), weekly (SC)	4 weeks (IV), weekly (SC)
Half-life in humans (days)	9.5	3	14	14	12	22	12	13
Target (s)	TNF	TNF and lymphotoxin	TNF	TNF	TNF	CD20	IL-6 receptor	CD80 & CD86

IL, interleukin; IV, intravenous; SC, subcutaneous; TNF, tumour necrosis factor.

Table 13.2 Structural classification of biological therapies

Molecular structure	Suffix	% Human sequence	Example
Monoclonal antibodies	-ximab	60–70	Infliximab
	-zumab	90+	Tocilizumab
	-mumab	100	Adalimumab
Receptor fusion proteins	-cept	100	Abatacept
			Etanercept

have been demonstrated to be efficacious in the treatment of RA on clinical, radiological and laboratory measures.

Interleukin-1 receptor antagonist

The next cytokine to be targeted for therapeutic use was IL-1 and anakinra is a recombinant human IL-1 receptor antagonist. Its short half-life means that subcutaneous injections have to be given on a daily basis. Used alone or in combination with methotrexate, anakinra produced significant if modest clinical improvement in RA. On the basis of the clinical study results, NICE does not recommend the use of anakinra for RA.

B-cell depletion

The B lymphocyte is not only the source of inflammatory cytokines and antibodies important to the pathogenesis of the disease such as rheumatoid factor and anticyclic citrullinated peptide, B-cell help is a vital contributor to T-cell activation and antigen presentation. It is therefore not surprising that the B-lymphocyte may be a suitable target for RA therapy despite previous dogma that RA is predominantly a T-cell-mediated disease. Rituximab targets the B-cell surface marker CD20, which is expressed from the pre-B-cell stage through to the mature memory B-cell. Binding of this chimeric monoclonal antibody depletes CD20+ B-cells in a transient manner. Rituximab, whether alone or in combination with methotrexate, is effective at suppressing inflammatory parameters and limiting structural joint damage in RA, although patients seronegative for rheumatoid factor and anti-CCP antibodies have responded less well. While the risk of infection remains a concern with B-cell depletion, this has not been a problem based on available clinical trial data. However,

clinicians should be alerted to reports of rare neurological diseases, such as progressive multifocal leucoencephalopathy caused by infection with the polyoma JC virus.

Abatacept

T-lymphocyte activation and proliferation requires a dual stimulatory signal that involves both the T-cell and the antigen presenting cell. Interruption of any individual part of this signalling complex, such as CTLA-4, the target of abatacept, disrupts T-cell contributions to the inflammatory environment. Abatacept has proven benefits in slowing disease activity and joint damage in RA, including in patients who have failed to respond to anti-TNF therapy. It can be given either intravenously or subcutaneously, frequently in combination with methotrexate.

Tocilizumab

Interleukin-6 is a broadly proinflammatory cytokine and is an important mediator of tissue damage in RA. Tocilizumab is an antibody targeting the IL-6 receptor that is highly effective and is given either intravenously or subcutaneously. In addition to side effects common to the biological therapies for RA, injection site reactions and infections, its use is associated with increased cholesterol and also abnormal liver enzyme levels in some patients.

Biosimilars

A biosimilar is a biological agent that has the same amino acid sequences as the original biological agent, but, because of the complex production methods, these are not exact copies. The differences arise from glycosylation patterns, these can potentially alter pharmacokinetic or pharmacodynamic properties. It is important to realize that these changes arise frequently in the original biological agents due to changes in manufacturing processes or purification techniques. Biosimilars of Remicade (infliximab) became available in Europe in early 2014 and of Enbrel (Etancercept) in 2016.

New small molecule DMARDs

Targeting signalling transduction pathways has been a major area of therapeutic endeavour but progress has been slowed by narrow therapeutic windows or lack of efficacy. Tofacitinib and

Baracitinib are drugs that is a drug that targets the Janus kinase-signal transducer and activator of transcription (JAK-STAT) pathway and has been approved for use in RA by the FDA, now approved by EMA also.

Identification of co-existing problems

Rheumatoid arthritis has long been regarded as an indolent disease until recently, when it has been recognized that RA may be associated with increased mortality. Life expectancy may be shortened by as much as 7 years in males and 3 years in females. Yet few studies have been able to attribute deaths directly to RA itself. Clinicians should therefore be constantly alert to the development of other co-morbidities in RA patients, of which cardiovascular disease is the most important.

Occurrence of cardiovascular disease has been reported in up to 42% of RA patients and scrupulous management and correction of cardiovascular risk factors are of the utmost importance to disease outlook. Although vasculitis, secondary amyloidosis and lymphoproliferative malignancies have been associated with the disease itself, these are rare and renal, pulmonary, gastrointestinal and infectious diseases are much more common because of the improved therapies outlined above. Furthermore, antirheumatic pharmacotherapy itself may compound these problems. The presence of co-morbidities is a known predictor for mortality in RA patients and due attention must be given to early identification.

Complementary therapy

Although our discussion has focused on the pharmacotherapy of RA, it should be remembered that one of the main goals of management is restoration of function. In this respect, the roles of physiotherapy and occupational therapy and meticulous footcare cannot be overlooked. Advances in orthopaedic surgery have also benefited situations such as atlantoaxial subluxation, arthroplasties, and tendon transfer and repair surgeries, although as mentioned previously the improved therapies has greatly reduced the need for surgical interventions.

Further reading

Blom M, van Riel PL. Management of established rheumatoid arthritis with an emphasis on pharmacotherapy. *Best Practice and Research: Clinical Rheumatology* 2007; **21**(1): 43–57.

Chan ESL, Cronstein BN. Drugs that modulate the immune response. In: *Samter's Immunologic Diseases*, 6th edn. Lippincott, Williams and Wilkins, Baltimore, 2001, pp. 1213–1223.

Fleischmann RM. Comparison of the efficacy of biologic therapy for rheumatoid arthritis: can the clinical trials be accurately compared? *Rheumatic Diseases Clinics of North America* 2006; **32**(Suppl 1): 21–28.

Goldblatt F, Isenberg DA. New therapies for rheumatoid arthritis. *Clinical and Experimental Immunology* 2005; **140**(2): 195–204.

Lee SJ, Kavanaugh A. Pharmacological treatment of established rheumatoid arthritis. *Best Practice and Research: Clinical Rheumatology* 2003; **17**(5): 811–29.

Schneider CK. Biosimilars in rheumatology: the wind of change. *Annals of the Rheumatic Diseases* 2013; **72**: 315–318.

Weise M, Bielsky M, de Smet K *et al.* Biosimilars: what clinicians should know. *Blood* 2012; **120**: 5111–5117.

CHAPTER 14

Spondyloarthritides

Andrew Keat[1] and Robert Inman[2]

[1] Arthritis Centre, Northwick Park Hospital, Harrow, UK
[2] Toronto Hospital –Western Division, Toronto, Canada

OVERVIEW

- Spondyloarthritides as a group occur with a similar prevalence to rheumatoid arthritis.
- The various spondyloarthritic syndromes share common clinical lesions, especially enthesitis, oligoarthritis, sacroiliitis, iritis, psoriasiform skin and mucosal lesions and overt or covert inflammatory bowel disease.
- Inheritance of HLA-B27 and other genes is common to all spondyloarthritides, the prevalence of these disorders varying with the local prevalence of HLA-B27.
- Diagnosis of ankylosing spondylitis is often long delayed; identification of inflammatory back pain in young adults is a key determinant in making the diagnosis early.
- Use of anti-TNF biologic drugs has revolutionized the treatment of severe ankylosing spondylitis.

The spondyloarthritides (SpA) comprise a group of syndromes which are distinct from rheumatoid arthritis and are characterized by inflammation of the spine in many but not all cases. Other key features include asymmetrical oligoarthritis, enthesitis, psoriatic skin and mucous membrane lesions and eye and bowel inflammation. Tests for rheumatoid factor, anticyclic citrullinated peptide (anti-CCP) antibody and other autoantibodies are negative but there is a strong association with the human leucocyte antigen (HLA) B27. Spondyloarthritides occur in both adults and children although spinal involvement is rare in children.

The SpA may be considered either as axial or peripheral (or a combination of the two) or as a set of semi-discrete syndromes (Figure 14.1). The classic forms of spondyloarthritis (also called spondyloarthropathies) and the key physical features are listed in Table 14.1.

Together, SpA are roughly as common as rheumatoid arthritis in Europe and North America although their prevalence varies in other areas, generally reflecting the prevalence of HLA-B27 in that population. Their prevalence and that of associated conditions is presented in Table 14.2.

Axial spondyloarthritis/ankylosing spondylitis

Axial spondyloarthritis (Axial SpA) is a spectrum of aseptic inflammatory disease of the joints and entheses of the spine. When there is clear radiographic change at the sacroiliac joints and the modified New York criteria are met, the term ankylosing spondylitis (AS) is used, whilst for individuals in whom inflammatory changes can only be demonstrated by magnetic resonance imaging (MRI), the term non-radiographic axial SpA (nr-axSpA) is applied. Most current data are derived from studies of AS.

Ankylosing spondylitis occurs in 0.2% of the general population, in 2% of the B27-positive population, and in 20% of B27-positive individuals with an affected family member. Males predominate with a male/female ratio ranging from 2.5:1 to 5:1 whereas in nr-axSpA the sex ratio is equal. AS typically begins in young adulthood, but symptoms may arise in adolescence or earlier. Up to 15% of children with juvenile idiopathic arthritis are classified as having juvenile-onset spondyloarthritis (JoSpA). Such children present with pauciarticular peripheral arthritis with a predilection for the tarsal joints; axial complaints, with the development of radiographic sacroiliitis, tend only to develop in late teenage or later.

The first symptom of AS is usually inflammatory back pain (Box 14.1) – the insidious onset of low back pain and/or buttock pain which persists more than 3 months, awakens the patient from sleep, is accompanied by early morning stiffness and is typically improved by exercise. Fatigue often accompanies inflammatory back pain but may also be present in fibromyalgia and other conditions. Persistent uncontrolled disease leads to persistent stiffness and progressive loss of spinal mobility.

The diagnosis of axial SpA is based on the ASAS classification criteria (Figure 14.2) which require characteristic SpA features combined with evidence of sacroiliitis demonstrated either by MRI scanning or X-ray. The modified New York criteria (Box 14.2), requiring radiographic sacroiliitis, describe AS: classic radiographic changes in the sacroiliac joints include erosions in the joint line, pseudo-widening, subchondral sclerosis and finally ankylosis, reflected as obliteration of the sacroiliac joint. Radiographic and

---

ABC of Rheumatology, Fifth Edition. Edited by Ade Adebajo and Lisa Dunkley.
© 2018 John Wiley & Sons Ltd. Published 2018 by John Wiley & Sons Ltd.

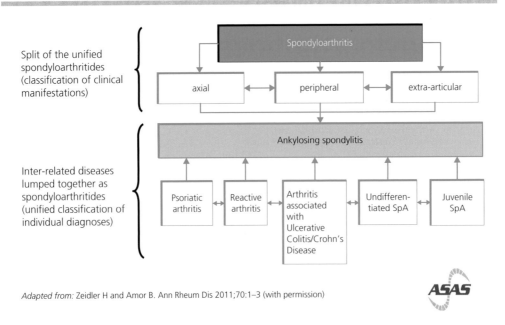

Split of the unified spondyloarthritides (classification of clinical manifestations)

Inter-related diseases lumped together as spondyloarthritides (unified classification of individual diagnoses)

Adapted from: Zeidler H and Amor B. Ann Rheum Dis 2011;70:1–3 (with permission)

Figure 14.1 Inter-relationship between the ASAS classification criteria and the disorders lumped together in the unified concept of SpA. Source: Adapted from Zeidler and Amor (2011)

Table 14.1 Examples of spondyloarthropathies

Syndromes	Features
Ankylosing spondylitis	Sacroiliitis
	Enthesitis
	Spondylitis
Psoriatic arthritis	Oligoarthritis
	Dactylitis
	Skin and membrane inflammation
Reactive arthritis (Reiter's syndrome)	Genitourinary inflammation, iritis
Enteropathic arthritis	Small and large bowel inflammation
Undifferentiated spondyloarthritis	Possible infectious trigger
Childhood spondyloarthritis	Associated with HLA-B27

Table 14.2 Prevalence of spondyloarthropathies

	Prevalence (%) per 100 000	Male:female
Ankylosing spondylitis	0.2	3.5
Psoriasis	2000	1.0
Psoriatic arthritis	20–100	1.3
Reactive arthritis	16	3.0
Crohn's disease	30–75	1.0
Ulcerative disease	50–100	0.8
Enteropathic arthritis	1–20% of inflammatory bowel disease	*

*Peripheral arthritis occurs

Box 14.1 **ASAS criteria for inflammatory back pain**

Back pain of more than 3 months duration is inflammatory if:

- Age at onset less than 40 years
- Insidious onset
- Improvement with exercise
- No improvement with rest
- Pain at night (with improvement on getting up)

The criteria are fulfilled if at least 4 of 5 parameters are present

Source: Sieper *et al.* (2009).

MRI changes of sacroiliitis are shown in Figure 14.3. Radiographs of the spine may reveal squaring and 'shiny corners' of the vertebral bodies (Figure 14.4a) and, later, syndesmophytes and facet joint fusion (Figure 14.4b). Not all patients with nr-axSpA will develop radiographic change so MRI is able to identify both patients who have not yet developed radiographic change and those who never will. HLA-B27 is also of diagnostic value when there is a high index of suspicion.

Up to 30% of patients with AxSpA also develop peripheral arthritis. Typically, this is asymmetrical oligoarthritis affecting leg joints, most commonly the knee. Involvement of the hip can occur at any point in the course of AS and may be highly destructive. Enthesitis – inflammation at attachments of tendon or ligament to bone – is also a characteristic feature of AS. Enthesitis at the calcaneal attachments of the Achilles tendon, usually accompanied by Achilles tendon bursitis (Figure 14.5) and plantar fascia, producing sometimes disabling heel pain, is highly characteristic of AxSpA, though it also occurs in other SpA. Dactylitis, usually affecting a toe (sausage toe – Figure 14.6), is also strongly suggestive of a SpA.

Ocular inflammation, usually acute anterior uveitis (iritis), occurs at some time in up to 40% of AS patients. Acute anterior uveitis typically causes pain, photophobia and, if untreated,

In patients with ≥3 months back pain and age at onset <45 years

| **Sacroiliitis on imaging***
 plus
 ≥1 SpA feature# | OR | **HLA-B27**
 plus
 ≥2 other SpA features# |

#SpA features
- inflammatory back pain
- arthritis
- enthesitis (heel)
- uveitis
- dactylitis
- psoriasis
- Crohn's/colitis
- good response to NSAIDs
- family history for SpA
- HLA-B27
- elevated CRP

*Sacroiliitis on imaging
- active (acute) inflammation on MRI highly suggestive of sacroiliitis associated with SpA
- definite radiographic sacroiliitis according to mod NY criteria

n=649 patients with back pain;
Sensitivity: 82.9%, Specificity: 84.4%
Imaging alone: Sensitivity: 66.2%, Specificity: 97.3%

Rudwaleit M et al. Ann Rheum Dis 2009;68:777–783 (with permission)

Figure 14.2 ASAS classification criteria for axial SpA. Source: Rudwaleit *et al.* (2009)

Box 14.2 **Modified New York criteria for ankylosing spondylitis (1984)**

A. Diagnosis
   1. Clinical criteria
      a. Low back pain and stiffness >3 months with improvement on exercise, not relieved by rest
      b. Limitation of spinal motion in both sagittal and frontal planes
      c. Limitation of chest expansion
   2. Radiologic criteria
      Sacroiliitis: Grade >2 bilaterally or Grade 3–4 unilaterally
B. Grading
   1. Definite ankylosing spondylitis if the radiologic criterion is associated with >1 clinical criterion
   2. Probable ankylosing spondylitis if:
      a. the three clinical criteria are present
      b. the radiologic criterion is present without any signs or symptoms satisfying the clinical criteria

---

impairment in visual acuity. Typically, it is unilateral and recurrent. Uncommon extra-articular manifestations of AS include aortic insufficiency, cardiac conduction defects and pulmonary fibrosis.

Assessment of ankylosing spondylitis

A range of instruments has been devised for measuring disease activity, overall function, severity and progression of AS. Those most widely used in clinical practice are listed below.

Disease activity – The Bath Ankylosing Spondylitis Disease Activity Index (BASDAI) is a patient-completed set of six visual analogue scales assessing symptoms. The erythrocyte sedimentation rate and C-reactive protein are typically elevated, but levels do not usefully indicate inflammatory activity of spinal disease.

Overall patient function – The Bath Ankylosing Spondylitis Functional Index (BASFI) is a similar patient-completed set of 10 visual analogue scales assessing normal daily activities. Assessments of work capacity and other socioeconomic aspects are also critical aspects of the measurement of function.

Spinal mobility – The Bath Ankylosing Spondylitis Metrology Index (BASMI) is a composite score derived from measurements of spinal mobility.

Many other measures are used in clinical studies, notably the modified Stoke AS Spinal Score (mSASSS) which measures radiographic progression. This uses lateral radiographs of the cervical and lumbosacral spine and can detect change over 2 years. It evaluates the anterior part of the lumbar spine and cervical spine and assesses chronic changes at each level with a score of 0 to 3 (0 = normal, 1 = erosion, sclerosis or squaring, 2 = syndesmophyte, 3 = bridging syndesmophyte).

The clinical course and disease severity of AS are highly variable. Inflammatory back pain and stiffness dominate the picture in the early stages, whereas chronic pain and deformity may develop over time. Osteoporosis tends to develop early in the disease, predisposing to spinal fractures later. One-third of AS sufferers give up work before retirement age because of their disease, though this may be changing thanks to biologic medication.

Psoriatic arthritis

Psoriatic arthritis is an inflammatory arthritis associated with psoriasis, usually with negative tests for rheumatoid factor. It is not a homogeneous clinical entity. In common with other spondyloarthritides, the key features are seronegative arthritis, enthesitis and, in a minority, sacroiliitis or spondylitis. It is the only SpA in which small joints of the hand are frequently affected. Five patterns of joint involvement are recognized (Box 14.3) though many patients have overlapping patterns of disease.

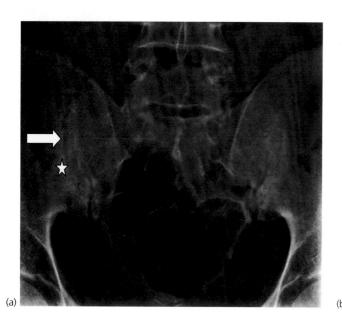

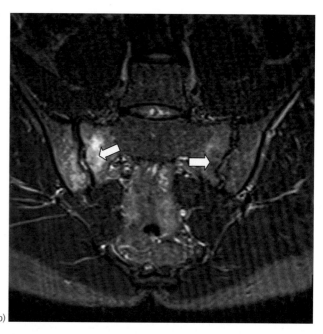

(a)

(b)

Figure 14.3 (a) AP radiograph of the sacroiliac joints showing grade 3 sacroiliitis on the right but less marked changes (grade 2) at the left SI joint. The right SI joint appears irregular with areas of 'erosions' (*arrow*) and juxta-articular sclerosis (*asterisk*). At the left SI joint there is juxta-articular sclerosis though the joint margins remain distinct. (b) MRI scan (STIR sequence) of the sacroiliac joints showing bilateral changes of sacroiliitis. At the right SI joint (*arrowed*), there is juxta-articular hyperdense change of active osteitis; at the left SI joint there is a hypodense area, possibly reflecting inactive disease, with a rim of hyperdense change on the sacral side

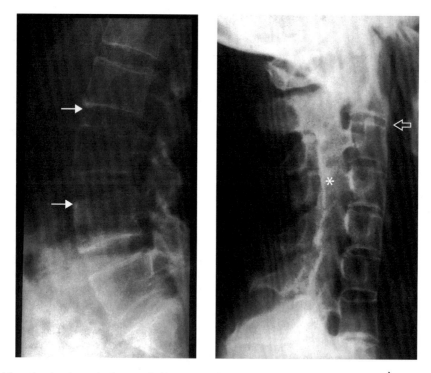

Figure 14.4 Radiographs of the spine showing early changes of 'shiny corners' (→), late changes of syndesmophytes (⇨) and facet joint fusion (*)

Psoriasis occurs in 5% of most Caucasian populations and 5–15% of sufferers develop one or another form of associated arthritis. In a small minority of patients, arthritis precedes the onset of psoriasis.

Typical psoriatic nail changes of pitting, onycholysis and hyperkeratosis are seen in over 80% of patients with psoriatic arthritis though skin lesions may be subtle and should be sought specifically in the scalp and natal cleft. Arthritis is characteristically oligoarticular and asymmetrical and may be associated with dactylitis of fingers or toes ('sausage digit' - see Figure 14.6). Distal interphalageal joint involvement at the fingers is uncommon but highly characteristic

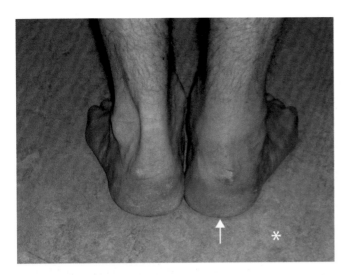

Figure 14.5 Achilles tendon bursitis

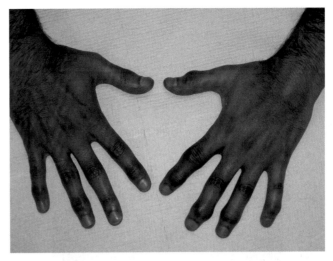

Figure 14.7 Distal interphalangeal joint involvement in psoriatic arthritis

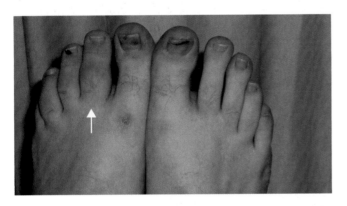

Figure 14.6 Sausage toe

Box 14.3 **Patterns of psoriatic arthritis**

- Asymmetrical oligoarthritis (50%); involvement of 1–5 joints
- Predominantly distal interphalangeal joint disease (5–10%); distinctive but unusual form of psoriatic arthritis
- Rheumatoid pattern (25%); symmetrical small joint arthritis particularly affecting metacarpophalangeal, wrist and proximal interphalangeal joints; may be indistinguishable from rheumatoid arthritis
- Arthritis mutilans (1–5%); osteolysis results in destruction of the small joints of the digits with shortening
- Spondyloarthritis (20%); may be isolated sacroiliitis, atypical or typical AS

(Figure 14.7). Enthesitis plays a role in dactylitis but may also occur at more typical sites around the patella or around the heel at the Achilles tendon or plantar fascia insertion. Twenty percent of patients with psoriatic arthritis develop low back pain with sacroiliitis and may develop typical or atypical spondylitis. Conjunctivitis and anterior uveitis may occur but less commonly than in AS.

Reactive arthritis

Reactive arthritis (ReA) is aseptic arthritis that occurs subsequent to an extra-articular infection, typically of the gastrointestinal (GI) or genitourinary (GU) tract. In the former, the key GI pathogens are *Salmonella typhimurium, Yersinia enterocolitica, Shigella flexneri* and *Campylobacter jejuni;* the most common GU pathogen is *Chlamydia trachomatis.* The true incidence and prevalence of ReA are not well defined. In epidemics involving *Salmonella* or *Yersinia,* ReA develops in up to 7% of infected individuals, but in as many as 20% of B27+ infected individuals. In such epidemic studies, B27 confers risk not only for the onset of arthritis but also for axial involvement and chronicity. Typically, arthritis begins 1–3 weeks after the GI or GU infection.

As with other SpA syndromes, the pattern of joint involvement in ReA is one of asymmetrical oligoarthritis mainly affecting joints of the leg. As in AS, enthesitis may arise as Achilles tendonitis or plantar fasciitis and dactylitis may occur at one or more toes. Sacroiliitis, with buttock pain, may occur in the acute phase but radiographic changes are seen largely in the patients with a chronic course.

When ReA is accompanied by urethritis, conjunctivitis and/or mucocutaneous lesions, the term Reiter's syndrome may be applied. Urethritis may be manifest as dysuria or discharge and psoriasiform skin and mucosal lesions include circinate balanitis and keratoderma blennorrhagicum (Figure 14.8), a painless papulosquamous eruption on the palms or soles. Painless lingual or oral ulcers may also be seen. Conjunctivitis is usually bilateral; acute anterior uveitis is usually unilateral and may not be synchronous with the acute episode but may be clinically indistinguishable from conjunctivitis.

The most important differential diagnosis for ReA is septic arthritis, so appropriate culture of synovial fluid should precede the diagnosis of ReA whenever possible. The course of ReA is variable, and few prognostic markers are available for the clinician to predict the course in any individual case. The majority of patients have an initial episode lasting 2–3 months, but synovitis may

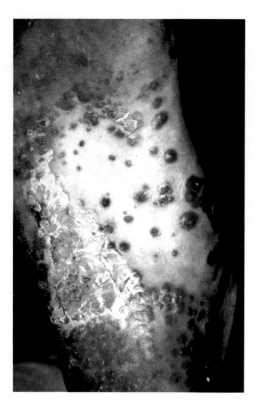

Figure 14.8 Keratoderma blennorhagicum

persist for a year or longer. In patients with chronic disease, a significant minority develop some degree of functional disability.

Enteropathic arthritis

Enteropathic arthritis is an inflammatory arthritis associated with inflammatory bowel disease, particularly ulcerative colitis and Crohn's disease. Two patterns of peripheral joint involvement are recognized, designated type 1 and type 2. Usually bowel and joint symptoms occur independently and arthritis may wax and wane over many years. Non-specific arthralgia and myalgia without an inflammatory component, similar to that seen in fibromyalgia, is not uncommon in people with inflammatory bowel disease (IBD).

Type 1 arthropathy affects approximately 5% of patients with IBD. Typically, the peripheral arthritis is oligoarticular and principally affects the knees. It is usually self-limiting without leading to joint deformities. Joint symptoms can occur early in the course of bowel disease and may precede the onset of bowel symptoms. Enthesitis of the Achilles tendon and plantar fascia and dactylitis may also occur.

Type 2 arthropathy affects approximately 3% of patients with IBD. Arthritis is usually polyarticular and may resemble rheumatoid arthritis. The metacarpophalangeal joints are principally affected; knees, ankles, elbows, shoulders, wrists, proximal interphalangeal and metatarsophalangeal joints may also be affected, sometimes in a migratory fashion.

Sacroiliitis and spondylitis occur in up to 20% of patients with either form of IBD. The course of spinal involvement is completely independent of the course of the IBD and may precede by years the first manifestations of bowel disease.

Undifferentiated spondyloarthritis

The development of inflammatory back pain or peripheral large joint arthritis, often in individuals who are HLA B27 positive, with or without other SpA features but without fulfilling criteria for any particular subtype, is referred to as undifferentiated SpA. Most patients are young adults, though children may be affected; a proportion of cases will evolve over time into a classifiable subset, particularly AS.

It is not unusual for the first feature of a spondyloarthritis to be an enthesitis, especially at the Achilles tendon or plantar fascia. These lesions may also occur independent of any arthritic conditions, especially in athletes. In spondyloarthritis, Achilles tendonitis typically affects the actual entheseal junction, often with marked bone oedema visible on MRI scanning and sometimes with Achilles tendon bursitis; in athletes, pain and tendon swelling occur higher up in the tendon close to the muscle belly. Plantar fasciitis is not so easily differentiated although it often occurs in overweight older adults.

There are no diagnostic criteria for undifferentiated SpA *per se*, the diagnosis being based solely on the presence of likely SpA features, other diagnoses having been excluded.

Treatment

The goals of treatment are to relieve symptoms, improve function and delay or prevent structural damage. To some extent, treatment of spinal inflammation differs from that of peripheral joint synovitis and enthesitis so treatment must be tailored to the actual problems in the individual patient at the time.

Sacroiliitis and spondylitis

First-line treatment – Regular physiotherapy and encouragement to exercise regularly; use of non-steroidal anti-inflammatory drugs (NSAIDS) such as naproxen or diclofenac, or COX-2 inhibitors such as etoricoxib or celecoxib.

Second-line treatment – Oral and intramuscular corticosteroids may control spinal symptoms but long-term use should be avoided. Local corticosteroid injections into one or both sacroiliac joints under radiographic imaging may be helpful. Sulfasalazine has not been shown, in trials, to be effective for spinal symptoms. However, it is often used in clinical practice and may sometimes be helpful.

Third-line treatment – Anti-TNF and anti-IL-17 agents have been proven significantly to reduce spinal pain and stiffness and to increase spinal movement and patient function. Reduction of spinal inflammation has been demonstrated by MRI scanning although evidence of disease modification, in terms of prevention of new bone formation, is currently equivocal.

Adjunctive treatment – Bisphosphonates, calcium and vitamin D may improve bone density although fracture reduction has not been demonstrated in AS. Low-dose amitriptyline at night may improve sleep and reduce pain and fatigue.

Oligoarthritis and/or enthesitis

First-line treatment – Analgesics such as paracetamol/acetaminophen or codeine-based drugs may be helpful. Intra-articular or intralesional corticosteroid injection can be useful for single peripheral joint involvement or enthesitis. Injections into weight-bearing tendon insertions should be avoided. NSAIDs may provide symptomatic relief. They must be used with caution in patients with IBD as they may exacerbate the gut disease. Orthotics, including heel pads, and carefully chosen footwear, including suitable trainer/running shoes, may provide the best symptomatic relief for arthritis or enthesitis affecting the feet. In patients with reactive arthritis, genital tract infection should be treated as in uncomplicated infection, with treatment of sexual contacts. Antimicrobial treatment of gut infection is not usually indicated and there is no clear evidence for long-term antimicrobial treatment of established arthritis.

Second-line treatment – Disease-modifying antirheumatoid drugs may be effective for those patients with aggressive, erosive or polyarticular disease, as in the treatment of rheumatoid arthritis. Methotrexate may be effective for both skin and joint disease though the published evidence is scant. In individuals with enteropathic arthritis, sulfasalazine may be effective for both joint and bowel disease. Rigorous monitoring of DMARD therapy, according to established practice guidelines, should be undertaken. Oral or intramuscular corticosteroid treatment may be effective, especially in those with marked systemic features. Steroid withdrawal carries a risk of exacerbation of psoriasis.

Third-line treatment – In those patients who have an inadequate response to conventional DMARDs and in whom the diagnosis is well established, anti-TNF and anti-IL-17 therapy may be dramatically effective in the control of joint and skin disease. Etanercept has not been shown to be effective for IBD.

Reference

Sieper J, van der Heijde D, Landewe R *et al.* New criteria for inflammatory back pain in patients with chronic back pain: a real patient exercise by experts from the Assessment of SpondyloArthritis international Society (ASAS). *Annals of the Rheumatic Diseases* 2009; **68**: 784–788.

Further reading

Carlin EM, Ziza JM, Keat A, Janier M. European Guideline on the management of sexually acquired reactive arthritis. *International Journal of STD and AIDS* 2014; **25**(13): 901–912.

Hannu H, Inman RD, Granfors K, Leirisalo-Repo M. Reactive arthritis or postinfectious arthritis. *Best Practice and Research in Clinical Rheumatology* 2006; **20**: 419–433.

Holden W, Orchard T, Wordsworth P. Enteropathic arthritis. *Rheumatic Diseases Clinics of North America* 2003; **29**(3): 513–530.

Rudwaleit M, van der Heijde D, Landewe R *et al.* The Assessment of SpondyloArthritis International Society classification criteria for peripheral spondyloarthritis and for spondyloarthritis in general. *Annals of the Rheumatic Diseases* 2011; **70**: 25–31.

Zochling J, van der Heijde D, Burgos-Vargas R *et al.* ASAS/EULAR Recommendations for the management of ankylosing spondylitis. *Annals of the Rheumatic Diseases* 2006; **65**: 442–452.

CHAPTER 15

Juvenile Idiopathic Arthritis

Anne-Marie McMahon and Evdoxia Sapountzi

Sheffield Children's Hospital, Sheffield, UK

OVERVIEW

- Juvenile idiopathic arthritis (JIA) is the most common rheumatic disease in children and one of the most common chronic illnesses of childhood.

- It is characterized by chronic arthritis of unknown aetiology, lasting at least 6 weeks, with an onset before 16 years of age.

- JIA is a heterogeneous group of disorders whose manifestations range from relatively mild inflammation of a single joint to severe involvement of multiple joints lasting into adulthood, and potentially leading to structural joint damage and incapacity.

Box 15.1 **Criteria for classification of juvenile idiopathic arthritis**

Age at onset <16 years
   Arthritis (swelling or effusion, or the presence of 2 or more of the following signs: limitation of range of motion, tenderness or pain on motion, and increased heat) in one or more joints
   Duration of disease: 6 weeks or longer
Onset type defined by type of disease in first 6 months:

- Polyarthritis: >5 inflamed joints
- Oligoarthritis (pauciarticular disease): <5 inflamed joints
- Systemic onset: arthritis with rash and characteristic quotidian* fever

Exclusion of other forms of juvenile arthritis

*quotidian = occurring daily.
Source: Modified from Cassidy *et al.* (1986).

Epidemiology

The worldwide incidence and prevalence of JIA are unknown. Epidemiological studies have reported a wide variance in different regions of the world, with low rates in Asian populations and relatively higher frequencies in those of European descent. Considering all types of arthritis, the prevalence of JIA ranges from 16 to 150 per 100 000 children. In the UK, the prevalence is approximately 1 in 1000 children. These wide-ranging numbers are attributable to population differences, particularly environmental exposure and immunogenetic susceptibility.

Classification

The nomenclature used to define childhood arthritis has changed several times over the last 40 years (Box 15.1). The latest definition, as put forth by the International League of Associations for Rheumatology (ILAR) in 1977 and later revised in 2001, divides JIA into seven subgroups (Table 15.1). The intent of this current classification system was to create consistency amongst international providers in order to identify children with similar characteristics for the purpose of research towards epidemiology, pathogenesis and treatment strategies. However, debate is still ongoing as to

whether this scheme should be further redeveloped, with emphasis more on antibody presence, age of symptom onset and symmetry of arthritis.

Etiology

By definition, JIA is idiopathic with no identifiable cause. It is almost certainly multifactorial and probably differs from one onset type to another. As technology improves, as with the advent of genome-wide association studies, the underlying genetic susceptibility factors of JIA are beginning to be defined. Familial JIA itself is uncommon and does not follow any mendelian modes of inheritance. One American registry identified 200 sets of siblings with JIA over a 10-year period, of whom 21 sets were twins.

The major histocompatibility complex (MHC) is a diverse and complex genetic loci central to immunity and inflammatory processes. The MHC comprises genes related to antigen presentation,

---

ABC of Rheumatology, Fifth Edition. Edited by Ade Adebajo and Lisa Dunkley.
© 2018 John Wiley & Sons Ltd. Published 2018 by John Wiley & Sons Ltd.

Table 15.1 Classification of chronic arthritis of childhood

Organization	European League Against Rheumatism (EULAR)	American College of Rheumatology (ACR)	International League of Associations for Rheumatology (ILAR)
Criterion name	Juvenile chronic arthritis	Juvenile rheumatoid arthritis	Juvenile idiopathic arthritis
Year	1977	1986	1997, revised 2001
Age of onset	<16 years	<16 years	<16 years
Duration	≥3 months	>6 weeks	>6 weeks

Subsets	1. Pauciarticular: <5 joints
	2. Polyarticular: >4 joints, RF-
	3. Systemic arthritis with characteristic fever
	4. Juvenile rheumatoid arthritis: >4 joints
	5. Juvenile ankylosing spondylitis
	6. Juvenile psoriatic arthritis
		1. Polyarthritis: >5 inflamed joints
		2. Oligoarthritis: <5 inflamed joints
		3. Systemic onset: arthritis with characteristic fever
			1. Systemic
			2. Oligoarthritis
			  a. Persistent
			  b. Extended
			3. Polyarthritis RF-
			4. Polyarthritis RF+
			5. Psoriatic arthritis
			6. Enthesitis-related arthritis
			7. Undifferentiated
			  a. Fits no other category
			  b. Fits more than one category

including human leucocyte antigens (HLA) A, B, C, DR, DP and DQ, minor HLA antigens, as well as other genes important in immune function such as tumour necrosis factor (TNF), macrophage inhibitor factor (MIF), interleukin (IL)-6 and IL-1a. The HLA class I and II alleles have been identified as a major susceptibility locus for JIA.

Possible non-genetic triggers include bacterial and viral infections (parvovirus B19, rubella, Epstein–Barr, influenza A, *Mycoplasma pneumoniae*), enhanced immune responses to bacterial or mycobacterial heat shock proteins, abnormal reproductive hormone levels and joint trauma. Some studies have demonstrated persistence of infectious markers within synovial fluid. However, many reports rely on the identification of serological antibodies to viruses, and interpretation of seropositivity can be controversial.

Pathogenesis

Juvenile idiopathic arthritis is an autoimmune disease associated with alterations in both humoral and cell-mediated immunity. T-lymphocytes have a central role, releasing proinflammatory cytokines. Complement consumption, immune complex formation and B-cell activation also promote inflammation. Inheritance of specific cytokine alleles may predispose to upregulation of inflammatory networks, resulting in systemic-onset disease or more severe articular disease.

Systemic-onset JIA (SoJIA) may be more accurately classified as an autoinflammatory disorder, more like familial Mediterranean fever (FMF) than other subtypes of JIA. This theory is supported by work demonstrating similar expression patterns of phagocytic protein (S100A12) in SoJIA and FMF, as well as the same marked responsiveness to IL-1 receptor antagonists.

All these immunological abnormalities cause inflammatory synovitis, characterized pathologically by villous hypertrophy and hyperplasia with hyperaemia and oedema of the synovial tissue. Vascular endothelial hyperplasia is prominent and is characterized by infiltration of mononuclear and plasma cells with predominance

of T-lymphocytes. Advanced and uncontrolled disease leads to pannus formation (proliferative synovium that grows over the joint surface) and progressive erosion of articular cartilage and contiguous bone.

Oligoarthritis

According to the ILAR classification, there are two categories of oligoarthritis. 'Persistent' oligoarthritis is defined as a disease which starts in four or fewer joints and never involves more than four joints. The second category, 'extended' oligoarthritis, is a form in which the arthritis is oligoarticular for at least the first 6 months, but then extends to involve more than four joints (Table 15.2).

Persistent oligoarthritis

Oligoarthritis is the most common form of JIA, characterized by an age of onset less than 6 years, female predominance and a relatively high incidence of complicating uveitis. Progression to extended oligoarthritis has been reported to occur in 20–50% in different series. Extension beyond four joints usually occurs within 2 years of onset but the incidence increases until a plateau is reached by about 5 years after onset.

Clinical features

With the onset of oligoarthritis, the child may not always complain of pain and may not be brought to a physician until advanced changes are present. The parents are most likely to have noticed a limp or seen a swollen joint. A very young child may stop walking or standing, or be fussy and unhappy when doing so, especially first thing in the morning (morning stiffness) with improvement later in the day. On examination, there will be a joint effusion, swelling and local warmth, with or without mild or moderate tenderness. There will be pain on the extremes of motion, limitation of range of motion, and pain on weight bearing or resisted movement. An antalgic gait is likely. The most common joints involved at presentation are the knees. The small joints of the hands and feet are

Table 15.2 ILAR classification criteria for oligoarthritis

Definition	Exclusions
Arthritis affecting 1–4 joints during the first 6 months of disease. Two subcategories are recognized: 1. Persistent oligoarthritis: affects no more than 4 joints throughout the disease course 2. Extended oligoarthritis: affects more than 4 joints after the first 6 months of the disease	a. Psoriasis or a history of psoriasis in the patient or first-degree relative b. Arthritis in HLA+ boy beginning after the 6th birthday c. Ankylosing spondylitis, enthesitis-related arthritis, sacroiliitis with inflammatory bowel disease, Reiter's syndrome, or acute anterior uveitis, or one of these disorders in first-degree relative d. Positive rheumatoid factor on at least 2 occasions at least 3 months apart e. Presence of systemic JIA in the patient

Table 15.3 Differential diagnosis of monoarthritis

Acute monoarthritis	Chronic monoarthritis

1. Early rheumatic disease
   Oligoarthritis
   Enthesitis-related arthritis
   Psoriatic arthritis
2. Arthritis related to infection
   Septic arthritis
   Reactive arthritis
3. Malignancy
   Leukaemia
   Neuroblastoma
4. Haemophilia
5. Trauma
6. Familial Mediterranean fever
	1. Juvenile idiopathic arthritis
	   Oligoarthritis
	   Enthesitis-related arthritis
	   Psoriatic arthritis
	2. Villonodular synovitis
	3. Sarcoidosis, Blau syndrome
	4. Tuberculosis
	5. Haemophilia
	6. Pseudoarthritis
	   Hemangioma
	   Synovial chondromatosis
	   Lipoma arborescens
	7. Autoinflammatory syndromes
	   Mevalonate kinase deficiency
	   Chronic infantile neurocutaneous and articular syndrome
	   Neonatal-onset multisystem inflammatory disease

involved in 10% or less. Wrist and elbow involvement may predict extension to polyarticular disease in the long term. Hips are rarely involved. Arthritis isolated to one or both hips should prompt consideration of enthesitis-related arthritis in the differential.

Acute onset, particularly in association with marked tenderness, redness, fever or severe pain and refusal to weight bear requires care to exclude infection or neoplasm, most often leukaemia. A history of tick bite or rash, or intermittent episodes of arthritis, especially in the knee, in patients who have been in endemic areas suggests possible Lyme disease.

Growth abnormalities may be generalized or limited to one limb. Arthritis in large joints, especially knees, initially accelerates linear growth, causing the affected limb to be longer and resulting in limb length discrepancy. Continued inflammation stimulates rapid and premature closure of the growth plate, resulting in shortened bones. Generalized growth retardation is becoming much less frequent with the availability of effective treatment. Muscles around inflamed joints may quite quickly become atrophic.

Diagnosis

Juvenile idiopathic arthritis is a clinical diagnosis of exclusion with many mimics and without diagnostic laboratory tests. The meticulous clinical exclusion of other diseases is therefore essential.

Laboratory tests in oligoarthritis are usually normal. Complete blood counts should be normal, but may show moderate increases in white blood cell (WBC) counts or mild anaemia. The ESR may be normal and is not usually greater than 30 mm/h, and higher values may predict progression to polyarthritis. Urinalysis and blood chemistries are normal. Positive rheumatoid factor (RF) is an exclusion for the classification of oligoarthritis. Antinuclear antibodies (ANA) are present in up to 70–80% of young girls with oligoarthritis and are a risk factor for uveitis.

Radiographs are usually normal and cannot make a diagnosis of oligoarthritis, but are necessary to rule out other diagnoses (Table 15.3). Magnetic resonance imaging (MRI) may show synovial hypertrophy and is not routinely necessary, but is helpful if there is suspicion of an underlying cause.

Most children presenting with monoarthritis do not need a joint fluid aspiration, but this is necessary if there is concern regarding joint sepsis.

Box 15.2 **Characteristics predicting disease extension in oligoarthritis**

Symmetrical joint involvement
Ankles and wrists disease
Elevated erythrocyte sedimentation rate
Presence of HLA-DR1

Extended oligoarthritis

The age of onset and sex ratios of the children who develop extended oligoarthritis are the same as those with persistent oligoarthritis. Extension to more than four joints occurs in the first 5 years of disease onset. The frequency of oligoarthritis becoming extended is unknown.

Clinical characteristics predictive of disease extension include ankle or wrist disease, symmetrical joint involvement and elevated ESR (Box 15.2). ANA positivity correlates with worse outcome in this group. The incidence of remission is lower and the potential degree of disability is greater than patients with persistent oligoarthritis.

Genetics

The principal differences between children with extended and persistent oligoarthritis are genetic. None of children with extended oligoarthritis have the HLA antigen DR6, although this antigen has a positive genetic association with oligoarthritis generally. Conversely, there is an association with DR1, which is predictive of progression to more joints, and to joint erosion.

Prognosis

The disease course and prognosis in children with oligoarthritis have improved considerably in the past 15 years. The frequency of significant joint contractures or leg length inequalities has diminished, probably as the result of prompt institution of pharmacological and physical therapy, in particular the use of intra-articular steroids.

Children with persistent oligoarthritis have a good chance for remission. Those in whom more extensive disease develops have a poorer prognosis. Children with oligo-arthritis, particularly girls who are ANA positive, with onset earlier than 6 years of age, are at risk for development of chronic uveitis. There is no association between the activity or severity of the arthritis and the chronic uveitis.

Uveitis

The most serious complication for all children with oligoarthritis is the potential blindness caused by uveitis. JIA-associated uveitis has a poor prognosis and a high rate of complications. Early diagnosis and rapid adequate interdisciplinary care are important for the long-term prognosis.

Epidemiology

The rates of uveitis in JIA (4–24%) vary because of the characteristics of different medical centres and geographical variations. The risk of uveitis is higher in north Europeans than in Asian populations. Meta-analysis estimates that the worldwide incidence is 8.3%.

The intraocular inflammation is mostly diagnosed between the fourth and sixth years of life. In half of patients, the uveitis manifests shortly before or more than 5 years after the onset of JIA, in some 75% within a year, in 90% within 4 years and later in only 3–5%.

In 75% of children the inflammation affects both eyes. Children with unilateral uveitis very rarely develop uveitis in the contralateral eye once more than 12 months have passed. However, there are exceptions, and unilateral uveitis may persist for many years in a few children before the other eye is involved.

Insidious-onset (chronic) uveitis

According to the classification of the International Standardization of Uveitis Nomenclature (SUN), which seeks to classify intraocular disorders, JIA-associated uveitis is typically a recurrent, non-granulomatous, anterior uveitis. Uveitis that occurs in association with JIA presents as chronic anterior uveitis, typically with an asymptomatic 'white eye'. Uveitis is detected in less than 10% of patients before the onset of arthritis, usually during a routine ophthalmic examination. The early detection of chronic uveitis requires slit-lamp biomicroscopy, which should be performed at the time of diagnosis in every child with JIA. The recommended frequency of ophthalmological examination is influenced by the level of risk of uveitis.

The diagnostic signs of anterior uveitis on slit-lamp examination are the presence of inflammatory cells and increased protein concentration 'flare' in the aqueous humour of the anterior chamber of the eye. Deposition of inflammatory cells on the inner surface of the cornea (keratic precipitate) may be detected at presentation or develop later.

Complications of chronic anterior uveitis are frequent and increase with increasing duration of active disease. A recent series reported the frequency of complications as lower than in earlier studies, presumably due to earlier treatment (Box 15.3).

Box 15.3 **Complications of chronic anterior uveitis**

Bilateral disease 67–85%
Cataract
Glaucoma
Posterior synechiae
Band keratopathy
Retinal detachment
Macular oedema
Hypotony
Visual loss

Sudden-onset (acute) uveitis

Sudden-onset (acute) uveitis differs in several ways from chronic anterior uveitis and is strongly associated with HLA-B27 and enthesitis-related arthritis (ERA). Boys are more commonly affected, it is more often unilateral, and is characterized by a painful, red, photophobic eye. The symptoms are often mistakenly attributed to a foreign body, infection or allergy. Because of the symptomatic nature of this uveitis, the process is usually identified and treated soon after onset. Therefore, long-term sequelae are less common.

Management of JIA-associated uveitis

The treatment of uveitis should be supervised by an ophthalmologist experienced in the management of children with this disease. The goal of therapy is to achieve normal vision by controlling inflammation in the eye (no cells) and surgical approaches to its complications, particularly cataract. The most exciting development in the medical treatment of JIA-associated uveitis has been the application of biological drugs in cases resistant to conventional systemic immunosuppressive therapy or cases in which conventional agents cannot be used.

In mild disease, treatment may be limited to corticosteroid eye drops. Non-steroidal anti-inflammatory drugs (NSAIDs) should not be used as monotherapy in active uveitis. Systemic immunosuppression is required, if using topical steroids does not result in uveitis inactivity within 3 months, if new complications arise, if the dosage of the corticosteroids has to be excessively high or if medication-related adverse effects develop.

In patients with severe inflammation, the treatment can be intensified at an earlier stage. Immunomodulating and disease-modifying substances (DMARDs) not only make it possible to use lower doses of corticosteroids but also improve the long-term outcome of uveitis. The most commonly used immunosuppressant is methotrexate. If after 4 months the effect is unsatisfactory, a second conventional or biological DMARD may be considered. Close liaison with paediatric rheumatology centres ensures access to the latest evidence and guidelines in the management of childhood uveitis.

Systemic juvenile idiopathic arthritis

Systemic arthritis (SoJIA) represents the childhood-onset equivalent of adult-onset Still's disease. Its onset can be quite non-specific and may suggest infection, malignancy or another inflammatory disease.

Table 15.4 Systemic juvenile idiopathic arthritis (ILAR)

Criteria	Exclusions
Arthritis with or preceded by daily fever of at least 2 weeks duration, that is documented to be quotidian (24 hours apart) for at least 3 days, and accompanied by one or more of the following: 1. Evanescent*, non-fixed, erythematous rash 2. Generalized lymphadenopathy 3. Hepatomegaly and/or splenomegaly 4. Serositis	a. Psoriasis or a history of psoriasis in the patient or first-degree relative b. Arthritis in HLA-B27+ boy beginning after the 6th birthday c. Ankylosing spondylitis, enthesitis-related arthritis, sacroiliitis with inflammatory bowel disease, Reiter's syndrome, acute anterior uveitis, or a history of one of these disorders in first-degree relative d. Presence of immunoglobulin M RF on at least 2 occasions at least 3 months apart

*Evanescent = transient, usually a few hours.

The disease is defined as systemic arthritis in the ILAR classification of juvenile idiopathic arthritis, based on the following criteria: presence of arthritis and of documented quotidian fever of at least 2 weeks' duration, plus one of the following: typical rash, generalized lymphadenopathy, enlargement of liver or spleen or serositis. Criteria and exclusions are shown in Table 15.4.

Systemic JIA accounts for 10% of children with JIA. The onset of the disease may occur at any time during childhood, with a broad peak of onset between 1 and 5 years of age, but there is a wide variation with a relatively similar frequency of onset at all age groups. Males and females are affected with approximately equal frequency or very minimal female excess 1.1:1.

Pathogenesis

The genetic factors associated with SoJIA are unclear. SoJIA is rarely familial, which is consistent with the hypothesis that the genetic background of the disease is complex. In contrast to classic autoimmune disease, genetic association with HLA class I or II alleles is weak. The most consistently reported associations include polymorphisms in the regulatory sequences of genes coding for cytokines of the innate immune response such as MIF, TNF-alpha, IL-6 genes, and the IL-1 and IL-1 receptor loci. Autoantibodies and autoreactive T-cells are not present in SoJIA. However, the number of innate immune cells such as monocytes and neutrophils is increased. Studies of gene expression profiles in blood cells provide evidence of disregulated innate immune response with increased production of inflammatory cytokines.

Extra-articular clinical features
Fever

High spiking daily fever is the most important clinical criterion, as it always present at the onset of the disease. Occasionally, it can start later after the development of arthritis. According to the Edmonton criteria for JIA, fever must have been present for at least 2 weeks, and documented to have a quotidian pattern (a single spike of fever per day) for at least 3 days. Typically, fever occurs in the afternoon or early evening, reaching 39 °C or more. The peak is followed by a sharp decrease under 37 °C. Chills are frequent at the time of fever, but rigors are rare. These children are often quite ill while febrile but may be surprisingly well during the rest of the day. The fever usually lasts for several months, may recur with flares of disease, and occasionally persists for years.

Rash

The rash is the second typical extra-articular manifestation and is present in more than 90% of cases at onset. The classic rash is evanescent, erythematous macules 2–5 mm in size that may appear in linear streaks, or more discrete occurring in areas of exposure to air or touch (Koebner phenomenon). The rash is usually described as salmon pink. It occurs typically with fever spikes, but may persist when fever is resolved. Sometimes, it can resemble urticaria, and can be quite pruritic.

Organomegaly and lymphadenopathy

Hepatomegaly is often present but it is mild and not tender. Chronic liver disease generally does not occur but there are reports of hepatic nodular regenerative hyperplasia, which can lead to portal hypertension.

Spleen enlargement occurs in 30% of cases and is usually mild. Massive splenomegaly is uncommon and raises suspicion for another diagnosis, particularly malignancy. Lymphadenopathy is found in up to 50% of cases, usually painless, freely mobile in the cervical, axillary and inguinal area. Mesenteric lymphadenopathy may cause abdominal pain, sometimes leading to a debate about possible surgical emergency in an undiagnosed child.

Serositis and other visceral manifestations

Pericarditis with or without pleural effusion is common and usually asymptomatic. However, chest pain with or without dyspnoea, especially in supine position, is a classic symptom of acute pericarditis. Tamponade is rare but some children will require drainage of pericardial fluid. Pericarditis is not a poor prognostic factor and is not related to gender or severity of joint disease, but appears to be more common in children with disease onset who are younger than 18 months of age.

Myocarditis is not common, although it may occur in the absence of pericarditis, leading to cardiomegaly and congestive heart failure. Endocarditis is very rare.

Pleural effusion is the most common respiratory manifestation, usually asymptomatic and an incidental finding on chest radiographs. Parenchymal pulmonary disease is rare.

Central nervous system disease

Acute neurological events are rare. Encephalopathy, seizures and intracranial haemorrhages are serious manifestations of central nervous system involvement in macrophage activation syndrome (MAS) (see below), and associated with significant mortality risk.

Musculoskeletal manifestations

Arthritis is absent at onset in about one-third of the cases, rendering the diagnosis difficult. Even if it is not present at onset, it usually develops within the next few months, or one or more years. Arthritis is generally symmetrical, affecting more than four joints in about one-quarter of the patients. The most commonly affected joints are knees, ankles and wrists but small joints, hips and cervical spine can be affected. The arthritis in SoJIA can involve any site that contains synovial membrane. Myalgia is common, especially during the febrile phase of disease, but there is no elevation in muscle enzymes.

Diagnosis and differential diagnosis

The diagnosis of SoJIA is made clinically, supported by typical laboratory findings, but it is a diagnosis of exclusion. The presence of characteristic rash and quotidian fever are very suggestive but the diagnosis may be difficult. Infections and septicaemia may mimic the disease initially, and the possibility of malignancy, other connective tissue diseases or vasculitis should be considered (Box 15.4).

When the constellation of clinical and laboratory findings is not typical for the diagnosis, more extensive investigations may be necessary, including chest and abdomen imaging, examination of bone marrow and biopsies of lymph nodes or affected organs.

Laboratory examination

Chronic anaemia is almost always present, but it can take some time to occur.

Box 15.4 Differential diagnosis of systemic JIA

Infections
- Bacterial endocarditis
- Acute rheumatic fever
- Cat scratch disease
- Lyme disease
- Brucellosis
- Mycoplasma
- Others

Malignancy
Rheumatic and inflammatory diseases
- Systemic lupus erythematosus
- Dermatomyositis
- Polyarteritis nodosa
- Kawasaki's disease
- Serum sickness
- Sarcoidosis
- Castleman's disease

Inflammatory bowel disease
- Familial Mediterranean fever
- Autoinflammatory syndromes
- Mevalonate kinase deficiency
- TNF receptor-associated periodic syndrome (TRAPS)
- Muckle–Wells syndrome
- Chronic infantile neurological cutaneous and articular syndrome (CINCA)
- Neonatal-onset multisystem inflammatory disease (NOMID)

Leucocytosis (neutrophilic) is characteristic of active SJIA. If leucocyte counts are normal or low, other diagnoses such as leukaemia, viral infection or a complication such as MAS should be considered. This complication is described in more detail below.

Thrombocytosis may reach high levels, reflecting the inflammation process. There is no risk of thrombosis. Normal or low platelets should lead to consideration of malignancy or MAS. Bone marrow aspiration and biopsy may help to rule out leukaemia or neuroblastoma.

Acute-phase reactants are also elevated. Elevated erythrocyte sedimentation (ESR) is constant and often reaches more than 100 mm/h. High levels of CRP are also characteristic. Fibrinogen and serum complement levels tend to be high. Extremely elevated ferritin levels are a feature of MAS. Autoantibodies are not generally present. A high ESR without significant thrombocytosis, or associated with high lactate dehydrogenase (LDH) levels, is highly suggestive of malignancy.

Features seen during the course of the disease

There are three patterns seen in the clinical course of patients with systemic arthritis

Monocyclic course

Children present with all typical features of disease but eventually remit completely. The treatment administered initially can be withdrawn gradually and the symptoms do not recur. This pattern of disease occurs in about 11% of cases.

Polycyclic course

These patients have relapses of disease with intervals of remission. The periods of remission can vary, sometimes lasting many years with a relapse in adulthood. This pattern of disease appears in approximately 34% of patients.

Unremitting course

Approximately 55% of children with SoJIA never go into remission and continue to require treatment.

Systemic complications
Macrophage activation syndrome

Macrophage activation syndrome is a serious, potentially fatal complication of rheumatic diseases, and is seen most frequently in SoJIA. It bears close resemblance to haemophagocytic lymphohistiocytosis (HLH). MAS may occur spontaneously, as a complication of active underlying disease, or may be triggered by an infection, a change in drug therapy or a toxic effect of medications, such as biologics. The hallmark of this syndrome is the finding on bone marrow aspiration of numerous non-malignant macrophages actively phagocytosing haematopoietic elements. Unfortunately, this bone marrow appearance does not occur until very late in the course of disease, by which time treatment may be too late.

Clinically, patients with MAS present with non-remitting high fever, pancytopenia, hepatosplenomegaly, hepatic dysfunction, encephalopathy, coagulation abnormalities and sharply increased levels of ferritin (often >5000 g/L) (Box 15.5).

Box 15.5 **Clinical and laboratory findings in patients with MAS**

- Persistent fever
- Splenomegaly
- Cytopenias (affecting at least two lineages in the peripheral blood)
  o Haemoglobin <90 g/L (in infants <4 weeks: <100 g/L)
  o Platelets <100 × 10⁹/L
  o Neutrophils <1.0 × 10⁹/L
- Falling ESR/CRP (in patient where previously elevated)
- Hypertriglyceridaemia and/or hypofibrinogenaemia
  o Fasting triglycerides ≥3.0 mmol/L
  o Fibrinogen ≤1.5 g/L
- Hemophagocytosis in bone marrow, spleen or lymph nodes; no evidence of malignancy
- Serum ferritin ≥500 µg/L (often >5000)
- Coagulopathy

Treatment

Macrophage activation syndrome is a life -threatening condition with high mortality rates so early recognition of the syndrome and immediate therapeutic intervention are critical. First-line therapy is high-dose corticosteroids (intravenous methylprednisolone pulse therapy 30 mg/kg for three consecutive days with a maximum dose of 1 g). Many patients need further pulse therapy within the following weeks, followed by maintenance oral prednisolone of at least 1 mg/kg/day. Supportive treatment is very important in all cases. After normalization of haematological abnormalities and resolution of coagulopathy, steroids are tapered slowly to avoid relapse of MAS.

However, MAS appears to be corticosteroid resistant in some patients, with deaths reported even among patients treated with massive doses of steroids. In these patients, therapy with additional agents including parenteral ciclosporin A (CsA), intravenous immunoglobulin (IVIG), etoposide (chemotherapeutic agent, but toxicity may limit its use), anakinra (IL-1 receptor antagonist) and tocilizumab (IL-6 receptor monoclonal antibody) should be considered.

Infections

Infections are common, due mainly to chronic immunosuppressive treatment. Therefore, high suspicion for this complication is required and rapid appropriate antibiotic therapy should be instituted.

Secondary amyloidosis

Secondary deposition of the fibrillar protein amyloid A is a rare complication since more aggressive treatment has been used. It is not a specific complication for SoJIA, since it can also be seen in chronic infections and other chronic inflammation. The deposits affect kidneys (including proteinuria and nephrotic syndrome) and digestive tract (causing diarrhoea, malabsorption and hepatomegaly). Amyloidosis can be preceded with high CRP levels and it is a life-threatening complication, which is resistant to most therapies.

Box 15.6 **ILAR classification of polyarthritis**

Polyarthritis RF-negative
Arthritis affecting more than 5 joints in the first 6 months of disease
RF is negative
Exclusions
a. Psoriasis or a history of psoriasis in the patient or first-degree relative
b. Arthritis in HLA-B27 positive boy beginning after the 6th birthday
c. Ankylosing spondylitis, enthesitis-related arthritis, sacroiliitis with inflammatory bowel disease, Reiter's syndrome, or acute anterior uveitis, or a history of one of these disorders in first-degree relative
d. Presence of immunoglobulin M RF on at least 2 occasions at least 3 months apart
e. Presence of systemic JIA in the patient

Polyarthritis RF-positive
Arthritis affecting more than 5 joints in the first 6 months of disease
>2 tests for RF at least 3 months apart during the first 6 months of disease are positive
Exclusions
a, b, c, e

Prognosis

The outcome of children with SoJIA has been reported in a number of studies. One-third or more of the patients develop significant disability. Patients with a polycyclic course and especially those with unremitting disease are at particularly high risk of an extremely poor outcome. Death is still an issue, being more frequently seen in patients with systemic arthritis than in other forms of JIA. The cause of death is most commonly a complication such as MAS, infection or secondary amyloidosis. Rare cases of sudden death have been reported, and some of them may be unrecognized MAS.

Polyarticular juvenile idiopathic arthritis

Chronic childhood arthritis affecting more than four joints in the first 6 months of disease is defined as polyarthritis. Polyarthritis accounts for approximately 20% of JIA patients; of these patients, 85% have negative RF (Box 15.6).

Rheumatoid factor-negative polyarthritis

Rheumatoid factor-negative polyarticular JIA can begin at any age before 16 years. The age of onset displays a biphasic trend with a peak at ages 1–3 years and another in later childhood and adolescence. Girls are affected four times more frequently than boys. Younger patients are more likely to be ANA positive with a greater risk of uveitis and poorer outcome.

Clinical features

The onset of RF-negative polyarthritis may be acute or insidious. Systemic features are absent by definition. Arthritis may be symmetrical or asymmetrical and both large and small joints may be affected. Knees, ankles, wrists, elbows, shoulders, cervical spine, the small joints of the hands and feet, and the temporomandibular joints may all be progressively affected (Box 15.7). Involvement of the hips is not common at the early stage of the disease but can occur later in patients with persistent disease. Tenosynovitis is common. Subcutaneous nodules are much rarer than in RF-positive polyarthritis. Chronic anterior uveitis is present in 5–20% of patients, and is strongly associated with early age at onset, female sex and ANA positivity.

Prognosis

The outcome of RF-negative polyarthritis is variable. Joint deformities do not differ compared to the other types of JIA. These may include:

- growth disturbances
- subluxation
- joint space narrowing and osseous erosion
- bone ankylosis.

Symmetrical arthritis and hand involvement appear to predict future disability and poorer overall well-being. Several studies have shown that the overall prognosis in RF-negative polyarthritis is worse than in oligoarthritis but better than in RF-positive polyarthritis.

Rheumatoid factor-positive polyarthritis

Rheumatoid factor-positive polyarthritis is the smallest category of JIA, making up to 5% of cases. It is most common in teenage girls with ratios between 5.7 and 12.8:1 (F:M). The incidence rate also varies with ethnicity and it is more common in non-Caucasian populations. RF-positive polyarthritis is associated with poor prognosis and may be considered the youngest end of the distribution of rheumatoid arthritis (RA). RF-positive polyarthritis has a mean age of onset around 9–12 years. It is strongly associated with HLA-DR4.

Clinical features

Rheumatoid factor-positive polyarthritis is characterized by symmetrical polyarthritis affecting large and small joints and often associated with rheumatoid nodules. Arthritis is typically aggressive,

with wrists, MCP and PIP joints usually affected early, with significant functional impact. Hip involvement is also critical, leading often to the need for early hip replacement.

Fatigue and weight loss may occur in active disease. Fever is rare and rash does not occur. Uveitis is present in up to 4.5% of patients.

The most common extra-articular signs in patients with RF-positive polyarthritis are rheumatoid nodules. In one series, 30% of patients had rheumatoid nodules in the first year of the disease. Rheumatoid nodules often occur distal to the olecranon, on flexor tendon sheaths, Achilles tendon and the soles of the feet. They are firm, mobile and usually non-tender and are poor prognostic factors.

Rheumatoid vasculitis and Felty's syndrome (persistent neutropenia, splenomegaly, frequent infections) have been reported rarely in adolescents with RF-positive polyarthritis.

Low-grade pericardial or pleural effusions are rarely reported. Asymptomatic and low-grade impaired lung function can be associated with active disease, but progressive fibrosis and methotrexate-related lung fibrosis have not been reported in children.

Prognosis

Rheumatoid factor-positive polyarthritis has a poor long-term prognosis compared to other categories of JIA. Female sex, polyarticular disease, ongoing disease activity and a positive IgM RF are all identified as poor prognostic indicators. Arthritis persisting for 7 or more years is unlikely to go into remission.

Psoriatic arthritis

Juvenile psoriatic arthritis (JPsA), as classified by the ILAR criteria, is arthritis with onset before the 16th birthday, lasting for at least 6 weeks, and associated with either psoriasis or with two of nail pitting, onycholysis or psoriasis in a first-degree relative. This definition resembles that defined by the older Vancouver criteria (Table 15.5). Using the ILAR criteria, children with psoriatic arthritis represent approximately 7% of patients with JIA. Series employing the more inclusive Vancouver criteria find that JPsA represents 8–20% of JIA. In the paediatric population, the first peak of onset, mainly in girls, occurs during preschool years, and the second is seen during middle to late childhood. JPsA is very uncommon before the age of 1 year. Due to the female preponderance of early-onset JPsA, girls account for 60% of patients in larger series.

Pathogenesis

The pathogenesis of psoriatic arthritis is unclear. Genetic factors or an environmental trigger such as infection or trauma appears to unleash an inflammatory process involving infiltration of lymphocytes, neutrophils and other effectors of innate immunity into entheses and synovium. The target of this immune response remains unknown.

Clinical features

Juvenile psoriatic arthritis is clinically heterogeneous. Younger patients who develop the disease before 5 years of age are more commonly female, ANA positive and affected by dactylitis, the

Table 15.5 Vancouver and ILAR criteria for juvenile psoriatic arthritis

	Vancouver	ILAR (Edmonton revision)
Inclusion	Arthritis plus psoriasis or arthritis plus at least two of the following: Dactylitis Nail pits FHx of psoriasis in a 1st- or 2nd degree-relative Psoriasis-like rash	Arthritis plus psoriasis or arthritis plus at least two of the following: Dactylitis Nail pits or onycholysis FHx of psoriasis in 1st-degree relative
Exclusion	None	1. Arthritis in an HLA-B27-positive male onset >6y 2. AS, ERA, sacroiliitis with IBD, reactive arthritis, or acute anterior uveitis, FHx of one of these disorders in a 1st-degree relative 3. Presence of IgM RF on at least 2 occasions 4. The presence of systemic JIA in a patient 5. Arthritis fulfilling ≥2 JIA categories

AS, ankylosing spondylitis; FHx, family history; ERA, enthesitis-related arthritis; IBD, inflammatory bowel disease; RF, rheumatoid factor.

sausage-like swelling of individual digits. This subgroup bears marked clinical and demographic similarity to early-onset oligoarticular JIA. However, clinical differences include the tendency to develop dactylitis, to involve the wrists and small joints of the hands and feet, and to progress to polyarticular disease in the absence of effective treatment.

By contrast, older children exhibit a gender ratio of 1:1, with a tendency to enthesitis and axial disease, more closely related to adult psoriatic arthritis.

Arthritis in JPsA begins as oligoarthritis in approximately 60–80% of children. Polyarticular onset is observed in 20–40% of cases. Joints affected in JPsA are often asymmetrical. The knee are affected more frequently, followed by the ankle and hip.

Axial arthritis in JPsA differs from most forms of JIA. JPsA is accompanied by an appreciable incidence of sacroiliitis, affecting 10–30% of patients in some series. Inflammatory disease of the lumbar spine occurs in less than 5% of children with JPsA. Axial disease in JPsA is generally milder than in ankylosing spondylitis, with a tendency for asymmetrical sacroiliac joint involvement and failure to progress to spinal ankylosis.

Enthesitis is defined as the inflammation localized to the insertion of a tendon, ligament, fascia or joint capsule into the bone. It is diagnosed clinically with specific tenderness and occasionally swelling at the specific sites, in the absence of other (i.e. traumatic) explanation. Suspected enthesitis can be confirmed by ultrasound or MRI. Using the ILAR criteria, most children with arthritis and enthesitis are classified as enthesitis-related arthritis (ERA), although patients with enthesitis may still diagnosed with JPsA if they fulfil the appropriate criteria.

Skin psoriasis occurs in 40–60% of patients with JPsA. It most commonly presents as the classic vulgaris form, although guttate psoriasis is also observed. Psoriasis in children tends to be subtle, with thin, soft plaques that may come and go. Lesions may be isolated to the hairline, umbilicus, behind the ears or in the intergluteal crease, and thereby escape ready notice.

Nail changes (pits, onycholysis, horizontal ridging and discolouration) accompany childhood psoriasis in up to 30% of cases. By contrast, the prevalence of nail changes in JPsA is approximately 50–80% of all cases.

Chronic uveitis occurs in 10–15% of patients with JPsA. As in other groups, younger age and ANA positivity are associated with highest risk. Acute anterior uveitis can occur in older children and is associated with the prevalence of HLA-B27.

Constitutional symptoms including anorexia, anaemia and poor growth may affect children with significant polyarticular JPsA. Fever can rarely occur in very severe cases but should not be ascribed to JPsA without a careful search for alternative causes.

Laboratory examination

Inflammation markers including ESR and CRP may be mildly elevated, but are frequently normal. Platelets have been noted to be elevated in younger patients. ANA is positive in 60% of younger patients and 30% of older patients. RF is typically negative.

Prognosis

The long-term prognosis in children with JPsA is incompletely defined. Patients followed for at least 15 years demonstrate worse outcome than patients with oligoarticular or polyarticular JIA, and 33% still required DMARD therapy. Another study which followed patients with JPsA for at least 5 years demonstrated active disease in 70%. More recent studies documented remission in approximately 60%, although only a minority achieve remission off medications.

Enthesitis-related arthritis

Enthesitis-related arthritis (ERA) is defined according to the ILAR classification as arthritis affecting joints and entheses of the lower extremities and can eventually affect sacroiliac (SI) joints or the spine (Box 15.8). It is characterized by the absence of RF and by a strong association with HLA-B27. In many instances, the disease evolves to closely resemble ankylosing spondylitis (AS), although spine and SI joint involvement at disease onset is seldom present in childhood and adolescence. The progression to AS is unpredictable but an early identification of individuals with axial disease is important so appropriate treatment can be initiated.

Epidemiology and pathogenesis

Among children with JIA, the proportion with ERA ranges from 8.6% to 18.9%. The mean age of disease onset is usually in late childhood and adolescence. There is a predominance of boys (7:1 to 9:1).

The aetiology of ERA is unknown. Clinical, genetic and epidemiological similarities suggest that infections may play a triggering role (e.g. enteric or genitourinary tract infections). No organisms have been isolated, however, from the joints of patients. Evidence of local inflammatory response to antigens is supported by some antibodies and cellular immune studies, but there is a lack of confirmation of these findings. While understanding of the role of infection is limited, the importance of the histocompatibility antigen HLA-B27 is clear.

Clinical features

The onset of ERA may be insidious or abrupt, and is characterized by intermittent musculoskeletal pain and stiffness or objective inflammation of peripheral joints. Symptoms suggestive of sacroiliac or lumbosacral inflammation are sometimes present at onset, but most commonly develop during the disease course.

Enthesitis

The most important clinical characteristic is the presence of enthesitis. Although this strongly suggests ERA, it must be noted that enthesitis occurs in other disorders, such as other types of JIA, other rheumatic diseases and occasionally in children without disease. Osgood–Schlatter disease should be excluded. Enthesitis is diagnosed clinically from the presence of marked localized tenderness or swelling at the entheseal insertion into the bone. Observation of stance and gait (including walking on the toes and heels) may reveal altered weight bearing as the child avoids pressure on inflamed entheses.

Arthritis

Arthritis most commonly affects the joints of the lower extremities, including the hips. The disease may be oligoarticular or polyarticular, symmetrical or asymmetrical. Large or small joints can also be affected. Joints of the upper extremities may be affected, but in the absence of lower extremity involvement, this is uncommon. The least commonly affected joints are the small joints of the hand. Symptoms include morning stiffness and sometimes night pain. The hallmark of the disease is restriction of the range of movement of the lumbosacral spine as determined by Schober's measurement. Tenderness can sometimes be elicited by direct pressure over the sacroiliac joint (Patrick test). Sacroiliac joint involvement may be unilateral initially and progress later to involve both joints.

Uveitis

The uveitis seen in ERA is characterized by an acutely red, painful and photophobic eye. It is usually unilateral and frequently recurrent, often in the other eye.

Systemic features

Systemic features are not common in ERA. Occasionally low-grade fever, fatigue and weight loss may be noted. The presence of gastrointestinal symptoms should raise the suspicion of arthritis related to inflammatory bowel disease. Poor weight gain and slow growth may be the first clues of gastrointestinal involvement.

Investigations (Box 15.9)

The ESR may be elevated. WBC is normal and mild anaemia could be present. ANA and RF are negative. HLA-B27 occurs in about 90% of children with ERA; it also occurs in 8–10% of the healthy north European Caucasian population. The presence of HLA-B27 *does not* indicate the presence of the disease.

Prognosis

In childhood, the prognosis is quite good. Poor prognostic factors include a family history of AS, high numbers of affected joints and failure to achieve remission in the first 6 months of disease onset. Long-term observation of patients with ERA is essential.

Undifferentiated arthritis

Undifferentiated arthritis accounts for 2–56% of patients in different studies, reflecting the insufficient criteria or overlapping criteria leading to an accurate diagnosis. The clinical manifestation of the disease may follow the clinical pattern of the other forms of JIA but at the same time do not fulfil all the criteria for the diagnosis or meet the exclusion criteria for this type.

Treatment of juvenile idiopathic arthritis

Juvenile idiopathic arthritis is a complex chronic disease and therefore should be managed by an experienced multidisciplinary team, including a rheumatology consultant, specialist nurse, paediatric physiotherapist, occupational therapist, ophthalmologist, pain specialist, orthopaedic surgeon, immunologist, endocrinologist, radiologist, pharmacist, psychology service and social worker to achieve the best possible outcome. Each member of the team contributes to the holistic management of the patient and family.

The Paediatric Gait, Arms, Legs, Spine screen (pGALS) is an excellent tool for the quick evaluation of a child with evidence of musculoskeletal disease.

The treatment approach is to achieve early diagnosis and rapid control of inflammation, minimize the side effects of treatment, and decrease the physical and emotional sequelae.

Lack of knowledge about aetiology and pathogenesis, and the variability of disease are limitations. However, recognition of the central role of cytokines has led to the development of biologic drugs, which have demonstrated positive outcomes in children with JIA resistant to conventional therapies. There is general agreement that there are fewer children with severely damaged joints and deformities than even a decade ago.

Furthermore, it is important that the child is involved as much as possible in the therapeutic decision making, especially adolescents, leading to better engagement with the disease and treatment. Issues like alcohol, drug use and pregnancy risk are more likely to be managed effectively if the adolescent is fully involved.

Non-steroidal anti-inflammatory drugs

Non-steroidal anti-inflammatory drugs continue to be the most commonly used class of medicine in JIA. NSAIDs block prostaglandin formation via inhibition of cyclo-oxygenase-1 and cyclo-oxygenase-2, leading to both analgesic and anti-inflammatory properties. NSAIDs as monotherapy are indicated by the ACR recommendations for up to 2 months, depending on disease activity. In addition, NSAIDs are often used in conjunction with disease-modifying antirheumatic drugs (DMARDs) and/or biologic therapy.

Corticosteroids
Systemic administration

Glucocorticoids represent a potent and rapidly effective therapeutic option for the management of JIA. High-dose 'pulses' of intravenous methylprednisolone (10–30 mg/kg/day) to a maximum 1 g/day on 1–3 consecutive days is effective but the effect is often short-lived. Therefore, continuing therapy with oral prednisolone 1–2 mg/kg/day to a maximum of 60 mg/day is frequently necessary. Short courses of low-dose (0.5 mg/kg/day) oral prednisolone may be considered to relieve symptoms while waiting for the therapeutic effect of a recently initiated DMARD. It is well known that steroids have significant side effects, therefore use is restricted to the first 3 months only if possible. Prolonged glucocorticoid therapy may lead to adrenal suppression.

Intra-articular administration

Intra-articular steroid injections (IAI) are widely used in the management of JIA. IAI lead to rapid decrease of joint inflammation, improving joint motion and minimizing the need for systemic steroids. Intra-articular steroids are used more frequently to treat oligoarticular JIA, but also all the other forms of arthritis during the clinical course of the disease.

Triamcinolone hexacetonide is a long-lasting preparation used by rheumatologists for intra-articular administration in JIA. Patients are advised to avoid high-impact physical activity for 24–48 hours after a joint injection. In case of relapse, reinjection may be considered.

Children younger than 8 years or with more than four joints affected should receive IAI under general anaesthesia. Older children can tolerate the procedure using Entonox as analgesia.

The most common side effect of IAI is subcutaneous atrophic skin changes at the site of injection, particularly of small joints, caused by extravasation of the injected medication from the joint space. Subcutaneous atrophy resolves over time for most patients, but persists in some. Therefore, careful injection technique by an experienced clinician must be performed.

Infection of the injected joint is not a common adverse event but patients are warned about this, and IAI will be deferred in a patient with intercurrent infection. Periarticular calcifications may occur in up to 5%.

DMARDs

Methotrexate has historically been second-line therapy for JIA following a course of NSAIDs. However, it may be indicated as first-line therapy for severe polyarticular disease. Methotrexate is an antimetabolite with anti-inflammatory and immunomodulatory properties. It is a folic acid analogue and inhibitor of dihydrofolate reductase that interferes with purine biosynthesis. Methotrexate also inhibits adenosine deaminase, leading to accumulation of adenosine. Usual starting dose is 10–15 mg/m^2/once weekly subcutaneously (SC), orally or intravenously. The SC route gives optimal bioavailability. Nausea, vomiting and anorexia are very common side effects. Transient elevation of liver enzymes is common so liver function monitoring is routinely performed.

Several other DMARDs have been studied in JIA patients, including sulfasalazine, hydroxychloroquine, penicillamine, azathioprine, ciclosporin, tacrolimus and thalidomide. The use of these medications is not routine therapy but they may be used in refractory disease or in non-polyarticular JIA in certain circumstances. Sulfasalazine in particular may benefit the enthesitis-related subtype of JIA.

Some of the similarities and differences in the specific management of the different subtypes are illustrated in Table 15.6 but this should only be regarded as a guide.

Biologic drugs

Biologic drugs are now widely used to treat JIA. Please see Table 15.7.

Table 15.6 Specific management of subtypes of JIA

	Systemic onset JIA	Oligoarthritis / Psoriatic arthritis	Polyarthritis	Established polyarthritis/ oligoarthritis	Enthesitis-related arthritis
Early/mild disease	Medium-dose CS	Intra-articular steroids NSAIDs	MTX Steroids (IACS or systemic)		NSAIDs IVMP/ high-dose CS followed by 2–4 weeks of low dose
Established/ severe disease	Pulsed IVMP* MTX Consider ciclosporin and biologics (anakinra)	See next column		MTX (ensure maximum dose, SC route) May need to add etanercept ± CS+IACS	Disease >2–4 months duration Sulfasalazine (may work better than other DMARDs) MTX / anti-TNF
Remission	Wean CS slowly Reduce other treatment with extreme caution – high risk of relapse	Ongoing monitoring	Wean CS first DMARDs continue longer then consider reduction or discontinuation	Continue treatment for several months Wean and discontinue steroids first Wait 1 year before weaning off DMARDs – off MTX last	Continue sulfasalazine 6 months–1 year
Relapse	Repeat high-dose CS Consider other biologic agents	If previous IACS effect >4 months, repeat injection If lasted <4 months, consider DMARD	Reintroduce all drugs on which remission was achieved	Reintroduce all drugs that induced remission Often requires step-up in treatment	Generally episodic course Short course of NSAIDs and sulfasalazine sufficient to obtain remission
Persistent disease	IL-6 and IL-1ra directed treatments		IAC targeted joints	Consider alternative biologic agent In severe cases consider BMT	

*If macrophage activation syndrome develops.
BMT, bone marrow transplant; CS, corticosteroid; DMARD, disease-modifying antirheumatic drug; IAC, intra-articular corticosteroid; MTX, methotrexate; NSAID, non-steroidal anti-inflammatory drug.
Source: Foster and Brogan (2018).

Table 15.7 Current use of biologics in juvenile idiopathic arthritis

Biologic agent	Mode of action	Administration	Commonly used doses	Indications
Abatacept	Humanized selective T-cell co-stimulatory modulator	IV infusion	10 mg/g at 0, 2, 4 wk then 4 weekly afterwards	Poly-JIA (exclude ERA and PsA), JIA-associated uveitis
Adalimumab	Humanized soluble anti-TNF monoclonal antibody	SC	24 mg/m^2 up to 40 mg fortnightly	Poly-JIA JIA-associated uveitis
Anakinra	Humanized anti-IL-1 receptor antagonist	SC	1–2 mg/kg daily (max. 100 mg)	SJIA
Canakinumab	Human anti-IL-1β monoclonal antibody	SC	2–4 mg/kg up to 150 mg 4 weekly	SJIA
Etanercept	Soluble TNF p75 receptor fusion protein	SC	0.4 mg/kg twice weekly up to 0.8 mg/kg in refractory disease (max. 25 mg twice weekly)	Poly-JIA Reduced efficacy in SJIA ERA, PsA
Infliximab	Chimeric human murine anti-TNF monoclonal antibody	IV infusion	6 mg/kg 0, 2, 6 weeks then interval 4–6 weekly depending on clinical response	Refractory poly-JIA JIA-associated uveitis ERA PsA
Rituximab	Anti-CD20 antibody (B-cell depleter)	IV infusion	750 mg/m^2 (max. 1 g) Day 0 and day 14	SJIA Refractory poly-JIA
Tocilizumab	Humanized anti-IL-6 receptor monoclonal antibody	IV infusion	>30 kg: 8 mg/kg <30 kg: 12 mg/kg fortnightly	SJIA

ERA, enthesitis-related arthritis; IV, intravenous; JIA, juvenile idiopathic arthritis; PSA, psoriatic arthritis; SC, subcutaneous; SJIA, systemic JIA.
Source: Foster and Brogan (2018).

References

Cassidy JT, Levinson JE, Bass JC *et al*. A study of classification criteria for diagnosis of juvenile idiopathic arthritis. *Arthritis and Rheumatism* 1986; **29**(2): 274–281.

Further reading

Al-Matar MJ, Petty RE, Tucker LB *et al*. The early pattern of joint involvement predicts disease progression in children with oligoarticular (pauciarticular) juvenile rheumatoid arthritis. *Arthritis and Rheumatism* 2002; **46**: 2708–15.

Arib N, Hyrich K, Thornton J *et al*. Association between duration of symptoms and severity of disease at first presentation to paediatric rheumatology: results from the Childhood Arthritis Prospective Study. *Rheumatology* 2008; **47**(7): 991–995.

European League Against Rheumatism. *EULAR Bulletin No 4: Nomenclature and Classification of Arthritis in Children*. EULAR, Basel, 1977.

Foster H, Brogan PA. NICE guidance on biologic therapies for JIA in the UK. In: *Paediatric Rheumatology*. Oxford University Press, Oxford, 2012, pp. 393–399.

Foster H, Brogan PA. *Paediatric Rheumatology*, 2nd edn. Oxford Specialist Handbooks in Paediatrics. Oxford University Press, Oxford, 2018.

Hinks A, Cobb J, Marion MC *et al*. Dense genotyping of immunerelated disease regions identifies 14 new susceptibility loci fot Juvenile idiopathic arthritis. *Nature Genetics* 2013; **45**(6): 664–669.

Martin A. JIA in 2011: new takes on categorisation and treatment. *Nature Reviews Rheumatology* 2012; **8**(2): 67–68.

Nigrovic PA, Sundel RP. Juvenile psoriatic arthritis. In: Petty R, Laxer R, Lindsley C, Wedderburn L (eds), *Textbook of Pediatric Rheumatology*, 7th edn. Elsevier, Philadelphia, 2016, pp. 256–267.

Oberle EJ, Harris JG, Verbsky JW. Polyarticular juvenile idiopathic arthritis–epidemiology and management approaches. *Clinical Epidemiology* 2014; **6**: 379–393

Ostrov BE. Systemic onset juvenile rheumatoid arthritis and adult onset Still's disease: comparison of clinical presentation at a single university centre. *Arthritis and Rheumatism* 2002; **46**: S326.

Petty RE, Southwood TR, Manners P *et al*. International League of Associations for Rheumatology classification of juvenile idiopathic arthritis: second revision, Edmonton, 2001. *Journal of Rheumatology* 2004; **31**(2): 390–392.

Prakken B, Albani S, Martini A. Juvenile idiopathic arthritis. *Lancet* 2011; **377**: 2138–2149.

Ravelli A, Grom AA, Behrens EM *et al*. Macrophage activation syndrome as part of systemic juvenile idiopathic arthritis: diagnosis, genetics, pathophysiology and treatment. *Genes and Immunity* 2012; **13**: 289–298.

Sabri K, Sauernmann RK, Silverman ED *et al*. Course, complications and outcome of juvenile idiopathic arthritis-related uveitis. *Journal of the American Association for Pediatric Ophthalmology and Strabismus* 2008; **12**: 539–545.

Schiappapietra B, Varnier G, Rosina S. Glucocorticoids in juvenile idiopathic arthritis. *Neuroimmunomodulation* 2015; **22**: 112–118.

Sen ES, Ramanan AV. New age of biological therapies in paediatric rheumatology. *Archives of Disease in Childhood* 2014; **99**: 679–685.

Webb K, Wedderburn LR. Advances in the treatment of polyarticular juvenile idiopathic arthritis. *Current Opinion in Rheumatology* 2015; **27**: 505–510.

Wells JM, Smith JR. Uveitis in juvenile arthritis: recent therapeutic advances. *Ophthalmic Research* 2015; **54**: 124–127.

CHAPTER 16

Musculoskeletal Disorders in Children and Adolescents

Helen Foster[1] and Lori Tucker[2]

[1] Newcastle University; Great North Children's Hospital; Newcastle upon Tyne Hospitals NHS Foundation Trust, Newcastle upon Tyne, UK
[2] British Columbia's Children's Hospital, Vancouver, Canada

OVERVIEW

- Musculoskeletal complaints in children are common, often benign and self-limiting, but can be presenting features of significant, severe and potentially life-threatening conditions.

- Making a diagnosis rests on competent clinical skills, knowledge of normal variants, knowledge of common clinical scenarios, 'red flags' to suggest severe conditions and judicious use and interpretation of investigations.

- Common clinical scenarios include the limping child, 'growing pains', back pain and knee pain.

- Knowledge of 'red flags' to suggest infection, malignancy, multisystem disease and inflammatory joint disorders is important.

- The management of musculoskeletal conditions involves a multidisciplinary approach.

- Many chronic conditions that begin in childhood continue into adult life, and the process of transitional care to adult services starts in early adolescence.

Musculoskeletal (MSK) presentations in childhood are common, with a spectrum of causes (Box 16.1), the majority of which are benign and self-limiting. It must be remembered, however, that severe, potentially life-threatening conditions such as malignancy, sepsis, vasculitis and non-accidental injury may also present with MSK complaints. Furthermore, MSK features are common in association with chronic conditions other than rheumatic disorders, such as inflammatory bowel disease and cystic fibrosis. Diagnosis relies on competent MSK clinical skills, with the minimum of pGALS as a basic MSK examination (Foster *et al.*, 2006), appropriate knowledge of normal variants (Box 16.2), 'red flags' to raise suspicion of malignancy or sepsis and clinical scenarios at different ages (Box 16.3).

The approach to MSK assessment in children is different to that of adults; as young children may have difficulty in localizing or describing symptoms, the history is often given by the parent/carer, and complaints may be non-specific, such as 'my child is limping'. Clinical assessment usually distinguishes between mechanical and inflammatory problems and an approach to assessment (Table 16.1) incorporates potential diagnoses according to whether pain is localized or diffuse, whether the child is 'well' or not and the presence or absence of 'red flags'. The presence of multisystem features broadens the differential to include connective tissue diseases.

The 'limping child'

This is a common presentation, with a spectrum of age-related causes (Box 16.4), and the site of the problem may be broad (from a foreign body in the sole of the foot to a tumour in the spine). Orthopaedic conditions at the hip are common and often present acutely, with a well (albeit limping) child, with possible diagnoses including slipped upper femoral epiphysis (usually the older, often overweight, child) and Perthes' disease (Figure 16.2) (which may follow a transient synovitis or 'irritable hip' in the younger child). The hip joint is unusual as a monoarthritis in juvenile idiopathic arthritis (JIA), and in isolation, sepsis (including mycobacterial infection) needs to be considered. The concept of referred pain from the hip or thigh, for example, must be sought in situations where the child has knee pain but there is no evidence of localized disease at the knee.

Back pain

Back pain is a common complaint, and is frequently mechanical with contributory factors such as poor posture, physical inactivity, overweight or abnormal loading (such as carrying heavy school bags on one shoulder). Certain sporting activities such as cricket, bowling or gymnastics pose increased risk of back pain, with possible consequences such as spondylolysis and spondylolisthesis. 'Red flags' for referral for a child with back pain include a painful scoliosis, neurological symptoms suggestive of

ABC of Rheumatology, Fifth Edition. Edited by Ade Adebajo and Lisa Dunkley.

Box 16.1 **Differential diagnosis of musculoskeletal pain**

Life-threatening conditions
- Malignancy (leukaemia, lymphoma, bone tumour)
- Sepsis (septic arthritis, osteomyelitis)
- Non-accidental injury

Joint pain with no swelling
- Hypermobility syndromes
- Idiopathic pain syndromes (reflex sympathetic dystrophy, fibromyalgia)
- Orthopaedic syndromes (e.g. Osgood–Schlatter disease, Perthes' disease)
- Metabolic (e.g. hypothyroidism, lysosomal storage diseases)

Joint pain with swelling
- Trauma
- Infection
  - Septic arthritis and osteomyelitis (viral, bacterial, mycobacterial)
  - Reactive arthritis (postenteric, sexually acquired)
  - Infection related (rheumatic fever, postvaccination)
- Juvenile idiopathic arthritis
- Arthritis related to inflammatory bowel disease
- Connective tissue diseases (SLE, scleroderma, dermatomyositis, vasculitis)
- Sarcoidosis
- Metabolic (e.g. osteomalacia, cystic fibrosis)
- Haematological (e.g. haemophilia, haemoglobinopathy)
- Tumour (benign and malignant)
- Chromosomal (e.g. Down's-related arthritis)
- Autoinflammatory syndromes, e.g. CINCA (Figure 16.1), periodic syndromes, CRMO)
- Developmental/congenital (e.g. spondyloepiphyseal dysplasia)

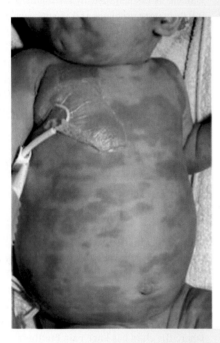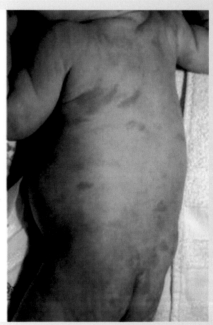

Figure 16.1 Chronic infantile neurological cutaneous arthritis (CINCA) syndrome: widespread rash

Box 16.2 **Normal variants in gait patterns and stance**

- Intoeing can be due to:
  - Hip: persistent femoral anteversion, commonly between ages of 3 and 8 years
  - Lower leg (internal tibial torsion): commonly from onset of walking to 3 years
  - Feet: metatarsus adductus – most resolve by the age of 6 years
- Bow legs (varus): birth to early toddler: most resolve by 3 years
- Knock knees (valgus): most resolve by age of 7 years
- Flat feet: most resolve by 6 years, and normal arches are evident on tiptoeing
- Crooked toes: most resolve with weight bearing

Indicators to cause concern
- Persistent changes that fail to resolve by the expected age
- Progressive changes
- Lack of symmetry
- Associated pain or functional disability
- Systemic upset
- Dysmorphic features/short stature

nerve root entrapment or cord compression and systemic findings to suggest malignancy or sepsis. Isolated back pain in a child under the age of 5 years is very unusual, and should warrant a referral for investigation. Inflammatory back pain may be a feature of enthesitis-related arthritis (a subtype of JIA), often presenting in late adolescence and with a strong association with expression of HLA-B27; however, it is important to note that few children or adolescents with JIA present solely with back pain as a presentation.

Mechanical pain

Osteochondritis of the knee (Osgood–Schlatter disease) is common, especially in adolescent boys who are physically active (particularly those who play football or basketball). Sever's disease (osteochondritis of the calcaneum) may present with a painful heel, and is also common in adolescent boys who play football or other running sports. Flat feet (Figure 16.3) are common, and standing on tiptoe should create a normal medial longitudinal arch; inability to do so or painful fixed flat feet warrant further investigation to exclude tarsal coalition. High fixed arches, or pes cavus, may suggest neurological disease.

Non-specific mechanical MSK pain in children is often labelled as 'growing pains'. Making a diagnosis of 'growing pains' requires careful assessment, and Box 16.5 suggests when alternative diagnoses need to be sought. Many children and adolescents with non-specific aches and pains, including growing pains, are found to have joint hypermobility, which is suggested by symmetrical hyperextension at the fingers, elbows and knees (genu recurvatum), and flat pronated feet. It is important, however, to consider and exclude 'non-benign' causes of hypermobility (e.g. Marfan's, Stickler's and Ehlers–Danlos syndromes), which are rare but important, as these children are at risk of retinal and cardiac complications.

Non-specific aches and pains are also a feature of idiopathic pain syndromes, which are mostly seen in older female children/adolescents; such patients are often markedly debilitated by their pain and fatigue – the pain can be incapacitating – but the child/adolescent is otherwise well, and physical examination is usually normal. Localized idiopathic pain syndromes most commonly affect the foot or hand, may be triggered by trauma (often mild) and are likened to reflex sympathetic dystrophy.

Box 16.4 **Common/significant causes of limping according to age**

Toddler/preschool
Infection (septic arthritis, osteomyelitis – hip, spine)
Mechanical (trauma and non-accidental injury)
Congenital/developmental problems (e.g. hip dysplasia, talipes)
Neurological disease (e.g. cerebral palsy, hereditary syndromes)
Inflammatory arthritis (JIA)
Malignant disease (e.g. leukaemia, neuroblastoma)

5–10 years
Mechanical (trauma, overuse injuries, sport injuries)
Reactive arthritis/transient synovitis – 'irritable hip'
Perthes' disease
Inflammatory arthritis (JIA)
Tarsal coalition
Idiopathic pain syndromes
Malignant disease

10–17 years
Mechanical (trauma, overuse injuries, sports injuries)
Slipped capital femoral epiphysis
Inflammatory arthritis (JIA)
Sever's disease (osteochondritis of the calcaneum)
Idiopathic pain syndromes
Osteochondritis dissecans
Tarsal coalition
Malignant disease (leukaemia, lymphoma, primary bone tumour)

Source: Reproduced by kind permission of Arthritis Research UK (www.arthritisresearchuk.org)

Box 16.3 **'Red flags' to warrant concern in children presenting with musculoskeletal symptoms**

- Systemic upset (fever, malaise, anorexia, weight loss or raised inflammatory markers)
- Bone pain and/or night pain
- Regression of achieved motor milestones
- Functional disability

Table 16.1 A strategy for characterizing musculoskeletal pain in children

Localized pain		Diffuse pain	
'Well' child	**'Unwell'** child	**'Well' child**	**'Unwell' child**
Strains and sprains	Septic arthritis	Hypermobility	Leukaemia
Bone tumours	Osteomyelitis	Diffuse idiopathic pain syndromes	Neuroblastoma
JIA (oligoarticular subtype)			JIA (systemic and polyarticular onset subtypes)
Localized idiopathic pain syndromes			SLE
'Growing pains'			Juvenile dermatomyositis
			Vasculitis

**Associated with one or more 'red flags', such as fever, anorexia, weight loss, malaise and raised inflammatory markers.
JIA, juvenile idiopathic arthritis; SLE, systemic lupus erythematosus.
Source: Adapted from Malleson and Beauchamp (2001).

Neoplasia

It is important to differentiate joint pain from bone pain. Bone pain is a 'red flag' and is a common feature of leukaemia, metastatic neuroblastoma and primary bone tumours (Figure 16.4). It is important to note that these malignancies may also present with frank arthritis. Osteoid osteomas (the most common benign bone tumour) are usually located in the femoral neck or posterior elements of the spine, and typically cause night pain that can be relieved by salicylates.

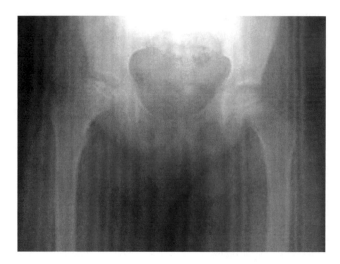

Figure 16.2 Perthes' disease, showing avascular necrosis of the right hip

Arthritis and infection

Children with septic arthritis are usually febrile, appear unwell and have severe pain with joint movement. Septic arthritis usually occurs in large joints, generally involving a single joint. Reactive arthritis is usually monoarticular or oligoarticular and follows bacterial infection in the gut (*Salmonella*, *Shigella*, *Campylobacter*, *Yersinia*), although in the older child and adolescent it is important to consider sexually acquired infection (*Chlamydia*, *Gonorrhoea*). Rheumatic fever (a form of reactive arthritis that follows pharyngeal streptococcal infection) is uncommon in the UK, but common in developing countries. Lyme disease following tick-transmitted infection with *Borrelia burgdorferi* is suggested by the presence of an oligoarthritis, history of a tick bite, erythema chronicum migrans, and a travel history to an endemic area.

Box 16.5 **The 'rules' of growing pains**

- Pains are not present at the start of the day after waking
- The child does not limp
- Physical activities are not limited by symptoms
- Pains are symmetrical in the lower limbs
- Pain is most frequent at night, or even waking from sleep
- Physical examination is normal (albeit evidence of joint hypermobility is common)
- The child is systemically well
- Gross motor milestones are normal
- Age range 3–11 years

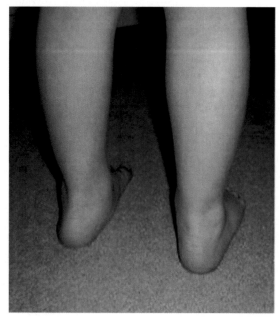
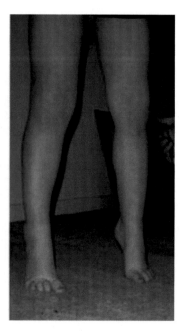

Figure 16.3 Normal variant: mobile flat feet are common

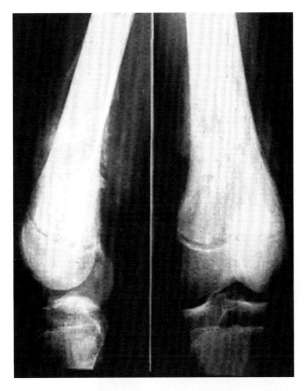

Figure 16.4 Periosteal elevation: soft tissue calcification in a malignant tumour of the distal femur

Mycobacterial disease must be considered in the context of the unwell child with joint pain or swelling and especially in the context of immunosuppression (through disease or treatment).

Chronic arthritis (JIA)

In the absence of sepsis or trauma, JIA is the most likely cause of a single swollen joint in a child and is covered in more detail in Chapter 15.

Connective tissue diseases

Systemic lupus erythematosus

Systemic lupus erythematosus (SLE) may be confused with chronic arthritis, because some patients present with arthritis as the primary clinical finding. SLE is rare but is more common in non-white individuals, with a predominance of girls affected in the adolescent group and a more equal sex distribution in young children.

The arthritis of SLE is usually polyarticular, and characterized by pain but often few inflammatory signs. In general, the arthritis of SLE is non-deforming and non-erosive. Extra-articular features are variable, and a diagnosis of SLE is made with a combination of clinical and laboratory features (Box 16.6). It is worth considering drug-induced SLE, which can develop from the use of anticonvulsants, oral contraceptives or minocycline.

The medical management of SLE is complex and requires specialist supervision, with nearly all patients requiring corticosteroid and immunosuppressive medications. In addition, patients often require antihypertensives, anticoagulation (related to antiphospholipid syndrome) and medications to control dyslipidaemias and avoid osteoporosis.

Juvenile dermatomyositis

Juvenile dermatomyositis (JDM) may present at any age, with characteristic skin involvement (Figure 16.5), and proximal muscle weakness which can present acutely or indolently. JDM has a broad range

---

Box 16.6 Systemic lupus erythematosus in children and adolescents

Common presenting symptoms
Malar rash
Arthritis
Fatigue
Fever
Weight loss
Oral ulcers
Alopecia
Pleuritis/pericarditis
Central nervous system findings
Photosensitivity
Raynaud's phenomenon
Lymphadenopathy
Hepatosplenomegaly

Laboratory findings
Anaemia (may be haemolytic with positive red cell autoantibodies)
Leukopenia, lymphopenia
Thrombocytopenia
Elevated liver enzymes
Elevated kidney function tests (blood urea nitrogen, creatinine)
Decreased complement components C3 and C4
Positive antinuclear antibody
High titre-positive antidouble-stranded DNA antibody
Positive autoantibodies to extractable antigens (anti-Ro (SSA); anti-La (SSB); anti-Sm; anti-RNP)
Positive antiphospholipid antibodies (anticardiolipin, lupus anticoagulant)

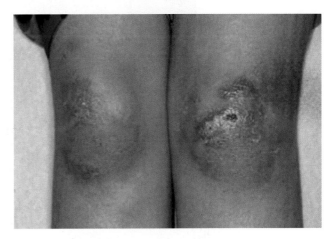

Figure 16.5 Gottron's rash over the knees in juvenile dermatomyositis

of severity and in contrary to adult-onset DM, there is no association with malignancy. Approximately one-third of children with DM may have concomitant arthritis, either early or later in the course of their disease. Severe complications at the time of active disease may include risk of aspiration pneumonia and interstitial lung disease.

Diagnosis usually rests on clinical assessment and elevated serum muscle enzymes; most children do not require electromyography or a muscle biopsy except in the absence of typical disease features. Magnetic resonance imaging of the muscles is very useful to demonstrate muscle involvement and monitor disease activity.

Treatment of JDM requires rapid initiation of high-dose corticosteroids, frequently accompanied by methotrexate, although other medications such as intravenous immunoglobulin, cyclophosphamide or anticytokine agents are used in severe or refractory disease. Physical therapy input is essential to optimize outcome. Patients with JDM may develop calcinosis as a late complication of poorly controlled disease (Figure 16.6).

Sclerodermas

Scleroderma in childhood is rare and heterogeneous, and subtypes are determined by the type and number of lesions, the area of involvement and serological abnormalities. Localized scleroderma (Figure 16.7) is the most common and can present at any age, with

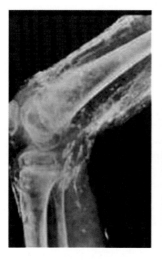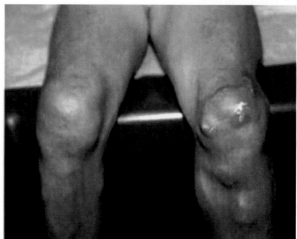

Figure 16.6 Calcinosis in juvenile dermatomyositis

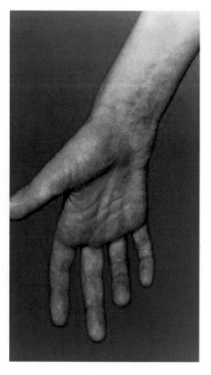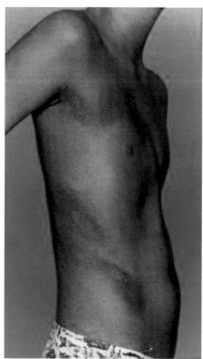

Figure 16.7 Localized scleroderma with morphoea (pigmented) skin lesions and underlying muscle wasting of the right hand

the appearance of a patch of abnormal skin, which when untreated generally follows a course of active expanding disease, fibrosis and eventual softening with some 'remission'. The functional and cosmetic impact can be profound, as the lesions may interfere with growth of a limb and subcutaneous tissues (of the face or a limb). Current practice advocates aggressive treatment regimes (corticosteroid and methotrexate) to control disease and limit severe disfigurement and disability.

Systemic scleroderma is very rare in children and includes progressive diffuse fibrous changes of the skin and fibrous changes involving internal organs – most commonly lungs, gastrointestinal tract, heart and kidneys – with a significant mortality. Systemic scleroderma is slowly progressive, has a guarded prognosis and requires potent immunosuppression, although clinical trials are lacking to guide practice.

Vasculitis

Vasculitis (Figure 16.8) encompasses a heterogeneous group of disorders, most commonly classified by the size of involved blood vessels. A diagnosis may be suggested by multisystem clinical involvement and laboratory features (Box 16.7). The common childhood vasculitides Henoch–Schönlein purpura (HSP) and Kawasaki's disease (KD) (Box 16.8) often include transient arthritis affecting large joints. HSP is characterized by palpable purpura (Figure 16.9) over the legs and buttocks, abdominal pain, haematuria and arthritis. In general, HSP resolves completely within 4 weeks of onset; however, some patients have recurrences of rash and gastrointestinal symptoms, and a small percentage of children who develop renal disease with HSP go on to renal failure.

Kawasaki's disease is an acute systemic vasculitis, predominantly in young children (less than 5 years); it is usually self-limiting but has the potential for causing severe long-term complications due to the involvement of coronary and other blood vessels with aneurysms. Prompt recognition of KD is essential in providing early treatment with intravenous immunoglobulin, which significantly decreases the risk of developing coronary aneurysms.

Box 16.7 **Vasculitides in childhood**

Type according to size of vessel

Large-vessel vasculitis
Takayasu's arteritis (giant cell (temporal) arteritis, rarely seen in adolescents/children)

Medium-vessel vasculitis
Polyarteritis nodosa
Kawasaki's disease

Small-vessel vasculitis
Granulomatosis with Polyangiitis
Eosinophilic Granulomatosis with Polyangiitis
Microscopic polyangiitis
Henoch–Schönlein purpura
Cutaneous leukocytoclastic vasculitis (cryoglobulinaemic vasculitis, rarely seen in adolescents/children)

Features suggesting a vasculitis in adolescents and children

Clinical
Fever, weight loss, persistent fatigue
Skin rash: palpable purpura, vasculitic urticaria, nodules, ulcers
Neurological signs: headache, mononeuritis multiplex, focal CNS lesions
Arthritis or arthralgia, myalgia or myositis
Hypertension
Pulmonary infiltrates or haemorrhage

Laboratory
Increased acute-phase reactants (ESR, CRP)
Anaemia, leukocytosis
Eosinophilia
Antineutrophil cytoplasmic antibodies (ANCA)*
Elevated factor VIII-related antigen (von Willebrand factor)
Haematuria

*ANCA: cytoplasmic (c-ANCA) associates specifically with Wegener's granulomatosis and perinuclear (p-ANCA) associates with microscopic polyangiitis and a variety of other vasculitides.
Source: Reproduced by kind permission of the Arthritis Research Campaign (www. arc.org.UK)

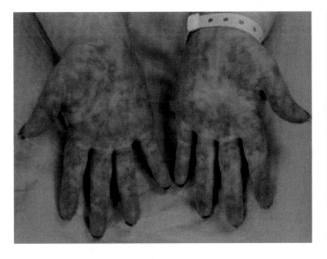
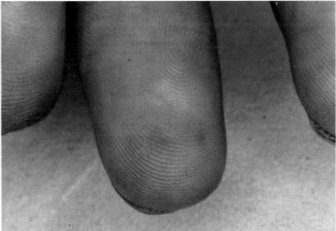

Figure 16.8 Vasculitis of the hands

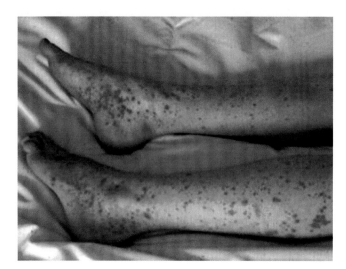

Figure 16.9 Palpable purpura in Henoch–Schönlein purpura

Reproduced by kind permission of Arthritis Research UK (www.arthritisresearchuk.org)

Rare inflammatory syndromes

Inherited autoinflammatory syndromes

These syndromes (Box 16.9) are rare, and children may present with repeated unexplained bouts of fever with a variety of clinical findings associated with the fevers, which may include rash (see Figure 16.1), MSK complaints, abdominal pain and ocular and neu-rological complaints. There is often a broad range of severity among patients with the same genetic disorder, making diagnosis on clini-cal grounds often challenging. New treatment options have become available for some patients with periodic fever syndromes, and patients require specialist supervision.

Chronic recurrent multifocal osteomyelitis (CRMO) is a condi-tion that presents similarly to bacterial osteomyelitis, but no organ-ism can be isolated and there are often multiple involved sites with recurring episodes. Children or adolescents present with bone pain, sometimes accompanied by swelling; the most common affected areas are long bones (tibia), but ribs, clavicle, vertebrae or mandible can be involved. Radiographs show osteolytic changes similar to osteomyelitis, and a bone scan may show lesions that are asymptomatic. Antibiotics are not effective, and many children with CRMO have good symptomatic relief with non-steroidal anti-inflammatory drugs. For those with persistent disease, bisphospho-nates are often effective.

The role of the multidisciplinary team

The paediatric rheumatology multidisciplinary team (MDT) is highly skilled in the provision and co-ordination of comprehensive and often complex management regimes for the child and family, providing education and support, with other specialist services as well as community services, schools and healthcare providers within shared care clinical networks. Many children with rheu-matic diseases have continuing disease activity or relapses in adult-hood, or sequelae from previous disease activity, which require ongoing medical treatment.

Healthcare transition for youths with childhood-onset rheumatic diseases describes the movement of patients from child- and family-centred paediatric care to adult-oriented healthcare systems. The MDT co-ordinates transitional care, addressing generic and disease-specific health issues (Box 16.10), and ultimately transfer to adult rheumatology services. Education and support are paramount, particularly with complex treatment regimes and the impact on adolescent behaviours, such as avoidance of pregnancy and excess alcohol in those taking methotrexate.

References

Foster HE, Kay LJ, Friswell M, Coady DA, Myers A. pGALS – a paediatric musculoskeletal screening examination for school aged children based on the adult GALS screen. *Arthritis Care and Research* 2006; **55**: 709–716.

Malleson PN, Beauchamp P. Diagnosing musculoskeletal pain in children. *Canadian Medical Association Journal* 2001; **165**: 183–188.

Further reading

Compeyrot-Lacassagne S, Feldman B. Inflammatory myopathies in children. *Pediatric Clinics of North America* 2005; **52**: 493–520.

Foster HE and Brogan PA. Handbook of Paediatric Rheumatology. Oxford Specialist Handbook series. Oxford University Press 2012 and second revision in press.

Foster HE, Cabral DA. Is musculoskeletal history and examination so different in paediatrics? *Best Practice and Research: Clinical Rheumatology* 2006; **20**: 241–262.

Foster HE, Jandial S. pGALS – paediatric Gait, Arms, legs and Spine: a simple examination of the musculoskeletal system. *Pediatric Rheumatology* 2013; **11**: 44.

Foster HE, Minden K, Clemente D, Leon L et al. EULAR / PRes Standards and Recommendations for Transitional care in Rheumatology, *Ann Rheum Dis* 2017 Apr **76**(4):639–646.

Klein-Gitelman M, Reiff A, Silverman ED. Systemic lupus erythematosus in childhood. *Rheumatic Disease Clinics of North America* 2002; **28**: 561–577.

McDonagh JE. Transition of care from adult to paediatric rheumatology. *Archives of Disease in Childhood* 2007; **97**: 802–807.

Murray KJ, Laxer RM. Scleroderma in children and adolescents. *Rheumatic Disease Clinics of North America* 2002; **28**: 603–624.

Ozen S. The spectrum of vasculitis in children. *Best Practice and Research: Clinical Rheumatology* 2002; **16**: 411–425.

Paediatric Musculoskeletal Matters – pmm – www.pmmonline.org – a free online resource covering essentials of musculoskeletal medicine, including video demonstrations of pGALS. Produced by Newcastle University, UK. pGALS app available - a free resource with multiple language translations.

Petty RE, Laxer R, Lindsley C, Wedderburn LR. *Textbook of Pediatric Rheumatology*, 7th Edition, Elsevier 2015.

CHAPTER 17

Polymyalgia Rheumatica and Giant Cell Arteritis

Christian D. Mallen[1] and Eric L. Matteson[2]

[1] Institute for Primary Care and Health Sciences, NIHR Research Professor in General Practice, NIHR CLAHRC West Midlands; NIHR School for Primary Care Research Training Lead, Honorary Professor in Rheumatology, University of Birmingham; Keele University, Keele, UK

[2] Division of Rheumatology, Department of Internal Medicine and Department of Health Sciences Research, Mayo Clinic College of Medicine, Rochester, USA

OVERVIEW

- Polymyalgia rheumatica and giant cell arteritis are the most inflammatory rheumatological disorders of older people, causing significant pain and stiffness of the shoulders and hips.
- Giant cell arteritis is the most common form of vasculitis and needs urgent assessment to prevent serious complications, including visual loss.
- Diagnosis of both conditions can be challenging and requires a systematic approach to exclude other potential causes of pathology.
- Treatment with glucocorticoids is successful for most patients but requires careful monitoring of potential adverse events.

Polymyalgia rheumatica (PMR) is characterized by bilateral pain and stiffness of the hips and shoulders, typically associated with elevated inflammatory markers. This highly disabling condition is the most common inflammatory rheumatological disorder of older people. Whilst most patients with PMR are exclusively managed in the community, diagnosis and management can be challenging, especially for those with an atypical presentation and those not responding classically to glucocorticoid treatment.

Giant cell arteritis (GCA) is a systemic vasculitis that frequently co-occurs with PMR. Whilst it may affect any large or medium-sized artery, it has a propensity to affect the branches of the external carotid artery, particularly the posterior ciliary arteries that supply the optic nerve and the superficial temporal artery (hence the use of the alternative name temporal arteritis). Prompt recognition and early treatment are essential to prevent long-term complications, including permanent loss of vision.

There are clinical and pathogenetic links between temporal arteritis, giant cell arteritis and polymyalgia rheumatica, which has led to the concept that they are manifestations of a disease spectrum that affects the same disease population. The two entities may occur in the same patient simultaneously, at different time points or independently. Polymyalgia rheumatica has been observed

in 40–60% of cases of giant cell arteritis, and 30–80% of patients with polymyalgia rheumatica have giant cell arteritis.

Epidemiology

Both PMR and GCA affect similar patient populations. Both conditions are rare below the age of 50 and peak in patients aged over 70 years. Women are affected three times more frequently than men, and whilst it can affect any ethnic group, it is more common in northern Europeans. The age-adjusted incidence rate is around 8.4 per 10 000 person-years for PMR and 2.2 per 10 000 person-years for GCA (Smeeth *et al.*, 2006). The lifetime risk of PMR is higher for women (2.4%) than for men (1.7%), as is the lifetime risk of GCA (1.0% for women and 0.5% for men) (Crowson *et al.*, 2011). Co-occurrence is common, with 3.8% of PMR patients having GCA previously and 8.2% of GCA patients having PMR previously.

Clinical features and diagnosis

Making a diagnosis of PMR can be challenging, especially given the absence of a 'gold standard' diagnostic test. Symptom onset is often rapid and dramatic, with bilateral pain and stiffness in the shoulders and hips causing marked functional impairment. Patients often report problems lifting heavy objects, getting off the toilet or rolling over in bed. Inflammatory markers (erythrocyte sedimentation rate (ESR) and C-reactive protein (CRP)) are usually elevated and patients may complain of systemic features including fatigue, weight loss, flu-like symptoms and depression. Atypical presentation may lead to diagnostic difficulty, and as such early referral for specialist assessment can be helpful in non-classic cases.

A wide range of rheumatological and non-rheumatological disorders mimic PMR (Table 17.1), making a careful clinical assessment essential to improve the accuracy of the diagnosis. The publication of provisional classification criteria, whilst not intended for diagnostic use (Table 17.2), usefully describes the core features of PMR (Dasgupta *et al.*, 2012).

Table 17.1 Differential diagnosis of PMR and GCA

Category	Example
Inflammatory rheumatological disorders	Rheumatoid arthritis Giant cell arteritis Spondyloarthropathy Crystal arthropathy
Non-inflammatory rheumatological disorders	Osteoarthritis Shoulder pathology (e.g. frozen shoulder, rotator cuff disease) Fibromyalgia
Infection	Bacterial endocarditis, osteomyelitis septic arthritis, tuberculosis and other infections
Malignancy	Leukaemia, lymphoma, myeloma Solid tumours (including prostate, renal, lung)
Endocrine	Diabetes Hypo/hyperthyroidism Hypo/hyperparathyroidism
Other disorders	Drug induced (e.g. statins) Motor neurone disease Parkinson's disease

Table 17.2 Provisional EULAR/ACR PMR classification criteria scoring algorithm – required criteria: age ≥50 years, bilateral shoulder aching and abnormal CRP and/or ESR

Criteria	Points without ultrasound (0–6)	Points with ultrasound* (0–8)
Morning stiffness duration >45 minutes	2	2
Hip pain or limited range of movement	1	1
Absence of RF or ACPA	2	2
Absence of other joint involvement	1	1
At least 1 shoulder with subdeltoid bursitis and/or biceps tenosynovitis and/or glenohumeral synovitis (either posterior or axillary) and at least 1 hip with synovitis and/or trochanteric bursitis	n/a	1
Both shoulders with subdeltoid bursitis, biceps tenosynovitis or glenohumeral synovitis	n/a	1

A score of 4 or more is categorized as PMR in the algorithm without ultrasound (US) and a score of 5 or more is categorized as PMR in the algorithm with US. ACPA, anticitrullinated protein antibody; n/a, not applicable; RF, rheumatoid factor.
* Optional ultrasound criteria.

Giant cell arteritis causes inflammation of the aorta and its major branches. Its clinical features are related to the affected arteries. The scalp is tender to the touch, and it can even hurt to wear spectacles. Jaw claudication may occur while chewing. Clinical signs vary according to the duration of the disease. In the early stages, the pulse is full and bounding, and the arteries tender (Figure 17.1). Later, fibrosis and repair may predominate, the artery may have a nodular indurated feel to it and the pulse is almost absent. Diplopia, partial or complete loss of vision and cranial nerve palsy may all occur if the condition remains untreated (Figure 17.2). It is important to consider atypical presentations as only half of patients report a temporal headache and 24% have no headache symptom at all. Systemic features, including polymyalgia symptoms, weight loss, fatigue and fever, may dominate, making diagnosis challenging.

Late complications of large vessel involvement including aortic aneurysm and stenosis may complicate the disease course. Patients should be followed long term for aortic disease with computed tomography and aortic magnetic resonance imaging, complemented by ultrasonography of the aortic root and abdominal

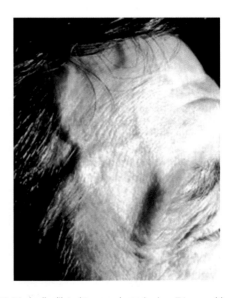

Figure 17.1 Markedly dilated temporal arteries in a 74-year-old man with giant cell arteritis. The arteries are visibly thickened and inflamed; palpation of the vessel is painful. Source: Courtesy of Lester Mertz, MD

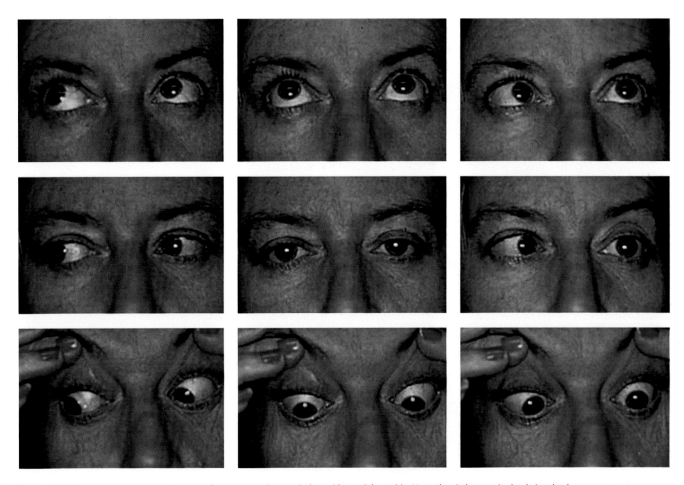

Figure 17.2 Temporary or permanent nerve palsy can occur in association with cranial arteritis. Here, the sixth nerve is clearly involved

aorta by clinical and imaging assessment, as aneurysmal rupture is a cause of premature mortality in these patients. Temporal artery biopsy remains the 'gold standard' diagnostic test (Box 17.1). Histologically, lesions are characterized by a mainly lymphocytic and macrophage infiltrate with the presence of giant and epithelioid cells (Figures 17.3, 17.4). The CD3+ and T-cell population comprises CD4+ or CD8+ subsets, in which CD4+ T-cells predominate.

Making the diagnosis

As highlighted in Table 17.1, making an accurate diagnosis of PMR and GCA can be challenging, even for specialists. Inflammatory markers (ESR/CRP) are elevated in more than 90% of patients and fall with effective treatment (although remember to treat the patient and not the blood test). Normal inflammatory markers do not exclude a diagnosis of PMR or GCA and should warrant prompt referral if the diagnosis is still suspected.

Other investigations (Box 17.2) are needed to exclude other potential diagnoses and commonly include a full blood count, liver function tests, urea and electrolytes, calcium, rheumatoid factor, thyroid function tests, creatine kinase and serum glucose (Dasgupta *et al.*, 2010a). A thorough clinical assessment is needed to exclude potential malignancy.

Box 17.1 **Biopsy for giant cell arteritis**

- Biopsy is most useful just before or within 24 hours of treatment initiation with steroids, but treatment should not be delayed for the sake of obtaining a biopsy
- Skip lesions occur, so a negative result does not exclude giant cell arteritis
- Temporal artery ultrasound may be a useful adjunct for diagnosis
- A positive result may resolve later doubt about diagnosis, particularly if the response to treatment is not rapid and classic
- It may not be possible to biopsy all patients; the decision depends on local resources
- One week after starting steroid treatment, the chance of obtaining positive biopsy falls to 10%, although the biopsy may still reveal evidence of inflammation more than 1 year after initiation of treatment

In a specialist setting, vascular assessment with ultrasound, computed tomography/magnetic resonance imaging or conventional angiography may be required to assess the activity and extent of vascular involvement. Ultrasound and magnetic resonance imaging may reveal a characteristic 'halo' around inflamed vessels, even of the calibre of the temporal arteries. Positron

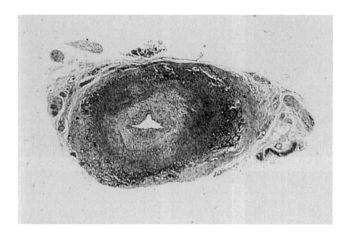

Figure 17.3 Histology of temporal arteritis. The elastic tissue appears black while various types of collagen stain yellow. Remnants of the internal elastic lamina are indicated by an arrow. An inflammatory infiltrate is found in the media and intimal fibrosis. Multinucleated giant cells and macrophages are attacking the elastic tissue and ingesting it. There is extensive intimal proliferation and fibrosis. Luminal narrowing has occurred almost completely. Involvement of other arteries may occur, including the ophthalmic artery, which results in loss of vision

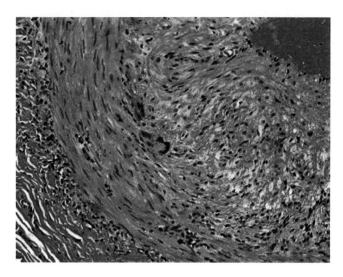

Figure 17.4 Photomicrographs of active arteritis in a temporal artery biopsy. Higher power view showing proliferation of intimal fibroblasts and transmural inflammation with multinucleated giant cells present at the media–intima junction (hematoxylin and eosin, 200×)

Box 17.2 **Investigations for PMR and GCA**

Basic investigations
- Full blood count with differential
- Liver function tests
- Blood glucose
- Acute-phase reactants (erythrocyte sedimentation rate and/or C-reactive protein)
- Urea, creatinine and electrolytes
- Blood lipids
- Thyroid function studies
- Creatine kinase
- Rheumatoid factor

Polymyalgia rheumatica
- Ultrasonography of hip and shoulder (where available and appropriate)

Giant cell arteritis
- Temporal artery biopsy
- Large vessel evaluation with echocardiography, ultrasound, computed tomography, magnetic resonance imaging of the vessel wall, and magnetic resonance or computed tomographic angiography as appropriate to the vessels of interest
- Positron emission tomography

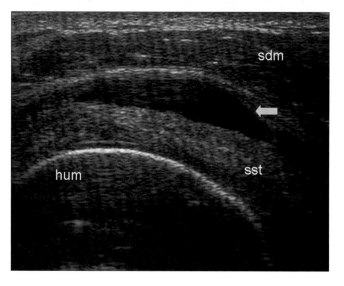

Figure 17.5 Ultrasound examination of a patient with polymyalgia rheumatica and subdeltoid bursitis. Anterior transverse ultrasound image of the right shoulder with maximum internal rotation of the arm. The dark area (arrow) between the subdeltoid muscle (SDM) and supraspinatus tendon (SST) represents subdeltoid bursitis. Source: Courtesy of Wolfgang Schmidt, MD

emission tomography may occasionally be useful in defining disease activity, but is not widely available. Musculoskeletal ultrasound of the hips and shoulders shows promise and has potential to improve the diagnostic accuracy for patients with PMR but it has yet to be widely evaluated outside specialist settings (Figure 17.5).

Treatment of PMR and GCA

The mainstay of treatment for both PMR and GCA is oral glucocorticoids. For patients with PMR, low-dose prednisolone at a starting dose of 15–20 mg per day is effective for around 80–90%, with patients usually reporting a significant improvement in symptoms within 3–5 days of starting treatment. There is limited trial evidence to support clinicians in reducing the dose of oral glucocorticoid and patients need to be counselled that treatment may last 2 years or more, and that they might experience a spike in symptoms as the glucocorticoid dose is reduced. Initially, the dose is reduced by 2.5 mg prednisolone every 2–4 weeks, slowing when 10 mg prednisolone is reached to 1 mg prednisolone reduction monthly (Dasgupta et al., 2010a).

Patients with GCA require a higher starting dose of glucocorticoids, usually in the range of 30–40 mg of prednisolone (60 mg prednisolone if the patient has jaw claudication as the risk of visual impairment is higher). The initial dose is maintained until symptoms have resolved and then reduced by 10 mg prednisolone every 2–4 weeks until the patient reaches 20 mg prednisolone a day, when reduction is slowed to 2.5 mg prednisolone every 2–4 weeks. When the patient reaches 10 mg, prednisolone reduction is slowed to 1 mg every 4–8 weeks (Dasgupta *et al.*, 2010b).

Patients with an incomplete response to glucocorticoids should be referred for specialist assessment. Whilst there is limited evidence from clinical trials to support the use of 'steroid-sparing agents' (usually methotrexate), they may be useful for some patients. There is a lack of trial evidence supporting the use of other drugs (such as leflunomide and tocilizumab) although they may be used by specialists under careful supervision for some patients not responding to usual treatment.

Monitoring PMR and GCA

A key role for clinicians is to regularly monitor patients, assessing the accuracy of the original diagnosis, checking for relapse (which is common) and for potential glucocorticoid complications. In particular, patients with PMR should be educated about and assessed regularly for GCA symptoms. Adverse events, usually related to glucocorticoid treatment, are a major concern to patients and commonly occur in those with PMR and GCA. Side effects include weight gain, bruising, infections, glaucoma, myopathy, osteoporosis, diabetes, hypertension, depression and dyspepsia. Patients should be fully informed about potential side effects and provided with a steroid information card. For patients at high risk of osteoporosis, baseline DEXA scan and prophylaxis with calcium, vitamin D and/or bisphosphonates should be considered (Dasgupta *et al.*, 2010a). Gastroprotection with a proton pump inhibitor should be considered, especially in older patients. Blood pressure and serum glucose should be monitored, especially in patients with pre-existing hypertension and diabetes. Advice on exercise and remaining physically active is important.

References

Crowson CS, Matteson EL, Myasoedova E *et al.* The lifetime risk of adult-onset rheumatoid arthritis and other inflammatory autoimmune rheumatic diseases. *Arthritis and Rheumatism* 2011; **63**: 633–639.

Dasgupta B, Borg FA, Hassan N *et al.* BSR and BHPR guidelines for the management of polymyalgia rheumatica. *Rheumatology* 2010a; **49**: 186–190.

Dasgupta B, Borg FA, Hassan N et al. BSR and BHPR guidelines for the management of giant cell arteritis. *Rheumatology* 2010b; **49**(8): 1594–1597.

Dasgupta B, Cimmino MA, Maradit-Kremers H *et al.* 2012 provisional classification criteria for polymyalgia rheumatica: a European League Against Rheumatism/American College of Rheumatology collaborative initiative. *Annals of the Rheumatic Diseases* 2012; **71**: 484–492.

Smeeth L, Cook C, Hall AJ. Incidence of diagnosed polymyalgia rheumatica and temporal arteritis in the United Kingdom, 1990–2001. *Annals of the Rheumatic Diseases* 2006; **65**: 1093–1098.

CHAPTER 18

Systemic Lupus Erythematosus and Lupus-Like Syndromes

Vijay Rao[1,3], Rosalind Ramsey-Goldman[2] and Caroline Gordon[1,3]

[1] University of Birmingham, Birmingham, UK
[2] Solovy Arthritis Research Society Research; Northwestern University Feinberg School of Medicine, Chicago, USA
[3] Department of Rheumatology; Sandwell and West Birmingham Hospitals NHS Trust, Birmingham, UK

OVERVIEW

- SLE is a multisystem autoimmune disease associated with genetic and environmental risk factors.
- SLE is most common in women and those from non-white ethnic backgrounds.
- Lupus nephritis occurs in up to 50% of SLE patients.
- SLE patients should receive pre-pregnancy counselling to ensure optimal disease control and drug therapy before conception.
- Premature cardiovascular disease is an increasing cause of death in SLE patients.

Systemic lupus erythematosus (SLE) is a multisystem autoimmune disease of unknown cause (Rahman and Isenberg, 2008), with a wide variety of manifestations that is usually characterized by remissions and relapses. SLE is part of a spectrum of autoimmune diseases that includes discoid lupus, drug-induced lupus, neonatal lupus, Sjögren's syndrome, antiphospholipid antibody syndrome, dermatomyositis/polymyositis and overlap syndromes. Antiphospholipid antibody may occur as a primary disorder or secondary to SLE or another autoimmune condition, such as autoimmune hypothyroidism or chronic active hepatitis. It is possible to achieve good disease control but lifelong follow-up is needed to prevent and treat flares, to limit the complications due to damage and reduce the risk of premature death. Thus, it is important that the primary care physician, patient and hospital specialists are involved closely in the management of these diseases.

Causes

Systemic lupus erythematosus is a multifactorial disease due to a complex interplay of genetic and environmental factors that vary between individuals (Boxes 18.1 and 18.2). SLE is characterized by

---

Box 18.1 Genetic factors involved in predisposition to SLE

- Major histocompatibility complex genes, e.g. HLA-DR2 and HLA-DR3
- Genes responsible for innate immune response in SLE are IR5, TNFAIP3 and TREX1
- Genes involved in lymphocyte activation/function are BANK1, BLK, FCGR2B, HLA, PTPN22 and TNFSF4
- Genes associated with innate immune response and lymphocyte activation/function are IRAK and STAT4
- Genes responsible for immune complex clearance are FCGR3A, FCGR3B, ITGAM, C1q, C2, C4A and C4B

Source: Bentham and Vyse (2013), reproduced with permission of SAGE Publications

---

Box 18.2 Environmental factors involved in susceptibility to or triggering of SLE

- Drugs, e.g. hydralazine, procainamide, minocycline
- UV light (UV-A and UV-B)
- Viral infections, e.g. EBV, CMV, retroviruses, parvovirus B19
- Hormones, e.g. oestrogens, prolactin
- Chemicals and heavy metals, e.g. silica and mercury
- Diet, e.g. L-canavanine in alfalfa (but still debatable)

---

multiple immune abnormalities including dendritic, B- and T-cell dysfunction, resulting in the development of autoantibodies and autoreactive T-cells. Defective clearance of apoptotic cells and immune complexes contributes to pathogenesis, with the activation of complement playing a major role in tissue damage. There is increasing evidence that the cytokine interferon-alpha (IFN-alpha) plays a role in activating genes involved in the disease, and that

---

interleukin (IL)-6 and Il-10 levels are increased in active disease. Antiphospholipid antibodies are a specific family of autoantibodies directed against anionic phospholipids located in cell membranes. The pathogenic mechanisms in antiphospholipid syndrome relate to the prothrombotic effects of these antibodies *in vivo*.

Neutrophil extracellular traps (NETs) are produced from low-density granulocytes (LDG) and are networks of extracellular decondensed chromatin fibres containing histones and several cytoplasmic proteins. Material produced from NETs stimulates plasmacytoid dendritic cells to release IFN-alpha, a critical cytokine in lupus pathogenesis. Some lupus patients lack the ability to efficiently degrade NETs. Lupus neutrophils are predisposed toward NETosis, with both IFN-alpha and autoantibodies serving as potential triggers. Elevated serum levels of matrix metalloproteinase-9 (MMP-9) are externalized from LDG-NETs and lead to endothelial dysfunction and atherosclerosis in SLE through activation of MMP-2 (Knight and Kaplan, 2012).

Epidemiology

There are significant disparities in the incidence and prevalence rates of SLE disease worldwide (Pons-Estel *et al.*, 2010; Somers *et al.*, 2014). This variability may be due to true population differences or to dissimilar methods of case ascertainment.

Nevertheless, the consistent trend reflects that the burden of disease is highest in women and higher among non-white ethnic groups (Table 18.1).

Clinical presentations

Systemic lupus erythematosus

The American Rheumatology Association's 1982 classification criteria for systemic lupus erythematosus were revised in 1997 (Box 18.3). These criteria were designed not for diagnosis but for classifying patients into studies and clinical trials. The diagnosis of SLE should be considered if a patient has characteristic features of lupus, even if they do not fulfil four of the 11 criteria. For example, a 25-year-old woman with malar rash, positive antinuclear antibody and histologically proven glomerulonephritis obviously has systemic lupus erythematosus, despite fulfilling only three criteria (Table 18.2).

The Systemic Lupus Collaborating Clinics (SLICC) revised and validated the American College of Rheumatology (ACR) SLE classification criteria (Table 18.3). The SLICC criteria for SLE classification require: (1) fulfilment of at least four criteria, with at least one clinical criterion AND one immunological criterion OR (2) lupus nephritis as the sole clinical criterion in the presence of ANA or anti-dsDNA antibodies (Petri *et al.*, 2012). These criteria are

Table 18.1 Prevalence and incidence of systemic lupus erythematosus worldwide

Country	Prevalence (per 100 000)	Incidence (per 100 000)
United Kingdom (Nottingham, Birmingham)		
• Adults	20.6–28.7	4.48–4.94
• Women	37.6–53.1	7.46–8.31
• White/Caucasians	20.2–36.3	2.5–3.4
• Black/Afro-Caribbeans	197.2–206.0	11.9–31.9
• Asians	64.0–96.5	4.1–15.2
Iceland	35.9	3.3
Spain	34.1	2.2
Sweden	38.9	4.8
USA		
• Adults	70.1–74.1	5–6.2
• Women	124.2–131.5	8.4–10.4
• White/Caucasians	46.6–50.9	3.2–4.4
• Black/ African-Americans	102.0–109.8	6.9–9.0
• Puerto Rican (New York only)	18.0	2.3
Canada	20.6–42.3	0.9–7.4
Australia (Aborigines)	11.0	13.4–89.3
Japan	3.7–19.3	0.9–2.9
Martinique	64.2	4.7

Box 18.3 **American College of Rheumatology (previously American Rheumatology Association) revised classification criteria for systemic lupus**

Malar rash	Renal disorder
Discoid rash	Haematological disorder
Photosensitivity	Immunological disorder
Mucosal ulcers	Positive antinuclear antibodies
Arthritis	
Serositis	
Neurological disorder (psychosis, seizures)	

Table 18.2 Cumulative percentage incidence of clinical features of systemic lupus erythematosus

Feature	(%)
Arthritis	72–94
Alopecia	52–80
Skin rash	74–90
Photosensitivity	10–62
Malar rash	37–90
Oral ulcers	30–61
Fever	74–91
Neuropsychiatric	19–63
Renal	35–73
Cardiac	10–29
Pleuropulmonary	9–54

Table 18.3 Clinical and immunological criteria used in the SLICC classification criteria.

Clinical criteria	Immunological criteria
Acute cutaneous lupus: malar rash, maculopapular rash, photosensitive rash and non-indurated psoriasiform rash	ANA
Chronic cutaneous lupus: discoid lupus, lupus panniculitis, mucosal lupus and chilblain lupus	Anti-dsDNA antibodies
Oral ulcers	Anti-Sm antibodies
Non-scarring alopecia	Antiphospholipid antibody
Synovitis: swelling or effusion OR tenderness in 2 or more joints and 30 minutes or more of morning stiffness	Low complement
Serositis: pleurisy for more than 1 day (symptoms/pleural effusions/rub) Pericardial pain for more than 1 day/pericardial effusion/rub/ECG evidence)	Direct Coombs test (in absence of haemolytic anemia)
Renal: urine protein/creatinine (or 24 h urine protein) representing 500 mg of protein/24 h Or red blood cell casts	
Neurological: seizures, psychosis, myelitis, mononeuritis multiplex, peripheral or cranial neuropathy, acute confusional state	
Haemolytic anaemia	
Leukopenia (<4000/mm^3 at least once) Or lymphopenia (<1000/mm^3 at least once)	
Thrombocytopenia (<100 000/mm^3 at least once)	

Source: Petri *et al.* (2012), reproduced with permission of John Wiley & Sons

meant to be clinically more relevant, allowing the inclusion of more patients with clinically defined lupus in studies and clinical trials than when using the current ACR criteria.

General features

Fatigue is common, troublesome and difficult to evaluate. It may be associated with depression or fibromyalgia secondary to SLE, hypothyroidism (often autoimmune in nature), anaemia, pulmonary or cardiovascular problems. Other constitutional symptoms of active disease include fever, malaise, anorexia, lymphadenopathy and weight loss.

The most common form of anaemia is a normochromic normocytic anaemia of chronic disease. Some patients develop an antibody-mediated haemolytic anaemia and others an iron deficiency anaemia secondary to peptic ulceration or gastritis (usually due to non-steroidal anti-inflammatory drugs.

Mucocutaneous manifestations

The most common mucocutaneous features are painful or painless mouth ulcers, diffuse alopecia (Figure 18.1), butterfly or malar rash (Figure 18.2) and photosensitivity. Nasal or vaginal ulcers may also occur. Mucocutaneous features are more prominent in Asians and whites. Subacute cutaneous lupus erythematosus is a non-scarring rash found in areas of the body exposed to the sun. Discoid lesions are chronic scarring lesions that heal with hypo- or hyperpigmentation. Non-scarring alopecia may be patchy or diffuse. Rapid, spontaneous hair loss indicates active disease. Raynaud's phenomenon is usually milder than in scleroderma.

Musculoskeletal manifestations

Generalized arthralgia with early morning stiffness and no swelling is very common. A non-erosive arthritis with joint tenderness and swelling may develop. Deformities are unusual but may occur due

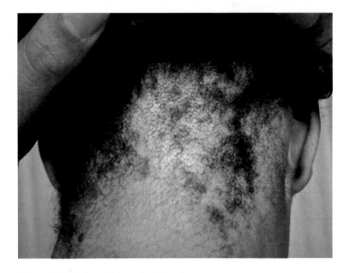

Figure 18.1 Patient with patchy alopecia

to ligamentous laxity (Jacoud's arthropathy) (Figure 18.3) compared with rheumatoid arthritis where the deformities are due to joint erosions. Myalgia is common but inflammatory myositis occurs in only 5% of patients. Indeed, secondary causes of myopathy are more common and can be caused by corticosteroids, antimalarials and lipid-lowering agents. Avascular necrosis and infection should be suspected if the patient complains of sudden-onset, severe pain in only one joint. In addition, the risk of osteoporosis and subsequent fracture due to minimal or no trauma can be increased in patients with SLE.

Haematological manifestations

Leucopenia may be an early clue to the diagnosis of SLE. Lymphopenia is the most common manifestation of SLE other than

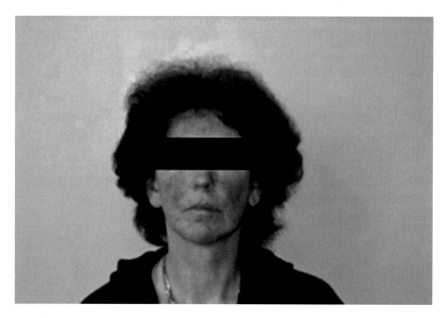

Figure 18.2 Malar rash in systemic lupus erythematosus

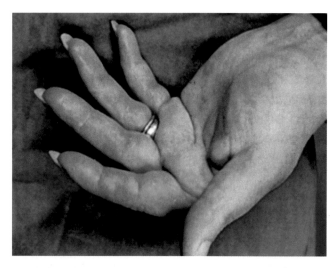

Figure 18.3 Jacoud's arthropathy

Box 18.4 **Central nervous system manifestations of systemic lupus erythematosus**

- Aseptic meningitis
- Cerebrovascular disease
- Demyelinating syndrome
- Headache (including migraine and benign intracranial hypertension)
- Movement disorders (including chorea)
- Myelopathy
- Seizure disorders
- Acute confusional state
- Anxiety disorder
- Cognitive dysfunction
- Mood disorder
- Psychosis

positive antinuclear antibodies and, in untreated patients, is caused by lymphocytotoxic antibodies. Mild neutropenia is relatively common in black people even without SLE, but values $<1.5 \times 10^9$/L are usually related to disease or drugs. Thrombocytopenia may occur as an immune-mediated condition associated with a risk of bleeding, as in idiopathic thrombocytopenic purpura, or as a milder abnormality with platelet counts $>70 \times 10^9$/L associated with a risk of thrombosis in the antiphospholipid syndrome (see below).

Renal manifestations

Renal disease is an important determinant of the outcome of SLE. It can occur in up to 50% of white patients and 75% of black patients. Studies have shown that renal disease is also more severe in non-white patients. Early nephritis is often asymptomatic, so regular urinalysis for protein, blood and casts is essential. Some patients present with nephrotic syndrome and a few with devastating accelerated hypertension and renal shutdown. Renal biopsy is helpful for assessing the severity, nature, extent and reversibility of the involvement and is an important guide to treatment and prognosis. For example, those with mesangial nephritis (class I) rarely progress to renal failure. In contrast, those with diffuse proliferative glomerulonephritis (class IV) are at risk for end-stage renal disease.

Nervous system manifestations

Systemic lupus erythematosus may affect the central and peripheral nervous systems. Definitions for these manifestations have been proposed by a consensus group (Boxes 18.4 and 18.5). The most common manifestations are headache, seizures, aseptic meningitis and cerebrovascular accidents. Antiphospholipid antibodies (including anticardiolipin antibodies) have been implicated in cerebrovascular accidents and chorea. It is often hard to determine whether the depression and headaches are due to lupus itself; in

Box 18.5 **Peripheral nervous system manifestations of systemic lupus erythematosus**

- Acute inflammatory demyelinating polyradiculoneuropathy (Guillain–Barré syndrome)
- Autonomic disorder
- Mononeuropathy (single or multiplex)
- Myasthenia gravis
- Neuropathy, cranial
- Plexopathy
- Polyneuropathy

many cases, they are related to psychosocial issues. Other possible causes such as sepsis, drugs, uraemia, severe hypertension and other metabolic causes must be sought and treated. Steroids are often blamed for inducing psychosis but if any doubt exists, patients should be given more, not less, steroid while under medical supervision, particularly if active lupus is evident in other systems.

Pulmonary and cardiovascular manifestations

Pleurisy, often without physical signs, is common in SLE. Less common manifestations are lupus pneumonitis, pulmonary haemorrhage, pulmonary embolism and pulmonary hypertension. Pulmonary haemorrhage can be sudden and acute and has high mortality. Pulmonary hypertension is associated with a poor prognosis, especially in pregnancy. Pericarditis is common but often asymptomatic. Other cardiac manifestations are myocarditis, endocarditis and rarely pericardial tamponade. Coronary artery disease is occasionally caused by vasculitis, but more often results from premature atherosclerosis.

Gastrointestinal manifestations

Abdominal pain, nausea, vomiting and diarrhoea occur in up to 50% of patients at some stage of disease. Although the presentation of greatest importance is mesenteric vasculitis, in which the patient presents with an acute abdomen and is at high risk of death, there have been reports of patients with subacute abdominal pain or aseptic peritonitis. This is usually associated with other serological signs of active disease and generally improves with steroid therapy. Other abdominal manifestations include subacute bowel obstruction, hepatitis, sclerosing cholangitis, protein-losing enteropathy, pancreatitis and ascites. Exclusion or treatment of infection is essential in patients with these conditions.

Pregnancy and systemic lupus erythematosus

No evidence suggests that SLE reduces fertility, but active disease and the presence of antiphospholipid antibody syndrome (see below) may increase the risk of intrauterine growth restriction, premature delivery, miscarriages and stillbirth (Jain and Gordon, 2011). Doses of prednisolone >10 mg/day predispose to preeclampsia, isolated hypertension in pregnancy, premature rupture of membranes and maternal infection. Minimal amounts of prednisolone cross the placenta due to enzymatic degradation in the placenta and there is very little evidence that non-fluorinated corticosteroids cause congenital abnormalities in humans.

Increasing evidence shows that azathioprine (<2 mg/kg/day) can be continued in pregnancy. Hydroxychloroquine is compatible with pregnancy and breastfeeding and may even improve outcomes (Jain and Gordon, 2011). If patients are on an angiotension converting enzyme inhibitor or mycophenolate mofetil for renal disease, then these medications must be discontinued due to their association with congenital malformations in the exposed fetus. Other antihypertensive medications such as methyldopa, labetalol and nifedipine are used most widely to control blood pressure control. Hydroxychloroquine, corticosteroids such as prednisolone and azathioprine can be added for lupus manifestations needing ongoing treatment. Pulmonary hypertension is associated with a 50% risk of mortality, particularly in the first 72 hours after delivery. This is usually a contraindication to planned pregnancy and needs specialist multidisciplinary care if diagnosed in pregnancy.

Pregnant women with lupus need close monitoring for optimal fetal and maternal outcome and are best managed in specialist units

Most babies born with congenital heart block need a pacemaker during the first year of life

Neonatal lupus syndrome

This is a syndrome that occurs in about 10% of babies born to mothers with anti-Ro or anti-La antibodies. The most common manifestation is a rash induced by ultraviolet light a few days or up to about 4 months after birth. It resolves spontaneously if the babies are removed from sunlight or ultraviolet light. A more serious, but much rarer manifestation of this syndrome is congenital heart block (CHB) that occurs in 1–2% of babies born to mothers with anti-Ro or anti-La antibodies. This is usually detected *in utero* between 16 and 28 weeks into the pregnancy. Babies born with CHB frequently need a pacemaker during the first year of life (Jain and Gordon, 2011).

Sjögren's syndrome

This clinical syndrome is characterized by sicca symptoms: dry eyes and dry mouth due to failure of salivary and mucosal glands, often preceded by salivary gland swelling, and is associated with autoantibody formation as described below. It may occur as a secondary disorder in patients with SLE or other conditions, including rheumatoid arthritis, systemic sclerosis and primary biliary cirrhosis, or as a primary disorder with features that resemble a mild form of SLE (mild symmetrical arthritis, photosensitivity, fatigue and diffuse alopecia). The primary syndrome is associated with hypergammaglobulinaemia with very high total immunoglobulin G levels and definitely positive antinuclear antibody, rheumatoid factor, and anti-Ro and anti-La antibody tests. Patients with these immunological abnormalities may benefit from specialist advice as they are at risk of systemic complications. Hydroxychloroquine and pilocarpine with other local symptomatic measures, such as artificial tears, are used to treat the condition.

> Sjögren's syndrome is often misdiagnosed as rheumatoid arthritis or systemic lupus erythematosus

Overlap syndromes and other lupus-like conditions

Up to 25% of patients with connective tissue disorders do not fit into classic descriptions and present with overlapping clinical features. Some may evolve into well-defined connective tissue disorders, while others have manifestations of more than one definite connective tissue disorder, for example systemic sclerosis combined with SLE and inflammatory myositis (see Chapter XX). Raynaud's phenomenon is often present and may occur in isolation as the first manifestation of a connective tissue disorder. Patients with mild undifferentiated connective tissue disorders may have inflammatory arthritis, oedema of hands and acrosclerosis. Generally, prognosis is good as long as patients do not develop pulmonary hypertension.

Polymyositis and dermatomyositis

Proximal muscle weakness, elevated muscle enzymes, myopathic changes on electromyography and inflammatory changes on muscle biopsy are diagositic criteria for polymyositis. The presence of a characteristic rash in the presence of the above features defines dermatomyositis. These diagnoses are made by fulfilling these criteria in combination and excluding other potential aetiologies for these test abnormalities.

Antiphospholipid syndrome

Antiphospholipid syndrome is an important cause of recurrent arterial and venous thrombosis and miscarriages (Ruiz-Irastorza *et al.*, 2010) (Box 18.6).

Thrombosis

The most common presentation of antiphospholipid syndrome is venous thrombosis in the arms or legs, which is often recurrent, multiple and bilateral, with a propensity for pulmonary embolism. Arterial thrombosis is less common but most frequently manifested by features of ischaemia or infarction. The severity of presentation depends on the acuteness and extent of the occlusion. The brain is the most common site, where thrombosis presents as stroke and transient ischaemic attacks. Other sites for arterial occlusion are the coronary arteries, subclavian, renal, retinal and pedal arteries.

Obstetric syndromes

Recurrent pregnancy losses in the second or third trimester are typical. Patients should be monitored for intrauterine growth

> Box 18.6 **Criteria for classification of antiphospholipid syndrome**
>
> **Clinical features**
>
> **Thrombosis**
> - Confirmed episode of arterial and/or venous thrombosis in any organ or tissue
>
> **Morbidity in pregnancy**
> - Fetal death beyond 10 weeks' gestation with confirmed normal fetal morphology
> - Three or more spontaneous abortions before 10 weeks' gestation in the absence of other maternal causes
> - More than one premature birth due to presence of severe placental insufficiency, pre-eclampsia or eclampsia before 34 weeks' gestation
>
> **Laboratory criteria**
> - Immunoglobulin G and/or immunoglobulin M anticardiolipin antibodies in medium to high titre on at least two different occasions more than 12 weeks apart (using a standard enzyme-linked immunosorbent assay for beta-2-glycoprotein I-dependent anticardiolipin antibodies)
> - Lupus anticoagulant in plasma on two separate occasions at least 12 weeks apart
>
> Antiphospholipid syndrome definitely is present if at least one of the clinical features and one of the laboratory criteria are met.

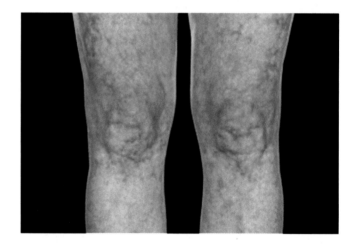

Figure 18.4 Livedo reticularis

restriction due to placental insufficiency and pre-eclampsia in a specialist unit. Planned early delivery is often required. (See below for treatment during pregnancy in the setting of antiphospholipid antibody syndrome.)

Other manifestations

Other prominent features include thrombocytopenia (up to 50% of patients), haemolytic anaemia, livedo reticularis (Figure 18.4), chronic ulcers, typically near the medial malleolus, and cutaneous vasculitis.

Catastrophic antiphospholipid syndrome

This is an acute and devastating syndrome characterized by multiple simultaneous vascular occlusions throughout the body which are often fatal. The kidney is affected most often, followed by the lungs, central nervous system, heart and skin.

Outcome of systemic lupus erythematosus and antiphospholipid syndrome

Although survival has improved substantially over the last 50 years (98% survival at 5 years and 95% survival at 10 years) (Pons-Estel *et al.*, 2010), awareness is increasing that these patients succumb to late complications of the disease or its therapy. Patients with renal involvement have a risk of end-stage renal disease and increased mortality, particularly in the black population (Somers *et al.*, 2014). Many lupus patients still die prematurely from infection or cardiovascular disease. Prevention and prompt management of infection, hyperlipidaemia, hypertension, ischaemic heart disease, diabetes mellitus and osteoporotic fractures are essential. Compliance with medications, clinic visits and lifestyle modifications are essential to prevent or reduce the risk of these associated problems, which may be iatrogenic or disease related in origin. It is important that phyisicans check that patients have received appropriate immunizations and screening for cancer (Mosca *et al.*, 2010).

Tests for antiphospholipid antibodies must be positive on two separate occasions, at least six weeks apart, before a confident diagnosis of antiphospholipid syndrome can be made (Box 18.7).

The long-term prognosis of antiphospholipid syndrome is poor, with organ damage in about one-third and functional impairment in up to one-fifth of patients about 10 years after diagnosis.

> Survival and disease control have improved in patients with systemic lupus erythematosus, but complications of premature vascular disease are recognized increasingly. The relative risk for myocardial infarction in women with systemic lupus erythematosus aged 35–44 years was 52.3 times the risk for women without lupus

Investigations

Investigations in systemic lupus erythematosus

A full blood count with differential white count, urinalysis and serum creatinine should be done for diagnosis and monitoring of the activity of SLE. Estimated glomerular filtration rate is more reliable than serum creatinine for detecting early impairment of renal function. Patients with proteinuria or haematuria, or both, on dipstick should have microscopy done to look for casts if infection, stones and menstrual blood loss have been excluded, and referral for renal biopsy should be considered if these abnormalities potentially due to lupus nephritis are confirmed.

For diagnosis, antinuclear antibody and anti-extractable nuclear antigens tests (see Chapter XX) should be done. No value is gained by repeating these tests, unless a change in clinical features is noted. Anti-ribonucleoprotein is associated with overlap connective tissue disease. Anti-dsDNA antibodies are useful for predicting patients at risk of developing renal disease and for monitoring disease activity. Although levels usually rise before a disease flare, they may fall at the time of flare. Levels of C3 and C4 fall with disease activity because of complement consumption, particularly in patients with renal disease. Levels also relate to the rate of synthesis in the liver and may rise in infections and pregnancy. Measurement of complement degradation products (for example, C3d, C4d) and C1q antibodies is less widely available but more reliable for monitoring disease activity, as these reflect complement consumption. In women planning pregnancy, it is important to check for anti-Ro and anti-La antibodies and for antiphospholipid antibodies and the lupus anticoagulant.

Investigations in antiphospholipid syndrome

Overall, 80–90% of patients with antiphospholipid syndrome are positive for antibodies to a complex of anticardiolipin antibodies and beta-2-glycoprotein I. Lupus anticoagulant is only found in 20% of patients with antiphospholipid syndrome but is associated with a high risk of thrombosis. Low levels of antiphospholipid antibodies of no clinical consequence may develop transiently after infections.

Management

General measures

Patients must be educated about the nature of their disease and the need for therapy (Table 18.4). Leaflets from patient support organizations and references to reliable internet websites are useful. More than just drug therapy is required. Patients with sun-induced rashes should use sunblock regularly for at least 6 months over the summer months but all year can be helpful. Other patients with SLE should be aware that sun exposure may precipitate a disease flare.

Lifestyle should be adjusted to ensure adequate rest, appropriate exercise and a well-balanced diet. Measures for reducing stress should be considered and career plans reviewed. Patients with Raynaud's phenomenon should wear appropriate warm clothing, including hats and gloves.

Raynaud's phenomenon is best treated with calcium channel blockers, local nitrate creams if mild to moderate, and intravenous prostacyclin infusions in severe cases. Angiotensin converting enzyme inhibitors may be tried if calcium channel blockers are not tolerated.

Box 18.7 Tests for antiphospholipid antibodies

- Anticardiolipin antibodies
- Antibodies against co-factors associated with anionic phospholipids, for example, beta-2-glycoprotein
- Lupus anticoagulant
- Biological false-positive serological tests for syphilis

Table 18.4 Management of systemic lupus erythematosus

Risk factor advice	Further management
Avoid sun and other ultraviolet light	Wear sun block, hat and protective clothing
Avoid infection	Treat bacterial infections early with antibiotics and prevent infections with immunizations
Avoid unplanned pregnancy	Advise appropriate contraception
Use non-steroidal anti-inflammatory drugs with care	Use other analgesics as needed
Use oral steroids with care	Consider local and intramuscular or intravenous steroids and cytotoxic agents
Monitor for active disease	Urinalysis, full blood count, creatinine, anti-dsDNA antibodies, C3, C4
Screen for hypertension	Treat with calcium channel blockers or angiotensin converting enzyme inhibitors
Screen for diabetes and lipids	Advise on diet and give drugs if needed
Assess osteoporosis risk	Give postmenopausal women bisphosphonates

Infections should be avoided and treated promptly if appropriate, as they can precipitate flares. Similarly, contraceptive pills that contain oestrogen may exacerbate lupus disease or thrombosis and should be used with caution. In general, barrier methods or progesterone-only contraception are preferred. Pregnancy should be planned, as the outcome is better, with fewer complications in both mother and fetus, if the mother has inactive disease at the time of conception. Drug therapy should be reviewed before conception.

Overlap and lupus-like conditions are managed much the same as mild SLE. Dry eyes should be managed by the frequent use of artificial tears. Dry mouth is best managed by taking sips of plain water, sucking ice cubes or eating sugar-free sweets. Artificial saliva preparations are disappointing.

Drug therapy in systemic lupus erythematosus (Bertsias *et al.*, 2012; Mosca *et al.*, 2010)

Milder cases with intermittent rashes, arthritis and other mucocutaneous features can usually be treated with steroid creams, short courses of non-steroidal anti-inflammatory drugs and hydroxychloroquine (<6.5 mg/kg/day). These drugs are also widely used in overlap syndromes, with the exception of non-steroidal anti-inflammatory drugs, which are contraindicated in patients with features of systemic sclerosis or renal disease. More severe cases of SLE usually require oral corticosteroids. Patients who need 10 mg/day of prednisolone or more despite hydroxychloroquine, or those who present with more severe manifestations (such as nephritis, gastrointestinal vasculitis or CNS disease) that need higher initial doses of prednisolone (0.5–1 mg/kg/day) are likely to need azathioprine, methotrexate or mycophenolate mofetil as steroid-sparing immunosuppressive agents (Table 18.5).

Cyclophosphamide is often given as intermittent intravenous 'pulse therapy' and is used predominantly for proliferative glomerulonephritis and systemic vasculitis.

Lefluonamide or belimumab (where funding is available) may be considered for patients intolerant or resistant to these agents. Steroids should always be reduced slowly.

Ciclosporin A and tacrolimus are useful in patients with haematological involvement as they do not cause bone marrow suppression but renal function needs careful monitoring. Mycophenolate mofetil is now widely used for the treatment of lupus nephritis as an alternative to cyclophosphamide. Intravenous cyclophosphamide is also used for severe neurological lupus. Refractory renal and CNS

Table 18.5 Steroid-sparing and cytotoxic drugs used in systemic lupus erythematosus

Drug Range (mg/kg/day)
Hydroxychloroquine ≤6.5
Azathioprine 1–2.5
Methotrexate 7.5–25 mg per week
Ciclosporin A 1–2.5
Lefluonamide 10–20 mg daily
Cyclophosphamide Intravenous pulses or ≤2 mg/kg/day orally
Mycophenolate mofetil 1–3 g/day

disease has been shown to respond to rituximab in open label studies but not controlled trials.

In pregnancy, patients may be given prednisolone, hydroxychloroquine and/or azathioprine as the advantages are now considered to outweigh the risks. During lactation, prednisolone and hydroxychloroquine are acceptable, and azathioprine rarely causes problems at low doses. Methotrexate, mycophenolate, lefluonamide, cyclophosphamide, rituximab and belimumab are contraindicated in pregnancy and while breastfeeding. Ciclosporin A has been used in pregnancy in patients who have undergone transplants.

Meticulous screening and treatment of blood pressure, diabetes, hyperlipidaemia and osteoporosis are essential.

In general, calcium channel blockers, angiotensin converting enzyme inhibitors and angiotensin receptor blockers are the preferred antihypertensive agents, because beta-blockers aggravate Raynaud's phenomenon. Bisphosphonates are often required in postmenopausal women, but they should be used with care in women who may want to become pregnant in the future. Bisphosphonates, statins, ACE inhibitors and angiotensin receptor blockers should be stopped before a planned pregnancy. Calcium and vitamin D can be used in all age groups. Treatment with anticoagulation and antiepileptic, antidepressant or antipsychotic drugs should be considered early in the management of patients with neuropsychiatric disease.

Oestrogen-containing contraceptives and hormone replacement therapy should be used with care in women with stable mild/moderate lupus and should be avoided in women with antiphospholipid antibodies, especially those with a history of thrombosis or pregnancy loss. Progesterone-only contraception is acceptable but is associated with a theoretical risk of increasing osteoporotic risk. Intrauterine devices can be used in women in stable relationships with a low risk of infection.

Biologic treatments currently used in lupus

Belimumab – Monoclonal antibody that inhibits B-lymphocyte stimulation and has been shown to be effective in lupus patients, especially those with high dsDNA antibodies and low complement. Usually given 4 weekly by intravenous infusion.

Rituximab – This monoclonal antibody targets CD20 and causes B-cell depletion. It has been used successfully in refractory lupus nephritis and cerebral lupus. Given as two infusions 15 days apart which may be repeated after 6–12 months if necessary.

Therapy in antiphospholipid antibody syndrome (Box 18.8)

There is no evidence for prophylactic treatment of patients serologically positive for antiphospholipid antibody syndrome but without a history of thrombosis, although aspirin is often given in practice. Oestrogen-containing contraceptives and hormone replacement therapy are best avoided in patients with antiphospholipid syndrome and those with antiphospholipid antibodies without thrombosis or fetal loss.

Treatment for thrombosis is usually initiated with intravenous or subcutaneous heparin and is soon changed to oral anticoagulation with warfarin. Most doctors recommend maintaining the international normalized ratio (INR) at 2–3 to prevent venous thrombosis and between 3 and 4 to prevent arterial thrombosis, as studies suggesting that INR in the range 2–3 was sufficient for patients after arterial thrombosis were flawed. Anticoagulation is usually lifelong unless a contraindication, such as poorly controlled hypertension, is present (Ruiz-Irastorza *et al*, 2010).

Pregnancy – A combination of low molecular weight heparin and low-dose aspirin is preferred. Pregnant women need close monitoring by the obstetrician, haematologist and rheumatologist, preferably in combined clinics at specialist units. Heparin dosage will depend on the clinical circumstances (Ruiz-Irastorza *et al*, 2010).

Box 18.8 **Goals of treatment in antiphospholipid syndrome**

- Prophylaxis
- Treatment of acute thromboses
- Prevention of further thrombotic events
- Management of pregnancy in antiphospholipid syndrome

Conclusion

Systemic lupus erythematosus is more common than many people realize. The presentations are diverse, and it may take a few years to realize that a variety of symptoms and signs can all be attributed to SLE, Sjögren's syndrome or an overlap syndrome. Antiphospholipid antibody syndrome should be sought actively in patients with a history of recurrent fetal loss or thrombosis, or both, because of the risk of future thrombotic complications. These diagnoses should not be made without appropriate clinical and serological features as there are many social consequences of these diagnoses, such as implications for obtaining insurance and mortgages.

With appropriate treatment, the outcome of these conditions is good, but the risk of late complications, particularly of atherosclerosis, is important. In the future, management of patients with these conditions should seek to reduce these risks as well as control active disease.

References

Bentham J, Vyse TJ. The development of genome-wide association studies and their application to complex diseases, including lupus. *Lupus* 2013; **22**(12): 1205–1213.

Bertsias GK, Tektonidou M, Amoura Z *et al*. Joint European League Against Rheumatism and European Renal Association-European Dialysis and Transplant Association (EULAR/ERA-EDTA) recommendations for the management of adult and paediatric lupus nephritis. *Annals of the Rheumatic Diseases* 2012; **71**(11): 1771–1782.

Jain V, Gordon C. Managing pregnancy in inflammatory rheumatological diseases. *Arthritis Research and Therapy* 2011; **13**(1): 206.

Knight JS, Kaplan MJ. Lupus neutrophils: 'NET' gain in understanding lupus pathogenesis. *Current Opinion in Rheumatology* 2012; **24**(5): 441–450.

Mosca M, Tani C, Aringer M *et al*. European League Against Rheumatism recommendations for monitoring patients with systemic lupus erythematosus in clinical practice and in observational studies. *Annals of the Rheumatic Diseases* 2010; **69**(7): 1269–1274.

Petri M, Orbai A, Alarcon G *et al*. Derivation and validation of the Systemic Lupus International Collaborating Clinics classification criteria for systemic lupus erythematosus. *Arthritis and Rheumatism* 2012; **64**(8): 2677–2686.

Pons-Estel GJ, Alarcon G, Scofield L *et al*. Understanding the epidemiology and progression of systemic lupus erythematosus. *Seminars in Arthritis and Rheumatism* 2010; **39**(4): 257–268.

Rahman A, Isenberg DA. Systemic lupus erythematosus. *New England Journal of Medicine* 2008; **358**(9): 929–939.

Ruiz-Irastorza G, Crowther M, Branch W, Khamashta M. Antiphospholipid syndrome. *Lancet* 2010; **376**(9751): 1498–1509.

Somers EC, Marder W, Cagnoli P *et al*. Population-based incidence and prevalence of systemic lupus erythematosus: the Michigan Lupus Epidemiology and Surveillance program. *Arthritis and Rheumatology* 2014; **66**(2): 369–378.

CHAPTER 19

Raynaud's Phenomenon and Scleroderma

Christopher P. Denton, Carol M. Black and Voon H. Ong

Royal Free Hospital and UCL Medical School, London, UK

OVERVIEW

- Survival from systemic sclerosis is improving due to earlier identification of major complications and more effective treatment of vascular complications, including scleroderma renal crisis and pulmonary arterial hypertension

- Lung fibrosis is common but not always severe or progressive. Patients who are at risk of progression should be treated with intravenous cyclophosphamide.

- Any of the major complications can occur in either of the two systemic sclerosis subsets, limited or diffuse, based upon the extent of skin disease. Most complications are more frequent in early diffuse systemic sclerosis.

- New classification criteria have recently been developed by the ACR and EULAR and these allow cases with milder disease to be included in systemic sclerosis cohorts.

- In diffuse disease, the extent of skin sclerosis may be maximal within 18–24 months of onset of disease and then plateau or improve.

- Almost all patients with systemic sclerosis have Raynaud's phenomenon but only a small proportion of patients with RP progress to connective tissue disease (and these can be identified by positive ANA and abnormal nailfold capillaroscopy).

Diagnosis, classification and epidemiology of scleroderma

Scleroderma is a collective term that applies to several related disorders that share key clinical features. It is useful to consider a spectrum of conditions that include a number of different forms of scleroderma. Localized forms of scleroderma occur most often in childhood and include morphea and linear scleroderma. In adults, these conditions may also occur. Some rare forms such as pansclerotic morphea or generalized morphea can be very severe and although not life-threatening, warrant intensive treatment.

The systemic forms of scleroderma comprise forms of systemic sclerosis (SSc). These are autoimmune rheumatic diseases that lead to inflammation and thickening of the skin, vascular disturbance, notably Raynaud's phenomenon, and a number of potentially lethal

internal organ manifestations. It is notable that some features, such as upper gastrointestinal dysmotility or secondary Raynaud's phenomenon, occur in all cases whereas other manifestations affect only a minority. The timing and frequency of these major complications are now well established and have recently been highlighted in a large consecutive patient series.

There are other forms of systemic sclerosis, including those cases with additional features of another autoimmune rheumatic disease such as myositis, arthritis, lupus or Sjögren's syndrome and also a rare subset that has internal organ and vascular features but no skin sclerosis, termed systemic sclerosis sine scleroderma. It is useful to also include some cases of Raynaud's phenomenon that have serological or other features of SSc within the scleroderma spectrum as some of these may progress to SSc.

There are newly established classification criteria for SSc that are likely to facilitate clinical care and research as they correct a number of limitations of previously developed preliminary criteria. In practice, although developed for classification, these criteria are likely to be used widely to confirm the diagnosis of cases of suspected SSc.

The prevalence of SSc has been difficult to ascertain due to the clinical heterogeneity and rarity of the condition and the spectrum of severity outlined above. Current best estimates suggest approximately 1 in 10 000 prevalence of SSc in the UK, with similar frequency in most European populations that have been examined. In the USA, it is believed that SSc is rather more common and that up to 1 in 5000 of the population may be affected.

The main focus of this chapter is on systemic sclerosis and the other forms of the condition will not be considered further as they are of less relevance to general rheumatology practice.

Raynaud's phenomenon and connective tissue disease

Episodic cold-induced vasospasm (Figure 19.1), triggered by cold or emotional stress, affects around 5% of the adult population, especially young females. In primary Raynaud's (90%), there are no other clinical or investigational abnormalities. Secondary Raynaud's

---

ABC of Rheumatology, Fifth Edition. Edited by Ade Adebajo and Lisa Dunkley.
© 2018 John Wiley & Sons Ltd. Published 2018 by John Wiley & Sons Ltd.

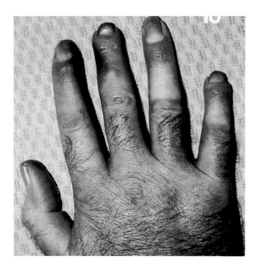

Figure 19.1 Well-defined blanching of skin, characteristic of Raynaud's phenomenon

---

Box 19.1 Points to consider when looking for underlying cause of Raynaud's phenomenon

- Occupation: working outdoors, fishing industry, using vibrating tools, exposure to chemicals such as vinyl chloride
- Examination of peripheral and central vascular system for proximal vascular occlusion
- Drugs: such as beta-blockers, oral contraceptives, bleomycin, migraine therapy
- Symptoms of other autoimmune rheumatic disorders:
  ○ Arthralgia or arthritis
  ○ Cerebral symptoms
  ○ Mouth ulcers
  ○ Alopecia
  ○ Photosensitivity
  ○ Muscle weakness
  ○ Skin rashes
  ○ Dry eyes or mouth
  ○ Respiratory or cardiac problems

(10%) implies there are other features, usually an underlying autoimmune rheumatic disease.

Investigation of Raynaud's symptoms includes the identification of secondary causes (Box 19.1). Such causes of Raynaud's, or acrocyanosis, include vibrating machine tools, thoracic outlet obstruction, drugs such as beta-blockers and haematological abnormalities such as cryoglobulinaemia. Macrovascular arterial disease, embolization and systemic vasculitis, including Berger's disease, are important but rare differential diagnoses. Some patients with isolated Raynaud's phenomenon have positive antinuclear antibodies and abnormal nailfold capillaroscopy. These cases are at increased risk of developing a defined connective tissue disease, with up to 50% of such cases progressing within 10 years. The negative predictive value of normal nailfold capillaroscopy and negative autoantibody screening is powerful, allowing robust reassurance.

The vast majority of patients with RP have isolated symptoms that typically develop in the teenage years and become more troublesome in adulthood. These cases are female predominant and often run in families. These include the majority of cases of primary Raynaud's phenomenon in which there are no clinical features of an associated condition and, more specifically, no alteration in microvascular structure, evidenced by normal nailfold video-capillaroscopy and absence of antinuclear autoantibodies. Thus, patients with possible RP need to be carefully and appropriately evaluated. Some cases of isolated RP are identified in which there are features that point to the development of a connective tissue disease, in particular, altered nailfold capillaries and positive ANA. The pattern of capillaroscopy can be helpful in determining significance and likely associated or future connective tissue disease and ANA patterns can be similarly informative. A landmark study has shown that up to 50% of cases develop SSc if they have an SSc hallmark ANA and scleroderma pattern capillary alterations. This forms an important group of cases that may facilitate very early diagnosis of SSc (VEDOSS).

It is helpful to perform systematic assessment in all cases to determine any underlying cause or associated condition (summarized in Figure 19.2).

In addition to defined autoimmune rheumatic diseases, there are many patients with overlap syndromes or undifferentiated connective tissue disease who have Raynaud's and also features such as arthralgia, malaise or photosensitivity but who do not fulfil classification criteria for a defined disease. These may later evolve into more significant diseases (see also Chapters 18 and 20).

Systemic sclerosis

The most important disease within the scleroderma spectrum is SSc (Table 19.1). This has high mortality, and approximately 60% of patients diagnosed with SSc will ultimately die from the disease. Most often, this is due to cardiorespiratory complications. Nevertheless, there has been significant improvement in survival recently due to better treatment of organ-based complications, and the overall 5-year survival now approaches 80%. Cardinal features of SSc are the association of skin sclerosis with Raynaud's phenomenon, which is almost always present, and with internal organ involvement, which varies in extent between patients. The majority of cases fall into one of two major subsets. The characteristics of patients with each subset at different times in their disease are summarized in Boxes 19.2 and 19.3.

Diffuse cutaneous systemic sclerosis (dcSSc)

The dcSSc subset is determined by involvement of skin proximal to the knees and elbows and may actually be confused with an inflammatory arthropathy in its early stages. Most of the important complications develop within the first 3 years of dcSSc, and skin sclerosis tends to be maximal at around 18–30 months. Thereafter, skin involvement tends to stabilize or improve. Despite stabilization or improvement in skin sclerosis, internal organ complications may develop at a later stage, and so long-term follow-up is mandatory. In dcSSc, Raynaud's generally develops concurrently with the skin disease or shortly afterwards.

Proposed patient flow for diagnosis of systemic sclerosis (SSc) and other connective tissue diseases in patients presenting with isolated Raynaud's phenomenon

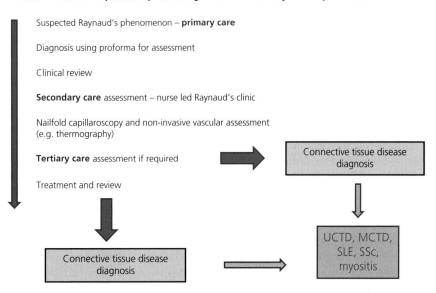

Suspected Raynaud's phenomenon – **primary care**

Diagnosis using proforma for assessment

Clinical review

Secondary care assessment – nurse led Raynaud's clinic

Nailfold capillaroscopy and non-invasive vascular assessment (e.g. thermography)

Tertiary care assessment if required

Treatment and review

Connective tissue disease diagnosis

Connective tissue disease diagnosis

UCTD, MCTD, SLE, SSc, myositis

Figure 19.2 Schematic summarizing investigation of cases of Raynaud's phenomenon to identify those with an associated connective tissue disease

Table 19.1 The spectrum of scleroderma and scleroderma-like disorders

Localised scleroderma (morphoea)	Dermal inflammation and fibrosis. No visceral disease, few vascular symptoms
Plaque morphoea	Fewer than four localised areas of involvement
Generalised morphoea	More than four localized areas of involvement
Linear morphoea	Skin sclerosis follows a dermatomal distribution; commonest form of childhood onset scleroderma
En coup de sabre	Scalp and facial linear lesion often with underlying bone changes
Systemic sclerosis	
Diffuse cutaneous systemic sclerosis	Skin involvement proximal to elbows or knees, short history of Raynaud's phenomenon associated with anti-topoisomerase-1 (Scle-70) or anti-RNA polymerase III antibodies
Limited cutaneous systemic sclerosis	Skin thickening affects extremities only, long history of Raynaud's phenomenon, associated with anti-centromere antibodies
Overlap syndromes	Clinical features of systemic sclerosis associated with those of another autoimmune rheumatic disease (SLE, myositis, arthritis)
Systemic sclerosis sine scleroderma	Serological, vascular and visceral features of SSc without detectable skin sclerosis
Isolated Raynaud's phenomenon	
Primary	Common, onset in adolescence, female predominance, normal nailfold capillaroscopy and negative autoantibody profile
Secondary	Raynaud's with abnormal nailfold capillaries and/or positive antinuclear autoantibody testing

Box 19.2 Characteristic findings and management approach for limited cutaneous systemic sclerosis

- Long-standing Raynaud's phenomenon is common and may be the presenting feature together with dysphagia or gastro-oesophageal reflux. These are treated symptomatically
- All patients should be screened at diagnosis for organ-based disease, including lung fibrosis and pulmonary hypertension. Regular assessment should be long term as complications, especially pulmonary hypertension, may occur at any stage of follow-up
- Constitutional symptoms including fatigue are common but associated diagnoses such as hypothyroidism or consequences of malnutrition should be excluded
- Skin involvement is generally mild but vascular complications can be severe and may require intravenous prostacyclin or other advanced therapies

Box 19.3 Characteristic findings and management approach for diffuse cutaneous systemic sclerosis

- Diffuse systemic sclerosis is generally associated with a shorter duration of pre-existing Raynaud's phenomenon and the vascular symptoms may develop after onset of skin or musculoskeletal inflammatory symptoms
- Weight loss is common in early disease which is also associated with severe skin itching and progressive skin sclerosis
- Presence of anti-RNA polymerase III pattern of ANA or tendon friction rubs point towards increased risk of scleroderma renal crisis but this usually occurs within the first 3 years of disease
- Immunosuppression should be considered for skin and lung involvement, if severe or progressive, with drugs such as mycophenolate mofetil, methotrexate or intravenous cyclophosphamide
- In later stages, the skin disease often stabilizes or improves but organ-based complications, including pulmonary hypertension, may occur at any stage and ongoing vigilance is essential with regular screening

Limited cutaneous systemic sclerosis (lcSSc)

The lcSSc subset of SSc (Figure 19.3) accounts for around 60% of cases in most North American or European series. Skin involvement is much less extensive and may be confined to the fingers (sclerodactyly), face or neck. Raynaud's phenomenon is very prominent and may precede development of SSc by several years. The designation 'CREST syndrome' is used to describe a subgroup of lcSSc in whom calcinosis, Raynaud's phenomenon, oesophageal [esophageal] dysmotility, sclerodactyly and telangiectasia occur. It is probably better not to distinguish such cases, as these manifestations are not universal and de-emphasize the life-threatening complications that develop in a significant proportion of lcSSc patients. These include pulmonary arterial hypertension, severe midgut disease and interstitial pulmonary fibrosis.

Other SSc cases include overlap syndromes with features of polyarthritis, myositis or systemic lupus erythematosus, and the small group of SSc sine scleroderma who have major visceral involvement, Raynaud's phenomenon and a hallmark autoantibody, typically antitopoisomerase 1. The term MCTD is widely used and refers to patients with overlap connective tissue disease that has specific features and is characterized by high-titre ANA with anti U1-RNP specificity. Although such patients can be identified, it is unclear whether they really represent a distinct subset of overlap syndrome, especially as many evolve over time into a predominant clinical phenotype of SSc or SLE, and the anti U1-RNP pattern of ANA can occur in either of these more defined connective tissue diseases. Major internal organ complications such as lung fibrosis, pulmonary arterial hypertension or renal involvement can occur in patients with a diagnosis of MCTD.

Aetiopathogenesis

Systemic sclerosis is rare and complex and like other uncommon diseases, this suggests that the factors that lead to the development of SSc occur infrequently. These include genetic and environmental factors, although interestingly, many of the genetic susceptibility loci that have been identified code for genes that are also implicated in the development of other autoimmune or rheumatic diseases.

In addition, the strongest genetic contributor is the major histocompatibility complex (MHC). This conclusion comes from many candidate gene and genome-wide association (GWAS) studies and confirms that SSc is undoubtedly an autoimmune disease in which innate and adaptive immune system dysfunction occurs.

However, there are also very clear environmental aspects to the aetiology. Thus, there are chemical triggers of SSc such as silica dust, organic solvents or cancer chemotherapies. Individual complications may also be triggered exogenously and the timing and frequency of some of the complications are consistent with multiple trigger mechanisms.

Recent intriguing data suggest that SSc can sometimes occur as a paraneoplastic condition and that this may relate to altered expression of target autoantigens in tumour tissue, notably variant RNA polymerase III. The association between anti-RNA polymerase III and cancer has recently been confirmed in a large series. The precise mechanism that leads to SSc remains unclear but undoubtedly there is interplay between immune, vascular and connective tissue dysfunction. Other cellular compartments are also implicated, including progenitor cells, the haemopoietic system and epithelial cells. The latter may be especially important in the gut, kidney and lung where specialized epithelial structures are in close juxtaposition with the endothelium and may be altered. Sequential pathogenesis linking immunological, microvascular and fibrotic processes is oversimple, based upon the likely shared mediators and signalling intermediates between these different processes that have emerged as molecular pathology is better understood from microarray and other detailed analyses. The description of pathology is now much more complete and allows more targeted approaches to therapy to be developed.

Autoantibody profiles

The SSc-associated patterns of autoantibody reactivity are summarized in Table 19.2. These are important as they may offer means for early prediction or diagnosis of complications and risk stratification. These major hallmark autoantibodies associated with SSc are mutually exclusive (Figure 19.4). Thus, if a patient has anticentromere

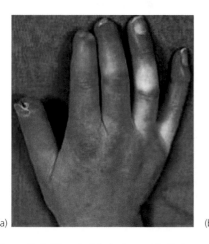
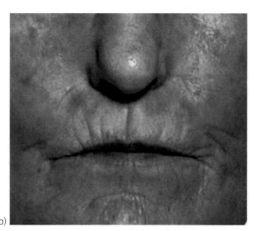
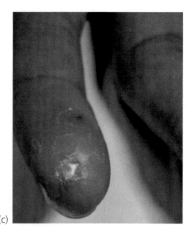

(a)　　　　　　　　　　(b)　　　　　　　　　　(c)

Figure 19.3 Characteristic features of limited cutaneous scleroderma. (a) Puffy fingers, tight skin, Raynaud's phenomenon, loss of distal digits and ulceration of tips of digits. (b) Microstomia and telangiectasia. (c) Calcinotic deposits typically occur over pressure areas, including the fingertips, and extensor surface of forearms and elbows.

antibodies they will almost never have antitopoisomerase 1 or another reactivity associated with SSc. This appears to reflect the immunogenetic background of these individuals and may explain the clinical differences between patients with hallmark reactivity.

Risk stratification in systemic sclerosis

The clinical heterogeneity of SSc and differences in natural history between the two major subsets and the life-threatening nature of some of the SSc-associated complications have led to attempts

Table 19.2 Autoimmune serology in SSc

Antibody target	Prevalence	Comments
Centromere	60% lcSSc	Associated with typical CREST pattern of disease
Scl-70 (topoisomerase-1)	40% dcSSc 15% lcSSc	Predictive of interstitial lung involvement in both SSc subsets
RNA polymerase III	20% SSc	Anti-RNA polymerase III associated with diffuse skin disease, scleroderma renal crisis and malignancy
U1-RNP	10% SSc	Associated with overlap features
U3 RNP (fibrillin)	5% SSc	Poor outcome, cardiac disease and pulmonary arterial hypertension
PM-Scl	3% SSc	Myositis overlap
Th/to	5% SSc	Lung fibrosis in lcSSc
Anti-M2	5–10% SSc	Especially in lcSSc with primary biliary cholangitis

to risk-stratify patients at diagnosis and initial assessment. Abnormalities reflecting systemic inflammation (elevated erythrocyte sedimentation rate), pulmonary disease (impaired diffusion capacity, DLCO) or renal involvement (proteinuria) identify patients with a poor 5-year survival. In addition, the clinical association of antibody profiles allows patients at increased risk of pulmonary or renal complications to be identified. In the future, such information is likely to direct management and screening. Antibodies can predict particular complications such as antitopoisomerase and lung fibrosis, anti-RNA polymerase and renal crisis or anti-Th/To and respiratory involvement in lcSSc. At present, the strongest genetic associations relate to SSc-specific autoantibodies, but other genetic factors that determine the disease profile are being sought.

Management of systemic sclerosis

A cornerstone of long-term management is proactive regular investigation to determine the presence of complications. This is important as these organ-based complications may be life threatening but treatable. Recent initiatives have focused on earlier detection of pulmonary artery hypertension (PAH) and have led to the development of the DETECT algorithm for identification of patients at high risk of PAH (see below). In addition to proactive investigation for complications, it is also important to address the symptoms of SSc that reflect non-life-threatening manifestations as these may be improved. Thus, musculoskeletal pain and inflammation and upper gastrointestinal dysmotility, together with other gastrointestinal

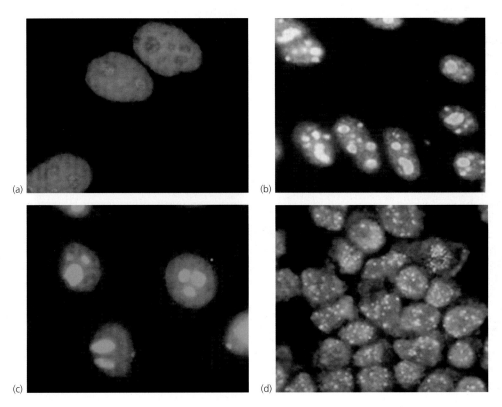

Figure 19.4 Common immunofluorescent patterns seen on testing for antinuclear antibodies. (a) Homogeneous – typical of antibodies to DNA, with or without histones. (b) Speckled – typical of antibodies to Ro, La, Sm and ribonucleotide protein. (c) Nucleolar – typical of scleroderma. (d) Centromere – mainly found with limited cutaneous scleroderma

manifestations such as constipation and small intestinal bacterial overgrowth, can be improved with standard therapies that are not SSc specific. Other non-life-threatening complications can be more challenging such as calcinosis, contractures and anorectal incontinence. Digital ulcer management has improved now that newer treatments are available and with greater appreciation of the importance of active therapy of ulcers and complications such as infection. More than half of SSc patients describe digital ulcers at some time in their disease course and around 20% have ulcers at any one time.

Unfortunately, at present there are no disease-modifying treatments of proven efficacy. Most patients benefit from vascular therapy, and a number of agents that suggest the potential for vascular remodelling have been used in trials (Box 19.4). Immunosuppressive treatment is generally reserved for patients with early and aggressive dcSSc or with a major organ-based complication such as interstitial lung disease or myositis. Two major studies suggest treatment benefit from cyclophosphamide for lung fibrosis in SSc and data also support use of immunomodulation to improve skin sclerosis including methotrexate, cyclophosphamide and even novel approaches such as hyperimmune goat serum or oral native collagen. The most compelling results have come from studies of high-intensity immunosuppression and autologous peripheral stem cell rescue.

Box 19.4 **Drugs to treat Raynaud's phenomenon**

Pharmaco-nutrients

Antioxidant vitamins: vitamins C and E at high dose may reduce oxidant stress in Raynaud's and SSc

Fish oils: maxepa, cod liver oil supplements may promote endothelial production of vasodilatory factors

Gamolenic acid: mechanism uncertain

Seredrin: Gingko biloba, vasodilator giving symptomatic relief in Raynaud's

Vasodilators

Calcium channel blockers: nifedipine and others may be effective; primary Raynaud's responds better than secondary; different agents may demonstrate varied effectiveness and side effects; side effects are frequent and often dose-limiting, including headache, ankle swelling and postural hypotension

Angiotensin receptor blockers: effective for SSc associated hypertension; may also help Raynaud's symptoms and have potential beneficial effect on vascular remodelling

Nitroglycerin: topical glyceryl tri-nitrate ointment or patches may benefit ischaemic digits, but limited by side effects; new micro-emulsions under evaluation with better tolerability

Other agents

5HT reuptake inhibitors: give well tolerated and effective symptom relief in many Raynaud's patients; mechanism of action probably involves depletion of platelet serotonin

Surgical options include lumbar sympathectomy for lower limb symptoms and digital sympathectomy (adventectomy) for severely affected digits; cervical sympathectomy disappointing and only temporarily beneficial

Lifestyle adjustments (especially cold avoidance and cessation of smoking), silk lined gloves and chemical hand warmers often provide substantial benefit

---

A number of other approaches are being evaluated in clinical trials, such as high-dose immunosuppression with autologous peripheral stem cell rescue. There are currently no effective antifibrotic agents for established SSc, but a number are under development. They include biological therapies that neutralize key potential cytokines driving SSc, including transforming growth factor beta 1 (TGF-beta-1) and connective tissue growth factor (CTGF). Other biological approaches to immunomodulation have been used in SSc, including rituximab, abatacept and basiliximab. Some benefit has been suggested and other biological antirheumatic agents including infliximab and tocilizumab, targeting TNF-alpha and IL-6 respectively, have been used in small trials and case series.

Organ-based complications

The outcome of SSc is largely determined by the extent and severity of organ-based complications. Some of these are almost universal, such as oesophageal reflux or secondary Raynaud's phenomenon, while many of the severe complications occur in only around 10–15% of cases overall.

Pulmonary hypertension – Pulmonary hypertension (PH) is one of the largest causes of death directly attributable to SSc. Recent estimates suggest that 1–2% of patients with SSc develop PH per annum and that this risk continues for the duration of disease. This explains some of the variation in estimated prevalence from earlier studies. PH is defined by mean PA pressure of at least 25 mmHg and an elevated pulmonary vascular resistance. Precapillary PH, termed pulmonary arterial hypertension (PAH), accounts for approximately two-thirds of PH in SSc and is associated with a pulmonary artery wedge pressure (PAWP) no greater than 15 mmHg. PAH is treatable and should be regularly screened for in SSc.

The DETECT screening tool has been developed based upon statistical analysis of non-invasive tests to identify patients at risk of PAH. These patients should be referred for diagnostic right heart catheterization. Treatment depends on the level of symptoms, defined mainly by the degree of dyspnoea. All symptomatic cases should have targeted therapy, such as a phosphodiesterase type 5 (PDE5) inhibitor or an endothelin receptor antagonist. These agents have improved symptoms and are associated with improved long-term outcome. Other patients may have postcapillary PH, due to cardiac disease or PH secondary to hypoxia from severe interstitial lung fibrosis. However, it should be remembered that some lung fibrosis is common in SSc and may co-exist with PAH. Thus, PAH management is specialized and should be shared in partnership with a designated specialist PH centre.

Lung fibrosis – Interstitial lung fibrosis is a common internal organ manifestation of SSc (Figures 19.5 and 19.6). It is present in more than 30% of cases but may not be extensive or progressive. All SSc cases should be evaluated at diagnosis using lung function tests and if these are abnormal, with a restrictive pattern, or if there are any other suspicions then an HRCT should be performed. This represents the current gold standard for detecting parenchymal lung disease and allows the extent and pattern to be ascertained. Studies suggest that extensive disease, defined as more than 20% involvement of the total lung volume, is associated with a high risk of progression and these cases should be actively treated.

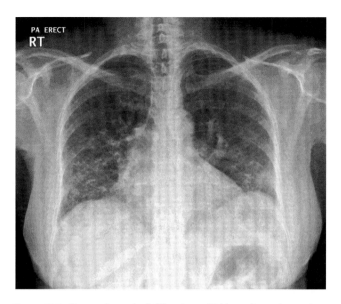

Figure 19.5 Chest radiograph of diffuse interstitial lung disease in a patient with scleroderma

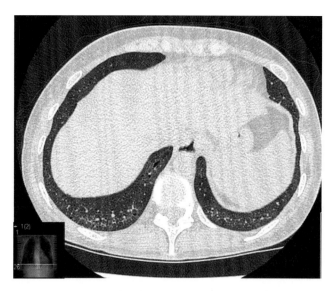

Figure 19.6 High-resolution computed tomography scan showing evidence of early interstitial lung disease

Management includes vigorous antireflux therapy that can reduce progression, possibly due to treatment of microaspiration. The cornerstone of treatment is immunosuppression and this is underpinned by supportive evidence from two placebo-controlled trials. These defined benefit for cyclophosphamide compared with placebo. Our practice is to add low-dose prednisolone, 10 mg daily, and other agents such as N-acetylcysteine may be useful. There is emerging evidence that rituximab may be used as a rescue treatment for cases that are refractory to treatment with other agents. Increasingly, mycophenolate mofetil (MMF) is used for maintenance treatment, mostly after a period of intravenous cyclophosphamide. Ongoing studies will determine whether MMF may be a reasonable first-line treatment in place of cyclophosphamide.

Some markers of lung disease are emerging. These include SSc-specific ANAs including antitopoisomerase 1 autoantibody, but also other reactivities such as anti-Th/To, especially in limited SSc and anti-U11/12. Levels of serum markers such as KL-6 may also be useful in assessing disease and add value to the HRCT in defined cases at increased risk of progression. Recently, IL-6 levels in serum have emerged as a potential additional marker of progression in SSc-associated lung fibrosis. Histologically, most cases of SSc-associated lung fibrosis are classified as non-specific interstitial pneumonia (NSIP), rather than the usual interstitial pneumonia (UIP) pattern of idiopathic lung fibrosis. This may explain the better outcome for most patients with SSc compared with idiopathic pulmonary fibrosis (IPF). Lung biopsy is not routinely performed in SSc-associated lung fibrosis with typical CT appearance although it may be useful in atypical cases or if there is concern about possible lung malignancy.

Scleroderma renal crisis (SRC) – There have been major advances in management of renal disease in SSc. The major problem is one of recognition, and education of both patients and physicians is important. SRC often presents non-specifically with headaches and visual disturbances before encephalopathy, cardiac failure or acute oliguric renal failure develop.

Treatment with angiotensin-converting enzyme (ACE) inhibition is mandatory. Patients should be admitted for blood pressure control and monitoring of renal function. Fifty percent of cases require dialysis, which is temporary in many individuals. There may be significant recovery in renal function for up to 2 years after renal crisis, and decisions regarding transplantation should be delayed until that time. There is no evidence that prophylactic administration of ACE inhibitors is helpful in preventing renal crisis or improving outcome. Three recent observational cohort studies suggest that cases have a worse long-term outcome if on ACE inhibitors at the time of SRC although the basis for this paradoxical finding is not clear.

The cornerstone of management, however, is patient education, vigilant blood pressure monitoring and avoidance of nephrotoxic drugs or high-dose corticosteroids, with prompt initiation of appropriate therapy early in the course of the SRC. When renal dysfunction occurs in SSc, it is important to consider other potential causes such as vasculitis or glomerulonephritis and a thorough serological and laboratory assessment is mandatory. ANCA positivity or serological features of SLE are important clues for an alternative renal pathology and should prompt early renal biopsy.

Gut disease – The gastrointestinal tract is the organ most frequently affected in SSc. Up to 90% of patients demonstrate oesophageal dysmotility with reflux, and the proton pump inhibitors have dramatically improved symptomatic disease. Strictures are now relatively rare, although vigilance for Barrett's metaplasia is required, with standard approaches to surveillance if confirmed histologically. Midgut disease with bacterial overgrowth may respond to broad-spectrum antibiotics, although maintenance treatment may be required. Paradoxically, colonic involvement may lead to severe constipation, and anorectal incontinence is prevalent. It is important that acute abdominal complications of SSc are managed conservatively as far as possible, because major abdominal surgery is poorly tolerated owing to SSc-related co-morbidity, prolonged postoperative ileus and poor healing.

Malignancy and systemic sclerosis – Although not a specific complication of SSc, it is important to be vigilant for the presence of concurrent malignant disease. Recently, a potential link between anti-RNA polymerase III ANA (ARA) and cancer has emerged. This may relate to altered expression of the antigen in tumours, especially breast or ovarian tumours. Interestingly, some of the hallmark 'red flags' for paraneoplastic scleroderma such as absence of a defined ANA (prior to testing for ARA), prominent finger contractures with palmar fibrosis and mild or absent Raynaud's at time of onset of skin disease (though often severe later) are hallmarks of ANA-positive SSc.

Conclusion

Scleroderma remains an important disease with high morbidity and mortality but one for which a number of treatments are now available and others are likely to be developed soon. Raynaud's phenomenon is an important clinical feature in SSc but more usually occurs in other contexts as a primary disease. It is a common and troublesome disorder that needs appropriate investigation and assessment. Outcomes are improving for SSc but still the worst forms of the disease are enormously challenging and greater focus is required for morbidity as well as mortality. Localized scleroderma should also be identified and treated.

Further reading

Burt RK, Shah SJ, Dill K *et al.* Autologous non-myeloablative haemopoietic stem-cell transplantation compared with pulse cyclophosphamide once per month for systemic sclerosis (ASSIST): an open-label, randomised phase 2 trial. *Lancet* 2011; **378**(9790): 498–506.

Coghlan JG, Denton CP, Grünig E *et al.*, on behalf of the DETECT Study Group. Evidence-based detection of pulmonary arterial hypertension in systemic sclerosis: the DETECT study. *Annals of the Rheumatic Diseases* 2014; **73**: 1340–1349.

Denton CP, Black CM. Scleroderma and related disorders: therapeutic aspects. *Baillière's Best Practice and Research: Clinical Rheumatology* 2000; **14**: 17–35.

Khanna D, Denton CP. Evidence-based management of rapidly progressing systemic sclerosis. *Best Practice and Research: Clinical Rheumatology* 2010; **24**(3): 387–400.

Koenig M, Joyal F, Fritzler MJ *et al.* Autoantibodies and microvascular damage are independent predictive factors for the progression of Raynaud's phenomenon to systemic sclerosis: a twenty-year prospective study of 586 patients, with validation of proposed criteria for early systemic sclerosis. *Arthritis and Rheumatism* 2008; **58**(12): 3902–3912.

LeRoy EC, Medsger TA Jr. Criteria for the classification of early systemic sclerosis. *Journal of Rheumatology* 2001; **28**: 1573–1576.

Nihtyanova SI, Denton CP. Autoantibodies as predictive tools in systemic sclerosis. *Nature Reviews Rheumatology* 2010; **6**(2): 112–116.

Van den Hoogen F, Khanna D, Fransen J *et al.* 2013 classification criteria for systemic sclerosis: an American College of Rheumatology/European League against Rheumatism collaborative initiative. *Arthritis and Rheumatism* 2013; **65**(11): 2737–2747.

Resource

Scleroderma and Raynaud's UK: www.sruk.co.uk

CHAPTER 20

Reflex Sympathetic Dystrophy

Chris Deighton[1] and Paul Davis[2]

[1] Derbyshire Royal Infirmary, Derby, UK
[2] University of Alberta, Edmonton, Canada

OVERVIEW

- Reflex sympathetic dystrophy (RSD) is a descriptive term for a condition mainly affecting the limbs, with severe pain, a preceding event that might be relatively trivial in traumatic terms, and abnormal blood flow and sweating in the affected area.

- Eventual structural changes to superficial and deep structures lead to atrophic, shiny skin, contractures and patchy osteoporosis around joints on X-rays.

- The cause is not clearly understood, but probably a variety of central and peripheral voluntary and involuntary neurological pathways play a part.

- The diagnosis is usually clinical, although X-rays and bone scans may show a characteristic appearance.

- Treatment is empirical, but relies on pain reduction, early mobilization and restoration of function. Further randomized controlled trials are needed to improve the therapeutics of this difficult condition.

Introduction

Reflex sympathetic (osteo)dystrophy (RSD) is a descriptive term for a poorly understood clinical condition of unknown aetiology. It has also been variously termed shoulder-hand syndrome, Sudeck's atrophy and algodystrophy. It has often been confused and compared with causalgia, a different condition with similar clinical symptoms. Generally speaking, the more words used in the description of a condition, the less we understand that condition. In 1993, it was suggested that reflex sympathetic dystrophy be renamed 'complex regional pain syndrome (CRPS) type I'. This change in nomenclature has done little to reassure the non-specialist that our understanding of the condition has substantially improved. The change in terminology has also failed to catch on, so that many specialists still refer to RSD, even though it is clear that the reflexes are not necessarily involved, and the sympathetic nervous system cannot be implicated in many patients (for example, sympathetic ganglia blockade only relieves the pain in some patients).

To have the 'full house' clinically, the following should be present: (a) severe pain, usually starting peripherally, and working more proximally over time in a non-dermatomal fashion (allodynia) – the pain is disproportionate to the triggering event and clinical findings (hyperpathia); (b) usually a preceding event that might be relatively trivial in traumatic terms; (c) abnormal blood flow to the affected area(usually a limb),with colour changes (blues, whites and reds) and oedema; (d) abnormal sweating in the area; (e) changes in the motor system, with weakness and some- times tremor; (f) eventual structural changes to superficial and deep structures leading to atrophic, shiny skin, contractures and patchy osteoporosis around joints on X-rays.

Although diagnostic criteria have been proposed, these have not been validated and are complicated by the fact that not all features may be present at the same time and may vary in their intensity. The condition tends to affect upper limbs more commonly than lower limbs. Usually one limb is affected, but it can become bilateral, or affect another limb. It is usually most evident distally (hand and wrist, or foot and ankle), but a whole limb can be affected, such as in 'shoulder-hand syndrome'.

This chapter explores the following areas: What causes RSD? How is RSD diagnosed? What is the treatment of RSD?

What causes RSD?

The cause of RSD is far from understood, but it appears to involve an exaggeration of normal physiological responses and involves changes at multiple levels in the central and peripheral nervous systems. Some epidemiological features of RSD are shown in Box 20.1. Taking total knee arthroplasty as an example, a prevalence of between 0.8% and 1.2% of persistent RSD has been quoted. However, a recent prospective study suggested that 21% of patients fulfilled diagnostic criteria 1 month after operation, falling to 12.7% at 6 months, suggesting that symptoms and signs of RSD are not uncommon after operation, but persistent full-blown disease is mercifully unusual. Figures of up to 35% and 5% have been reported for Colles' fracture and peripheral nerve injury, respectively. The pathology of RSD is bedevilled by the lack of tissue studies, either pre- or post-mortem. Limited histological investigations have suggested that microangiopathy or other

ABC of Rheumatology, Fifth Edition. Edited by Ade Adebajo and Lisa Dunkley.
© 2018 John Wiley & Sons Ltd. Published 2018 by John Wiley & Sons Ltd.

Box 20.1 **Some epidemiological factors in reflex sympathetic dystrophy**

Triggers	**Usually some noxious event such as:** Wrist and tibial fractures (about 30% may demonstrate mild features, but only a minority go on to severe disease) Trauma: mild or moderate Rotator cuff tendonitis or subacromial bursitis Surgery: carpal tunnel decompression, arthroscopy, arthroplasty, lumbar spine surgery Central nervous system disorders: head injury, hemiplegia, spinal cord injury, neuropathy Myocardial infarction Immobilization: in any of the above may be an important factor
Sex	More common in women than men, with a ratio of 3:1 quoted
Age	Any age, although the mean in some studies is quoted as 52 years; now well recognized in children
Genetics	Some evidence to support a familial predisposition
Personality traits	No convincing evidence to support an association
Psychological factors	Some patients can have motor weakness and movement disorders relieved by placebo, nerve blocks or infusions

Table 20.1 Treatment modalities for RSD.

Medical	Rehabilitation	Psychological
Medications NSAIDs	Motivation	Counselling
Opioids Tricyclics	Desensitization	Behaviour
Adrenoceptor	Isometric exercises	modification
antagonists	Mobilization Flexibility	Coping skills
Corticosteroids	Strength exercises	Relaxation therapy
Calcitonin		Hypnosis
Neurological blocks		
Sympathetic Regional		
Epidural		
Neurostimulation		
Peripheral Epidural		

Source: Modified and simplified from Stanton-Hicks et al. (2002)

vascular abnormalities may be a key driver. A crucial question that has not been satisfactorily answered is: Why do the majority of patients who suffer the potential triggers listed in Table 20.1 make a full and uneventful recovery, but a minority go on to develop RSD? A number of theories have been propounded, but revolve around peripheral mechanisms, central mechanisms and neurogenic inflammation with microvascular dysfunction. These interrelate in a series of vicious circles that result in the characteristic features of RSD, which are summarized below.

Peripheral mechanisms – Trauma to C fibres and A afferents is likely to be an initiating event. Many patients have sympathetically maintained pain, which may activate both mechanoreceptors and nociceptors. Some patients experience benefit from alpha block-ade, supporting a role for adrenoceptors in the pathogenesis of RSD. These receptors become expressed on nociceptors in some cases of soft tissue and nerve injury. Some patients demonstrate supersensitivity to catecholamines, consistent with increased adrenoceptor responsiveness.

Central mechanisms – In RSD an initial activation of nociceptors may lead to alteration of central information processes, resulting in central sensitization. Patients exhibit normal thresholds for the detection of cold and heat, but reduced thresholds for cold-pain and heat-pain, suggesting a central nervous disturbance. Activation of low-threshold mechanoreceptors is interpreted as noxious, and results in normal sensations being interpreted as painful ('allo-dynia'). There is a close similarity between the autonomic features of RSD and those of autonomic failure after stroke. The latter occur in the absence of pain, suggesting an uncoupling of the mecha-nisms that under pin the pain and sensory symptoms from the autonomic features. Tests on normal volunteers that create conflict between motor sensory central nervous processing can lead to pain and sensory disturbances, such as using mirrors during congruent and incongruent limb movements. It has been proposed that central processing of persistent sensory motor conflict may lead to chronic pain in some vulnerable individuals.

Neurogenic inflammation – Release of vasoactive peptides, including substance P and calcitonin gene-related peptide, from afferent nerve fibres causes vasodilatation, with increased vascular permeability and protein leakage. Neuropetides may also be released in response to impaired blood flow, oxygen deficiency and an increase in pro-tons and skin lactate levels. This might explain why some of the early clinical features of RSD appear to be inflammatory.

Microvascular dysfunction – A number of investigators have con-firmed microvascular dysfunction in RSD, although it remains unknown whether these changes, reflected by colour and tempera-ture changes, drive the disease process or are secondary to it.

Bringing these factors together, it has been suggested that RSD is initiated by trauma to C fibres and A afferents in soft tissue or nerves, resulting in neurogenic inflammation. Signs of inflammation pre-dominate in early disease, with redness, increased skin temperature due to inhibition of cutaneous vasoconstrictor neurons, with subse-quent loss of function and pain. Early in the disease, the sympathetic nervous system plays a role, but when central sensitization takes over, with changes at the dorsal root ganglion level, the pain becomes independent of sympathetic nerves. There is competition between the continued inhibition of vasoconstriction and supersensitivity of the peripheral vessels to circulating adrenaline. Late intractable disease can be characterized by a cold, painful limb with poor or no function, with disuse leading to immobility and contractures.

How is RSD diagnosed?

In the early stages of RSD the limb is swollen and tender, and the diagnosis may not be straightforward, as it can mimic many other diseases, such as inflammatory arthritis, cellulitis, osteomyelitis, deep venous thrombosis, lymphatic obstruction and malignancy. In the late intractable disease, when the limb becomes cold, chronic arterial insufficiency needs to be considered.

There is no diagnostic test for RSD, and tests are only required to rule out the other causes of a painful swollen limb as listed above. Routine investigations, such as a full blood count and erythrocyte sedimentation rate should be normal, and if not an explanation should be sought. In terms of positive features supporting RSD (Box 20.2), X-rays may show patchy osteoporosis, especially in the juxta-articular region. Joint space is usually preserved, but may be lost in late disease with ankylosis. On bone scanning there is increased uptake in early disease and reduced uptake in late disease. Patients with markedly increased uptake may have a better prognosis, possibly reflecting the fact that they have not yet progressed to late-stage disease. Thermography detects asymmetry in limb surface temperature, but is not widely available. Bone densitometry and magnetic resonance imaging (MRI) may show non-specific changes, such as reduced bone density, soft tissue swelling and bone marrow oedema, but nothing specific to positively diagnose RSD. The greatest value of MRI is to rule out other causes of a painful swollen limb.

How is RSD treated?

Owing to our limited understanding of the aetiology and pathogenesis of RSD, much of the therapeutics is empirical, and what helps one patient may not help others. Because established RSD can be very challenging to treat, emphasis has been placed on prevention where possible and, failing that, early intervention. The main aims are to reduce pain and restore function. Early mobilization following predisposing conditions is important, and graded physiotherapy may be very helpful. A trial in 1999 showed that vitamin C, a powerful antioxidant, may prevent RSD, supporting the growing evidence for the role of oxygen free radicals in RSD. This needs to be researched further.

Patients who are particularly vulnerable are those with a previous history of RSD, particularly if they require surgery on the previously affected part. A controlled study found that the risk of RSD could be reduced by a stellate ganglion block after the operation. An uncontrolled study suggested preoperative calcitonin may prevent recurrence.

Although many experts and committees have recommended physiotherapy, occupational therapy, vocational rehabilitation and behavioural therapy, the evidence base for these is weak or lacking. One study compared physiotherapy and occupational therapy with social work intervention as the control, and showed no differences in the three groups for pain at 12 months, with only small improvements in temperature and global impairment for the intervention arms of the trial. An algorithm of treatment has been proposed by Stanton-Hicks *et al.* (2002) with a cautious start (heat, massage and gentle movement to restore normal sensory processing), then isometric exercises for strengthening, treatment of secondary myofascial pain syndrome, aerobic conditioning, through to complete functional rehabilitation. Because pain can be the main rate-limiting factor in rehabilitation, medical and psychological therapies often have to run side by side (Table 20.1).

The mainstay of drug interventions is analgesics and non-steroidal anti-inflammatories. Low-dose antidepressants and anticonvulsants are commonly used, but the evidence base is sparse. A systematic review of therapies concluded that the only trial data that consistently demonstrated analgesia was with oral corticosteroids. However, many clinicians have understandable concerns about using steroids for disease that has the potential to become chronic, and where the evidence base for ongoing inflammation driving the disease is limited. A plethora of other drugs have been tried in RSD, which is testimony to the difficulties in treating the condition. Intranasal calcitonin has shown conflicting results. Drugs that do show promise are the bisphosphonates, justified initially on osteoporosis being a significant feature of RSD. A controlled trial of alendronate showed improved bone mineral content of the affected limb, but only small benefits to pain management. By contrast, a trial of intravenous clodronate showed substantial improvements in pain management at 6 months, with highly significant pain reduction compared with placebo.

The role of sympathetic blockade is controversial. For paravertebral blockade, the stellate ganglion for upper limb RSD is locked with a series of local anaesthetics, depending on response, and the lumbar sympathetic chain for lower limb RSD. Another technique is intravenous blockade, usually with guanethidine. However, a systematic review found this treatment to be ineffective, so its use may decline in future. Continuous blockade of the brachial or lumbar plexus has been advocated with drugs such as morphine, so that whenever the catheter is in place, the patient can take advantage of the pain relief to maximize their rehabilitation.

Intrathecal baclofen proved to be effective for the upper limb dystonias in six out of seven patients, but did not improve pain. Spinal cord stimulation has been shown to be effective in relieving pain in controlled trials. The procedure is, however, not without risk, as it involves placing an electrode on the dorsal aspect of the spinal cord, and an electric current produces paraesthesias that block the pain in the affected area. However, the average improvement in pain is sustained but not substantial, and functional and quality-of-life benefits have not been demonstrated. This leaves the dilemma of whether invasive and costly interventions that provide modest pain relief are justified. Clearly, these concerns and the risks involved mean that patients have to be carefully selected.

Reference

Stanton-Hicks MD, Burton AW, Bruehl SP et al. An updated interdisciplinary clinical pathway for CRPS: report of an expert panel. *Pain Practice* 2002; **2**(1): 1–16.

Further reading

Bean DJ, Johnson MH, Kydd RR. The outcome of complex regional pain type 1: a systematic review. *Journal of Pain* 2014; **15**: 677–690.

Cossins L, Okell RW, Cameron H, Simpson B, Poole HM, Goebel A. Treatment of complex regional pain syndrome in adults: a systematic review of randomized controlled trials published from June 2000 to February 2012. *European Journal of Pain* 2013; **17**: 158–173.

Field J. Complex regional pain syndrome: a review. *Journal of Hand Surgery* 2013; **38**: 616–626.

Freedman M, Greis AC, Marino L, Sinha AN, Henstenburg J. Complex regional pain syndrome: diagnosis and treatment. *Physical Medicine and Rehabilitation Clinics of North America* 2014; **25**: 291–303.

Harden RN, Oaklander AL, Burton AW *et al.* Complex regional pain syndrome: practical diagnostic and treatment guidelines, 4th edn. *Pain Medicine* 2013: **14**: 180–229.

Goebel A. Complex regional pain syndrome in adults. *Rheumatology* 2011; **50**: 1739–1750.

Wertli MM, Kessels AG, Perez RS, Bachmann LM, Brunner F. Rational pain management in complex regional pain syndrome 1 (CRPS 1) – a network meta-analysis. *Pain Medicine* 2014; **15**: 1575–1589.

CHAPTER 21

Is It an Autoimmune Rheumatic Disease?

Mohammed Tikly[1] and David D'Cruz[2]

[1] Chris Hani Baragwanath Academic Hospital and University of the Witwatersrand, Johannesburg, South Africa
[2] Louise Coote Lupus Unit, Guys and St Thomas' Hospitals, London, UK

OVERVIEW

- Raynaud's phenomenon, arthralgia and sicca symptoms are common presenting features of autoimmune rheumatic diseases.

- The indirect immunofluorescence test is sufficient as a screening test for antinuclear antibodies, which are the serological hallmark of autoimmune rheumatic diseases.

- Patients frequently present initially with non-specific features of an autoimmune rheumatic disease but do not fulfil criteria for any specific disorder.

- Less than one-third of patients with undifferentiated autoimmune rheumatic diseases evolve clinically to fulfil classification criteria for a classifiable autoimmune rheumatic disease.

- It is important to recognize and treat potentially aggressive disease, and to avoid overtreatment where the diagnosis is unclear or the disease has a potentially benign course.

Systemic autoimmune rheumatic diseases, also commonly referred to as connective tissue diseases, are immune-mediated inflammatory disorders associated with autoantibodies. The diagnosis of these disorders, such as systemic lupus erythematosus and scleroderma, can be challenging because many of the presenting clinical features are non-specific and this often results in delayed diagnosis. Classification criteria for the major systemic autoimmune rheumatic diseases (see Chapters 12 and 18) have been developed primarily as a means of standardizing patient populations for clinical research rather than for diagnosis in routine clinical practice. These classification criteria are extremely limited for the early diagnosis of these disorders as they were designed to be highly specific and therefore lack diagnostic sensitivity.

In patients presenting with non-specific symptoms and signs, such as Raynaud's phenomenon, inflammatory arthritis, sicca symptoms and constitutional symptoms of fever, malaise and fatigue, it is often not possible to make a definitive diagnosis of a specific autoimmune rheumatic disease, especially early in the course of the illness (Box 21.1, Figure 21.1). Most patients over a period of months, or sometimes, years, fulfil classification criteria for one or more of the major systemic autoimmune rheumatic diseases. From a management perspective, it is important not only to recognize and treat potentially aggressive disease, but also to avoid overtreatment in patients where either the diagnosis is unclear or the disease has a potentially benign course.

Autoantibody profile in diagnosis

Antinuclear antibodies are a hallmark of systemic autoimmune rheumatic diseases and can be found in a variety of clinical settings. However, their occurrence does not necessarily indicate the presence of any specific disease – they are thus sensitive but not specific diagnostically. Serology is of particular value in situations where clinical expression of the autoimmune rheumatic disease is incomplete, where the presence of a particular antinuclear antibody profile may be diagnostic. It is therefore imperative that requests for antinuclear antibody tests and the interpretation of the results be done in the light of clinical findings.

The indirect immunofluorescence test, using the HEp2 cell substrate, is the gold standard for detecting antinuclear antibodies (Table 21.1). In systemic lupus erythematosus and scleroderma, antinuclear antibodies can be detected in 95% or more of untreated patients with active disease by this method. In patients suspected of having an autoimmune rheumatic disease, the indirect immunoflourescence test is enough as a screening test for antinuclear antibodies. It is not cost-effective to test automatically for anti-dsDNA or other antibody specificities. The individual antinuclear antibody fluorescent patterns are of limited diagnostic utility but may provide guidance to more specific immunological tests. A false negative antinuclear antibody test result sometimes occurs if either the antigen is outside the nucleus (for example, anti Jo-1 and anti-ribosomal P protein antibodies, both often categorized under the umbrella term 'antinuclear antibodies') or if it is present in a form not recognized by a particular autoantibody (for example, when anti-Ro is directed exclusively to determinants on the native Ro molecule not expressed in cultured HEp2 cells). In such cases, the clinical picture dictates that specific autoantibody assays should be undertaken.

Having detected antinuclear antibodies with the screening test, it is important to determine their specificity. This is part of the standard

---

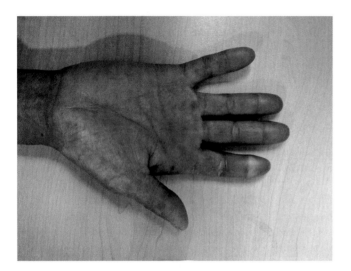

Figure 21.1 Raynaud's phenonenon with thumb involvement in scleroderma

Table 21.1 Antinuclear antibodies in various diseases detected by indirect immunofluorescence

Condition	Frequency of antinuclear antibodies (%)
Systemic autoimmune rheumatic diseases	
Drug-induced lupus	100
Systemic lupus erythematosus	98
Scleroderma	95
Sjögren's syndrome	80
Pauciarticular juvenile idiopathic arthritis	70
Polymyositis or dermatomyositis	60
Rheumatoid arthritis	20
Organ-specific autoimmune diseases	
Primary autoimmune cholangitis	100
Autoimmune hepatitis	70
Myasthenia gravis	50
Autoimmune thyroid disease	45
Idiopathic pulmonary hypertension	30
Other conditions	
Waldenstrom's macroglobulinaemia	20
Subacute bacterial endocarditis	20
Infectious mononucleosis	15
Leprosy	15
HIV	10
Normal population	
Children	8
Adults	15

operating procedure of serology laboratories, but the process is greatly facilitated by the clinician giving sufficient clinical information when requesting the antinuclear antibody test. Specific antinuclear antibody tests are often helpful in stratifying patients into clinical subsets, which may be useful in the further management of specific clinical manifestations and prognostication (Table 21.2). These autoantibodies are usually present from the beginning of the clinical presentation and are detectable throughout the course of the disease. Some studies have shown that autoantibodies may be present for many years prior to clinical presentation. In some instances, such as the anti-dsDNA test, autoantibody titres may fluctuate with disease activity. Many serology laboratories use commercial kits to detect specific autoantibodies and there is a move to using bead-based multiplex immunoassays. Although the newer tests are less labour intensive, they vary in sensitivity and sometimes produce false-positive results. This is especially the case with the anti-dsDNA, anti-Ro-52 and anti-Sm assays.

Which systemic autoimmune rheumatic disease?

Although the clinical presentation in the early stages can be similar between the systemic autoimmune rheumatic diseases, the evolution of typical clinical features over weeks or months usually distinguishes

the characteristic patterns associated with the different diseases. Early diagnosis is aided by recognition of distinctive serological profiles that are generally present with the earliest clinical manifestations. Diagnosis can also be facilitated by typical laboratory abnormalities and histological changes in the tissues involved. For example, microscopic polyangiitis presenting with weight loss, fever, polyarthritis and active urinary sediment can be distinguished from lupus by an autoimmune response characterized by p-ANCA antibodies directed against myeloperoxidase and the typical histological picture of pauci-immune focal necrotizing glomerulonephritis. Similarly, clinically amyopathic dermatomyositis that presents with photosensitive eruptions on the face, arms and hands and is associated with myalgia can be distinguished from lupus by the distribution of the skin eruption, a raised serum creatine kinase, anti-MDA5 and other myositis antibodies and typical changes on muscle biopsy, despite the absence of frank muscle weakness.

Diagnosis is often complicated if lupus is part of an overlap syndrome and the patient fulfils classification criteria for more than one systemic autoimmune rheumatic disease. Sometimes the overlap features are evident at initial presentation; at other times, the picture evolves sequentially. Patients who fulfil criteria for both systemic lupus erythematosus and rheumatoid arthritis are sometimes referred to as having 'rhupus'. These patients are usually diagnosed as having rheumatoid arthritis initially because of typical rheumatoid features

Table 21.2 Specificity of autoantibodies in diagnosis and disease expression

Disease	Antibody	Frequency (%)	Clinical association
Systemic lupus erythematous	Anti-dsDNA‡	70	Lupus nephritis
	Anti-nucleosome	70	Early disease, lupus nephritis, drug-induced lupus
	Anti-Sm	10–25*	Vasculitis, neuropsychiatric lupus
	Anti-U1RNP	30-50*	Raynaud's phenomenon, swollen fingers, arthritis, myositis, mixed connective tissue disease
	Anti-Ro	40	Photosensitive rash, subacute cutaneous lupus erythematosus, neonatal lupus, congenital heart block, Sjögren's syndrome
	Anti-La	15	As for anti-Ro
	Antiribosomal P protein	15	Neuropsychiatric lupus (psychosis or depression)
Sjögren's syndrome	Anti-Ro	60–90†	Extraglandular disease, vasculitis, lymphoma
	Anti-La	35–85†	As for anti-Ro
Systemic sclerosis	Anticentromere	5–30#	Limited cutaneous disease, microvascular or macrovascular disease, telangiectasia, pulmonary hypertension
	Antitopoisomerase 1 (anti-Scl-70)	25	Diffuse cutaneous disease, interstitial lung disease
	Anti-RNA polymerases	20	Rapidly progressive diffuse cutaneous disease, scleroderma renal crisis
	Antifibrillarin (anti-U3RNP)	5–20*	Diffuse cutaneous disease in blacks, pulmonary hypertension
	Anti-ThRNP	4	Limited cutaneous disease
	Anti-PM-Scl	5	Scleroderma-polymyositis overlap
	Anti-Ku	2	Scleroderma-polymyositis overlap
Dermatomyositis and polymyositis	Anti-Jo-1	30	Antisynthetase syndrome: mechanic's hands, interstitial lung disease
	(antibodies to other tRNA synthetases)	(3)	(antisynthetase syndrome)
	Anti-SRP	4	Severe necrotizing myositis
	Anti-Mi2	10	Dermatomyositis
	Anti-TIF-1	50	Cancer-associated myositis
	Anti-MDA5	50	Clinically amyopathic dermatomyositis with interstitial lung disease
Systemic ANCA-associated vasculitis**	cANCA/antiproteinase 3	80–90	Granulomatosis with polyangiitis (Wegener's granulomatosis)
	pANCA/antimyeloperoxidase	90	Microscopic polyangiitis

‡ Anti-double-stranded DNA antibody.
* Higher frequency in people of African or Indian origin.
† With sensitive enzyme-linked immunosorbent assays.
# Low frequency in people of African origin.
** Antineutrophil cytoplasmic antibodies.

such as erosive arthritis, subcutaneous nodules and rheumatoid factor. An overlap syndrome should be considered when these features are accompanied by cutaneous, renal, haematological or other clinical manifestations characteristic of systemic lupus erythematosus and the presence of anti-dsDNA antibodies.

Development of Sjögren's syndrome during the course of systemic lupus erythematosus is well established but occasionally, patients with primary Sjögren's syndrome develop typical features of lupus, especially photosensitive eruptions typical of subacute cutaneous lupus erythematosus, after many years of disease.

A distinctive type of overlap syndrome is that of 'mixed connective tissue disease' (Box 21.2). Here patients have an overlap of puffy fingers of early scleroderma (Figure 21.2), systemic lupus erythematosus, polymyositis, and a characteristic serological profile that includes high levels of antibodies to U1RNP. However, there is much controversy as to whether this is a distinct systemic rheumatic disease, with critics and protagonists.

The concept of 'undifferentiated connective tissue disease', as opposed to 'mixed connective tissue disease', was coined by LeRoy

Box 21.2 Terminology

Undifferentiated connective disease	Rheumatic symptoms and signs with autoantibodies, but not meeting the criteria for a specific systemic autoimmune rheumatic disease
Overlap syndrome	Patients meet criteria for two or more systemic autoimmune rheumatic diseases
Mixed connective tissue disease	Specific overlap syndrome of rheumatoid arthritis-like arthritis, systemic lupus erythematosus, scleroderma and inflammatory myositis with antibodies to U1RNP

and colleagues in 1980 (Box 21.3). It refers to patients who present with symptoms and laboratory features of systemic autoimmune disease but who do not fulfil criteria for any specific systemic autoimmune rheumatic disorder. Long-term, prospective follow-up

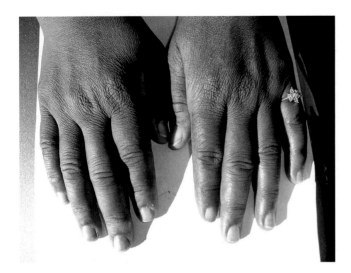

Figure 21.2 Swollen 'puffy' fingers of patient with undifferentiated autoimmune rheumatic disease

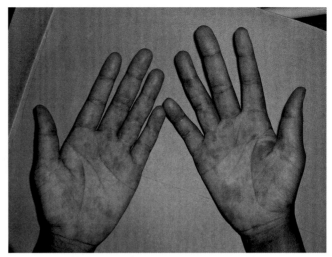

Figure 21.3 Hand vasculitis seen in systemic lupus erythematosus and dermatomyositis

> Box 21.3 **Characteristics of 'undifferentiated autoimmune rheumatic disease'**
>
> - Comprise 25–50% of referrals for autoimmune rheumatic disease
> - Common manifestations:
>   - Raynaud's phenomenon
>   - Arthralgia or myalgia
>   - Rash
>   - Sicca symptoms
>   - Constitutional symptoms (fever, malaise, and fatigue)
> - One-third evolve into a defined systemic autoimmune rheumatic disease, usually within 2 years

studies show that these patients represent a sizeable proportion (25–50%) of patients presenting to autoimmune rheumatic disease clinics. Only a minority of these patients, about 30% in the larger studies, evolve clinically to fulfil classification criteria of a defined autoimmune rheumatic disease. Spontaneous remission occurs in 5–10% of patients and in the majority of patients the undifferentiated connective disease state persists. Importantly, major organ involvement is rare in these patients.

Differential diagnosis

A common clinical conundrum is the distinction of systemic lupus erythematosus from other systemic autoimmune rheumatic diseases. A careful history and physical examination (Figures 21.3 and 21.4), urine analysis, chest X-ray, laboratory tests for an acute-phase response, blood count, serum biochemistry, complement levels, creatine kinase and serological profile, however, results in the correct diagnosis in a high proportion of cases.

Drug-induced lupus

A carefully elicited drug history is essential to exclude drug-induced lupus. The management of this is very straightforward, involving

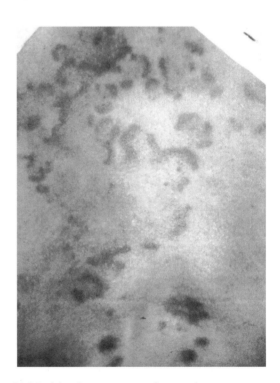

Figure 21.4 Rash in subacute cutaneous lupus erythematosus

discontinuation of the offending agent and short-term anti-inflammatory treatment. Procainamide and hydralazine carry the highest risk of inducing a lupus-like syndrome but are now seldom prescribed in clinical practice. In more recent years, several cases of drug-induced lupus have been reported in association with minocycline, which is often prescribed for acne, and sulfasalazine, a disease-modifying antirheumatic drug in rheumatoid arthritis, although the individual risk of drug-induced lupus is low with these agents.

In the context of rheumatoid arthritis, the diagnosis is sometimes difficult to make, particularly as antinuclear antibodies are present in up to 50% of patients with the condition. Drug-induced lupus is rare in people of African origin.

The clinical presentation is similar to that of idiopathic systemic lupus erythematosus, with systemic features including fever and weight loss, arthralgia or frank arthritis and serositis (particularly common with procainamide). Major organ involvement, such as nephritis and central nervous system manifestations, is less common, although renal disease can rarely occur in sulfasalazine-induced lupus. A high level of antinuclear antibodies usually shows a homogeneous pattern from the earliest presentation, and the typical preponderance of antihistone antibodies can be shown with specific assays. Antibodies to dsDNA and 'extractable nuclear antigens', commonly associated with idiopathic systemic lupus erythematosus, are invariably negative, except in the case of minocycline-induced lupus. The gold standard for diagnosis of drug-induced lupus, however, is that it resolves after the drug is stopped; the symptoms improve within days to weeks, although the antinuclear antibodies may take a year or two to disappear.

The anti-TNF agents, mainly when used in the treatment of rheumatoid arthritis but also for Crohn's disease and ankylosing spondylitis, can also rarely induce antinuclear antibody and anti-dsDNA antibody production. This phenomenon has been observed with all the anti-TNF agents currently on the market. Only a very small proportion of patients develop a lupus-like illness, manifesting mainly with skin changes, ranging from malar rash, discoid lupus and photosensitivity, worsening polyarthritis and serositis. The illness is usually mild, rarely associated with kidney disease, and resolves on discontinuation of the anti-TNF agent. As in the case of sulfasalazine-induced lupus, diagnosis can be challenging in patients with rheumatoid arthritis who have pre-existing antinuclear antibodies.

Other disorders of the skin

One of the most common conundrums is the patient referred with a history of photosensitivity or red face in association with musculoskeletal symptoms and, perhaps, systemic features such as fatigue. Photosensitive eruptions are common in the normal female population or may be induced by, for example, non-steroidal anti-inflammatory drugs. About 10% of women develop polymorphic light eruption, a pruritic papular eruption that occurs within hours of sun exposure, typically on normally covered sites, that spares the face and hands, and that resolves within days without epidermal change (Figure 21.5). In contrast, photosensitivity in systemic lupus erythematosus also affects the face and hands. The latent period after sun exposure is usually longer, the skin is less pruritic, and the eruption persists for longer.

Similarly, facial erythematous rashes that are seen typically in patients with systemic lupus erythematosus must be distinguished from other causes. Benign lymphocytic infiltration, such as Jessner's, may produce papular or annular lesions that are indistinguishable clinically from subacute cutaneous lupus erythematosus and papular lupus erythematosus (Figure 21.6). The typical histological appearance includes a dense dermal lymphocytic infiltrate without the characteristic epidermal changes of lupus. Typical rosacea consists of papulopustular lesions on a background of telangiectasia (Figure 21.7). Sometimes, light exposure aggravates this condition and a biopsy may be needed to distinguish atypical forms from lupus. Seborrhoeic dermatitis may affect the cheeks and

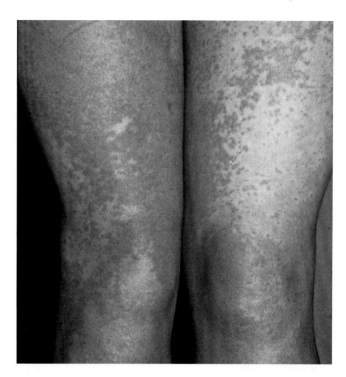

Figure 21.5 Polymorphic light eruption

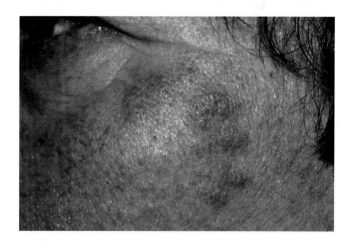

Figure 21.6 Papular light eruption and Jessner's

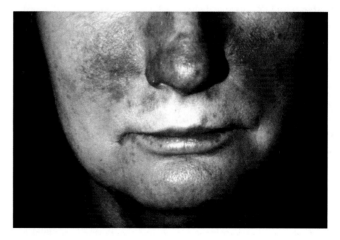

Figure 21.7 Rosacea papules and pustules

Table 21.3 Distinguishing features of systemic autoimmune rheumatic diseases and disorders that mimic them

Condition	Distinguishing features
Systemic autoimmune rheumatic diseases	
Rheumatoid arthritis	Erosive inflammatory polyarthritis; multisystem involvement uncommon at presentation; rarely antinuclear antibodies
Scleroderma	Pronounced Raynaud's phenomenon; digital ischaemia; sclerodactyly; nailfold capillary changes; characteristic serological profile
Dermatomyositis	Distinctive pattern of skin eruption; prominent muscle involvement; specific serological profile
Primary systemic vasculitis	Distinctive renal involvement; neutrophilia (sometimes eosinophilia); serological profile
Behçet's syndrome	Oral and genital ulcers; absence of autoantibodies
Adult-onset Still's disease	Intermittent late afternoon fever accompanied by transient erythematous maculopapular rash; absence of autoantibodies
Autoinflammatory syndromes (hereditary periodic fever syndromes, familial Mediterranean fever, hyperimmunoglobulin D)	Intermittent rashes, fever and serositis; raised CRP; absence of autoantibodies
Other systemic disorders	
Autoimmune hepatitis	Typical liver involvement; absence of typical lupus features; can be associated with primary Sjögren's syndrome
Sarcoidosis	Typical histology; absence of autoantibodies
Histiocytic necrotizing lymphadenitis (Kikuchi–Fujimoto's disease)	Typical histology; lymphadenopathy, fever, neutropenia and occasional antinuclear antibodies
IgG4 disease	Parotomegaly; pancreatitis; interstitial nephritis; aortitis; typical histology; absence of autoantibodies
Angioimmunoblastic lymphadenopathy	Typical histology; absence of autoantibodies
Other causes of photosensitivity and red face	
Polymorphic light eruption	Lack of systemic features; different histology; absence of autoantibodies
Rosacea	Papulopustular eruption; non-systemic; absence of autoantibodies
Seborrhoeic dermatitis	Different morphology and histology; non-systemic; absence of autoantibodies
Contact dermatitis	History of allergen contact; pseudovesicle; no autoantibodies
Jessner's benign lymphocytic infiltration	Typical histology; no autoantibodies
Erythrohepatic protoporphyria	Vesicobullous lesions; urinary and plasma porphyrin profile; no autoantibodies
Syphilis	Typical histology; diagnostic serology;
Lupus vulgaris	Painful nodular cutaneous form of tuberculosis
Other causes of fatigue and musculoskeletal pain	
Fibromyalgia	No objective inflammation; normal acute-phase reactants; absence of autoantibodies
Hypothyroidism	Little objective inflammation. May have Raynaud's phenomenon and carpal tunnel syndrome

paranasal folds and is usually pruritic and associated with desquamation. Contact dermatitis, which may be caused by cosmetics, produces superficial erythema, pseudovesicles and sometimes eyelid swelling. Lupus vulgaris, a painful nodular cutaneous form of tuberculosis, often affects skin over the nose and ears.

Fibromyalgia

Fibromyalgia syndrome (see Chapter XX) is often mistaken for lupus, especially if the antinuclear antibody test is also positive, and sometimes is treated inappropriately with, for example, corticosteroids. In addition, a significant proportion of people with fibromyalgia have other features that could be interpreted as manifestations of a systemic autoimmune rheumatic disease such as Raynaud's phenomenon, sicca symptoms and cognitive dysfunction. In those mistakenly treated with corticosteroids, although no evidence

shows therapeutic efficacy in fibromyalgia, corticosteroid withdrawal can make the symptoms worse. No evidence exists of an increased prevalence of positive antinuclear antibodies or the occurrence of autoimmune rheumatic disease in patients with fibromyalgia. It has become increasingly apparent, however, that systemic lupus erythematosus and Sjögren's syndrome may be associated with fibromyalgia which makes a considerable contribution to morbidity but is unrelated to the activity of the disease.

Endocrine disorders

Hypothyroidism can mimic an autoimmune rheumatic disease because of non-specific symptoms of malaise, arthralgia and myalgia, which may be further confounded by Raynaud's phenomenon and carpal tunnel syndrome. The diagnosis should be considered in the peri- and postmenopausal patient in whom acute-phase reactants are normal and rheumatoid factor and antinuclear antibody tests are negative.

Diabetic cheiropathy is seen especially in patients with longstanding, poorly controlled type 1 diabetes. It causes painless generalized puffiness and induration of the fingers resembling scleroderma. An inability to fully extend the fingers produces the so-called 'prayer sign'. Optimal glycaemic control and exercises may prevent worsening. Scleredema, another mimic of scleroderma in poorly controlled diabetes, presents as a thickened, indurated infiltrative skin disease. Unlike scleroderma, it occurs mostly on the upper back and is not associated with either Raynaud's phenomenon or antinuclear antibodies. It often clears spontaneously with good glyacaemic control.

Is it infection?

Some infections can mimic autoimmune rheumatic disease, especially systemic lupus erythematosus; these include HIV, syphilis, tuberculosis and persistent Epstein–Barr virus, parvovirus and cytomegalovirus infections (Table 21.3). They can present with mucocutaneous manifestations, fever, malaise, polyarthralgia, lymphadenopathy and serological abnormalities, such as positive tests for antinuclear antibodies and rheumatoid factor. Distinguishing systemic lupus erythematosus from HIV infection can be especially challenging because of the additional overlapping clinical features of neuropsychiatric complications, nephropathy and haematological abnormalities such as leucopenia and thrombocytopenia.

A common clinical problem is how to distinguish an acute infection from a disease flare in a patient with systemic lupus erythematosus. To complicate matters further, acute infections often trigger a lupus flare. Both bacterial infections and tuberculosis occur more commonly in lupus patients than in matched controls. Even patients in remission have an increased risk of infection, and this risk is enhanced by corticosteroids and other immunosuppressive agents such as cyclophosphamide. Bacterial infections involve the commonly occurring pyogenic organisms such as *Staphylococcus* species and *Escherichia coli*. Opportunistic infections also occur, especially in patients who take high-dose corticosteroids and immunosuppressive agents.

Measurement of C-reactive protein may be helpful in distinguishing between infection and a lupus flare. C-reactive protein levels are higher in patients with infection compared with those with active lupus; levels of CRP >60 mg/L strongly indicate infection while levels <30 mg/L make infection unlikely. Occasionally, high levels of CRP can be seen with lupus flares with arthritis or serositis in the absence of infection. Prospective longitudinal studies have, however, shown that CRP may be variable as a predictor of infection.

In the absence of useful surrogate markers of infection in systemic lupus erythematosus, exhaustive microbiological investigations and early and often repeated cultures, sometimes from affected tissues, are needed to make a definitive diagnosis.

Reference

LeRoy EC, Maricq HR, Kahaleh MB. Undifferentiated connective tissue syndromes. *Arthritis and Rheumatism* 1980; **23**: 341–343.

Further reading

Chikura B, Moore T, Manning J, Vail A, Herrick AL. Thumb involvement in Raynaud's phenomenon as an indicator of underlying connective tissue disease. *Journal of Rheumatology* 2010; **37**: 783–736.

Koenig M, Joyal F, Fritzler MJ *et al.* Autoantibodies and microvascular damage are independent predictive factors for the progression of Raynaud's phenomenon to systemic sclerosis: a twenty-year prospective study of 586 patients, with validation of proposed criteria for early systemic sclerosis. *Arthritis and Rheumatism* 2008; **58**: 3902–3912.

Louthrenoo W. Rheumatic manifestations of human immunodeficiency virus infection. *Current Opinion in Rheumatology* 2008; **20**: 92–99.

Perez-Alvarez R, Pérez-de-Lis M, Ramos-Casals M, for the BIOGEAS Study Group. Biologics-induced autoimmune diseases. *Current Opinion in Rheumatology* 2013; **25**: 56–64.

Sciascia S, Cuadrado MJ, Karim MY. Management of infection in systemic lupus erythematosus. *Best Practice and Research: Clinical Rheumatology* 2013; **27**: 377–389.

Solomon DH, Kavanaugh AJ, Schur PH, American College of Rheumatology Ad Hoc Committee on Immunologic Testing Guidelines. Evidence-based guidelines for the use of immunologic tests: antinuclear antibody testing. *Arthritis and Rheumatism* 2002; **47**: 434–444.

CHAPTER 22

Sport and Exercise Medicine

Cathy Speed

University of St Mark and St John, Plymouth; Centre for Health and Performance, Cambridge, UK

OVERVIEW

- Sport and exercise medicine is an established field that focuses upon the prevention and management of activity-related medical complaints, and the use of exercise for health-related benefit.

- Physical activity and structured exercise programmes have proven benefits in both the prevention and treatment of a wide range of conditions.

- All rheumatologists should have an awareness of the importance of exercise in the management of chronic rheumatological diseases.

- The assessment of sport-related injury requires an understanding of the potential intrinsic and extrinsic aetiological factors and a sound understanding of the opportunities for rehabilitation.

- Absolute rest is rarely if ever a component of a structured rehabilitation programme, which should aim to maintain physical fitness while restoring normal function.

Sport and exercise medicine is a field of medicine that addresses the prevention and management of sports and activity-related medical complaints, and the use of exercise for health-related benefit. Rheumatologists are often faced with sports injuries and also will have many patients who will benefit from an exercise prescription. Hence, this chapter is divided into two parts: sports injuries and exercise prescription.

Sports injuries

'Know the patient, know the sport, know the injury'

The key to managing sport-related injury is having an understanding of the patient and his/her expectations and concerns, as often there are high anxiety levels about the injury and its implications. An insight into the mechanics, training and techniques of the sport involved is also important, since this allows the underlying cause of the injury to be addressed (Figure 22.1).

Assessment

Consider both intrinsic and extrinsic factors.

Intrinsic factors encompass physical, physiological and psychological aspects of an individual that may contribute to injury (Table 22.1). Note that physical development is often different in athletes, and muscle development or joint range of motion may be asymmetrical depending upon the sport (e.g. tennis). Similarly, what is normal in the general population may be abnormal for an athlete; for example, flexibility that is typical of the general population would be considered inadequate in a gymnast.

Extrinsic factors play a significant role in the development of injury. Doing 'too much, too soon, too often' is a common factor. Consider other factors such as equipment errors, environmental conditions and hard/uneven surfaces.

A central concept in the development of an injury is a lack of functional control. This relates to the fine balance that exists between optimal mobility of the body or body area and its stability.

History – Take a history of the injury, training and competing habits, the potential role of other extrinsic factors, previous injury history and other medical issues. The mechanism of injury is important in elucidating the diagnosis, as it will implicate the structures involved and the severity of the injury.

Pain is typically the cardinal presenting symptom so a careful pain history should be recorded: the character of the pain, its site(s), radiation, timing of onset and subsequent temporal pattern, aggravating and relieving features and associated symptoms. The degree of swelling and its rapidity of onset after injury frequently correlate with the severity of injury. Instability or a feeling of 'pre-instability' are highly relevant in sport and may indicate a true structural deficit or a lack of neuromuscular control. Clicking and clunking of a joint is relevant particularly if new or painful. Neurological symptoms may be present and may indicate a true neurological deficit or, more frequently, neural irritation in association with a chronic soft tissue injury.

ABC of Rheumatology, Fifth Edition. Edited by Ade Adebajo and Lisa Dunkley.
© 2018 John Wiley & Sons Ltd. Published 2018 by John Wiley & Sons Ltd.

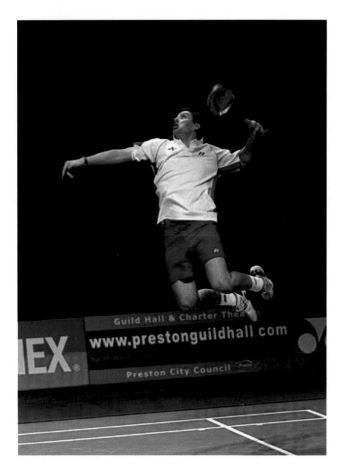

Figure 22.1 An insight into the mechanics, training and techniques of the sport is important in understanding sports injuries. This figure demonstrates the demands of a sport such as badminton, and the fine balance that exists between mobility and stability is a central concept in the consideration of sports injuries. Source: Figure courtesy of Badminton England

Table 22.1 Common extrinsic and intrinsic factors in sports injuries

Intrinsic	Extrinsic
Hypermobility	Training: too much, too soon, too often
Muscle weakness/imbalance	Technique
Poor flexibility (local, general)	Equipment
Femoral anteversion	Surface
Tibia varum/valgum	Environment
Pes planus/cavus	Drugs (e.g. anabolic/corticosteroids)
Presence of another injury	Poor nutrition
Chronic diseases (e.g. rheumatoid arthritis)	

Establish also the treatments used to date, medications (including supplements) and a general medical background. Always consider the possibility of an underlying medical complaint, such as a tumour or inflammatory arthritis/enthesitis. Note also that bone health issues are not uncommon in both male and female athletes.

The age of the patient is also very important: children have fragile skeletons with vulnerable growth plates and an increased risk of avulsion injuries. The senior population have an increased susceptibility to soft tissue injuries and arthritis and higher rates of co-morbidities that may influence the injury, and are slower to respond to treatment.

Examination – Examination commences with a general examination, in particular looking for stigmata of other disease, hypermobility and assessment of the spine, since dysfunction here can contribute to injury. Functional movements and core control are important. Assessment for asymmetry of muscle development and flexibility is important but must be interpreted carefully.

Regional assessment of the injury follows the usual strategy of 'look, feel, move, and special tests'. Identification of the site(s) of tenderness, swelling, instability and neurovascular status follows.

The clinician should seek to evaluate the patient dynamically, as at times only this will reproduce symptoms and functional control is so vitally important in injury causation and management. Part of this functional assessment is gait analysis (Figure 22.2).

Investigations – Investigations, in particular imaging, are frequently required in the assessment of the injury, but should be requested only after a clinical diagnosis is made, and interpreted carefully. No imaging is foolproof and it is vital to request the correct test for the suspected injury. Athletes may commonly have abnormalities on imaging that are not relevant to the clinical complaint.

Imaging includes plain X-rays, diagnostic ultrasound, MRI, CT and isotope bone scans. Plain X-rays assess for fractures, myositis ossificans, loose bodies and significant underlying joint damage but are not sensitive to early stress injuries, nor to many articular complaints. Stress views may be necessary to assess for instability. Diagnostic ultrasound demonstrates even subtle soft tissue pathologies and impingements and allows dynamic assessment of the joint in question. MRI provides further information of the surrounding anatomy, bone oedema, bone stress syndromes and some soft tissue injuries (Figure 22.3). MR arthrography may be necessary to evaluate the labra of shoulder and hip most accurately. CT is useful to detect loose bodies and to evaluate bone healing. SPECT may be used to evaluate bone stress injuries in particular. Serology for underlying medical complaints may be necessary.

Compartment studies measure intramuscular pressures before, during and after exercise, and are used to evaluate individuals with possible chronic exertional compartment syndromes.

Where there is a question about bone health in those with recurrent stress fractures, other investigations, such as DEXA scanning, may be warranted. The sites of low bone density in athletes may differ from the general population in view of the different patterns of skeletal loading; scanning of sites such as the forearm is often necessary.

Management (Box 22.1)

Management of sports injuries commences with an accurate diagnosis and identification of all the contributing factors. Education and counselling in relation to the injury, and discussion and agreement on an appropriate management strategy are vital. Ensuring the athlete has a clear understanding of the injury, its implications

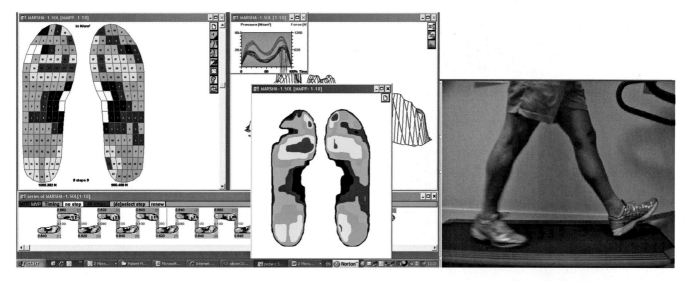

Figure 22.2 Gait analysis and shoe pressure measurement can be particularly helpful in the assessment of lower limb injuries

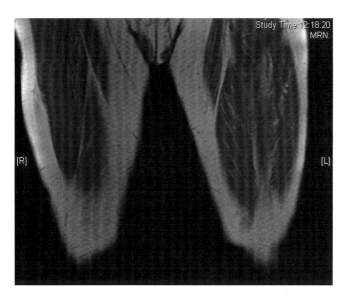

Figure 22.3 MRI of thighs showing left hamstrings muscle injury

---

Box 22.1 **Principles of management of sports injuries**

- Early diagnosis, to identify and correct the mechanism
- In the acute phase: PRICE
- Control pain in order to allow rehabilitation to proceed
- Rehabilitation addresses flexibility, strengthening, proprioception and sports-specific work such as agility, speed, power, technique
- Graduated return to sport

---

and treatment will enhance appropriate levels of compliance. Clear goals need to be set, and reviewed regularly.

Pain management is important principally to allow rehabilitation to proceed. In the acute injury, the classic PRICE regime (Protect, Rest, Ice, Compression (if necessary), Elevation) is followed. Rest is relative; the unaffected areas can and should continue to be exercised, for example swimming or aqua-jogging after a tibial stress fracture. Supports and braces, such as a splint in ankle sprain or boot in stress fractures of the foot, enable the individual to mobilize without overstressing the site of injury.

The most important aspect of management is rehabilitation, which addresses joint range of motion, proprioception, flexibility and strength issues initially. Underlying asymmetries in strength and flexibility are addressed, core stability is addressed and the patient then moves towards sports-specific rehabilitation to include power, agility and control during appropriate activities.

Pain control may be necessary in order to allow rehabilitation to proceed. This may be in the form of ice/heat modalities, simple analgesics or NSAIDs. Injections may be useful. For example, local anaesthetic may be used to identify the source of pain. Corticosteroid injections may be used for severe inflammation, and for chronic injuries where inflammation is ongoing. Injudicious loading under the influence of analgesia, and in particular corticosteroid, must be avoided. Other approaches include platelet-rich plasma injection for tennis elbow and extracorporeal shock wave therapy for tendon complaints.

Surgery may be required, either early or if other management approaches fail. The decision to intervene operatively will depend upon the nature of the injury and the circumstances of the athlete. Surgery is never an isolated treatment; rehabilitation remains an essential part of management. Examples of indications for early surgical intervention include fractures, acute traumatic tendon ruptures, significant loose bodies and labral injuries, and exertional compartment syndromes.

Even when surgery is likely to be indicated, many injuries may be managed in the intial phases with rehabilitation (Figure 22.4). This may be termed 'pre-habilitation', where strength and proprioception can be partly restored, enhancing the pace of postoperative recovery.

Common sports injuries – the acute injury

Sports injuries can be broadly divided into acute injury and chronic overuse injury. The most common acute injuries involve ligaments (sprain) or muscles (strain) and vary enormously in

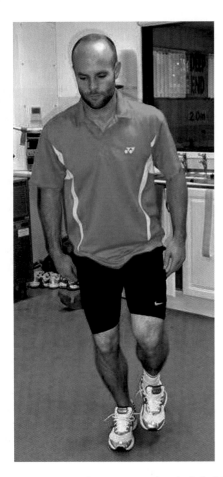

Figure 22.4 Rehabilitation involves progression from basic flexibility and strength exercises to sports-specific activities. Here, the athlete performs a single leg squat, a simple core stability exercise. Source: Figure courtesy of Badminton England

severity in terms of the extent of injury, the tissues affected and precise location (e.g. avulsion injury from bone versus midportion tendinopathy).

Ankle sprain – The most common acute sports injury is undoubtedly the lateral ankle sprain, which is damage to the lateral ankle ligaments, typically occurring with the foot in plantarflexion and slight inversion, such as at push-off (Figure 22.5). Such 'simple' injuries can result in long-term disability, often due to a lack of appropriate management. Without adequate treatment, recurrence is common and often with minimal trauma; this is more often due to functional instability rather than mechanical instability of the ligaments.

The degree of soft tissue damage is usually indicated by the extent of the swelling. Inability to bear weight and/or local bone tenderness suggests bone injury.

Many additional pathologies including tendinopathies and articular damage can occur.

Clinical assessment should evaluate balance and proprioception, mechanical stability of the ankle, distal tibiofibular joint and the foot, the sites and degree of tenderness and neurovascular status. Management of the acute injury should focus on early mobilization, range of motion and strengthening exercises (particularly the peroneals) and proprioceptive work. Use of an ankle brace helps in an earlier return to sport where that is indicated.

Common sports injuries – the chronic/overuse injury

Overuse injuries occur when a normal structure cannot cope with an excessive load. By comparison, an insufficiency injury occurs where a pathologically weak structure is unable to cope with a normal load. Overuse injuries can affect any tissue and common examples include tendinopathies, muscle injuries (e.g. myositis ossificans, chronic exertional compartment syndrome and medial tibial stress

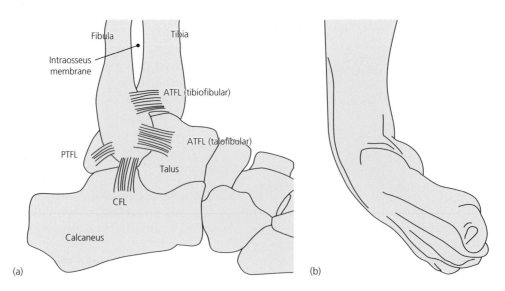

(a)   (b)

Figure 22.5 An ankle sprain involves a tear to one or more of the lateral ligaments of the ankle (a) and usually occurs with the foot in plantarflexion in slight inversion (b)

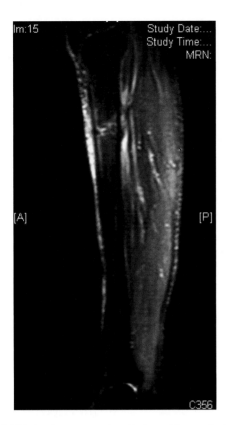

Figure 22.6 MRI showing a severe stress fracture of the proximal tibia

syndrome) and bone. Bone stress injuries are graded from minor periosteal reactions through to cortical breaches (stress fractures).

Bone stress injuries – While most bone stress injuries are fatigue related, the possibility of insufficiency fractures, particularly in lightweight athletes, must always be considered. Most stress fractures will respond to relative rest, support and correction of the underlying cause (training, biomechanics, equipment errors). However, certain stress fractures are associated with an increased risk of poor healing/completion, including the superior surface of the femoral neck, anterior tibial cortex and navicular (Figure 22.6). These are areas which are either under tension (rather than compression) and/or have poor vascular supply. They are managed either by non-weight bearing and close monitoring or early surgical intervention.

Exercise prescription

The benefits of exercise in the prevention and management of disease are well established. Many patients with rheumatological diseases should be given an exercise prescription as many are at

---

Box 22.2 **Components of an exercise prescription**

- Aerobic:
  - Activities selection
  - Duration
  - Frequency
  - Intensity
- Resistance training
- Flexibility training

Address issues such as adverse biomechanics from osteoarthritis prior to commencing. Counselling, supervision and progression of programme

---

increased risk of medical complications such as osteoporosis and cardiovascular events. Current recommendations are that adults aged 18–65 years need moderate-intensity aerobic physical activity for a minimum of 150 minutes per week, or vigorous-intensity aerobic physical activity for 75 minutes weekly, or a suitable mixture of the two. Strengthening exercises of major muscle groups should be performed 2–3 times weekly.

The exercise prescription has a number of components (Box 22.2) which are adjusted according to the individual's needs, characteristics (e.g. age) and preferences. Patients with moderate to severe cardiac risk should be assessed with an exercise test before commencing a programme. Compliance is enhanced by education and counselling, careful prescription in choice of activities, written information about the programme, goal setting and frequent follow-up, which may be done by telephone.

Summary

The evidence supporting the benefits of exercise and an active lifestyle in both preserving and restoring health is irrefutable. An active lifestyle will inevitably result in occasional musculoskeletal 'injury', and while sports and exercise medicine has now been recognized as a medical specialty and thus NHS provision should increase, the rheumatologist will still have a valuable role in contributing to the wider impact of activity-related musculoskeletal injury. It is therefore important that rheumatologists are confident in the assessment and rehabilitation of the exercising individual.

Further reading

American College of Sports Medicine. *ACSM's Guidelines for Exercise Testing and Prescription*, 10th edn. Wolters Kluwer, Philadelphia, 2017.

Brukner P, Kahn K. *Clinical Sports Medicine*, 4th edn. McGraw-Hill, Canberra, 2012.

CHAPTER 23

Vasculitis and Related Rashes

Richard A. Watts[1] and David G.I. Scott[2]

[1] Ipswich Hospital NHS Trust, Ipswich; Norwich Medical School, Norwich, UK
[2] Norfolk and Norwich University Hospital NHS Trust; Norwich Medical School, Norwich, UK

OVERVIEW

- Systemic vasculitis should be considered in the differential diagnosis of all patients presenting with multisystem illness.
- cANCA with proteinase 3 antibodies are associated with granulomatosis with polyangiitis (Wegener's), and pANCA with myeloperoxidase antibodies are associated with microscopic polyangiitis.
- Urinalysis is a key investigation as renal involvement is a major determinant of outcome.
- Treatment depends on the type of vasculitis following guidelines from the British Society for Rheumatology and European League against Rheumatism.
- Cyclophosphamide therapy should only be used for induction of remission; maintenance therapy should be with azathioprine or methotrexate in combination with glucocorticoids.
- Rituximab is becoming more widely used as an alternative to cyclophosphamide, especially for patients with AAV who relapse.

The vasculitides are a heterogeneous group of uncommon diseases characterized by inflammatory cell infiltration and necrosis of blood vessel walls. Systemic necrotizing vasculitis can be rapidly life-threatening, so early accurate diagnosis and treatment are vital. Vasculitis may be primary (granulomatosis with polyangiitis (Wegener's), eosinophilic granulomatosis with polyangiitis (EGPA; Churg–Strauss syndrome), microscopic polyangiitis, polyarteritis nodosa) or secondary to established connective tissue disease (such as rheumatoid arthritis), infection or malignancy. The severity of vasculitis is related to the size and site of the vessels affected. Classification is based on vessel size and determines the treatment approach (Table 23.1, Box 23.1).

Table 23.1 Classification of vasculitis

Dominant vessel	Idiopathic (primary)	Probable aetiology (secondary)
Large	Takayasu's	Syphilis
	Giant cell arteritis	Tuberculosis
		Aortitis – RA, AS
Medium	Polyarteritis nodosa (classic)	HBV-associated polyarteritis nodosa
	Kawasaki's disease	
Small		
ANCA	Microscopic polyangiitis	Drugs (propylthiouracil, hydralazine)*
	Granulomatosis with polyangiitis	
	Eosinophilic granulomatosis with polyangiitis	
Immune complex	Anti-GBM disease	Cryoglobulinaemic vasculitis (HCV)
	Cryoglobuinaemic vasculitis (non-HCV)	RA, SLE, Sjögren's syndrome
	IgA vasculitis	Serum sickness
	Hypocomplementaemic vasculitis	Drug induced ‡
Variable	Behçet's	
	Cogan's	

AS, ankylosing spondylitis; GBM, glomerular basement membrane; HBV, hepatitis B virus; HCV, hepatitis C virus; RA, rheumatoid arthritis; SLE, systemic lupus erythematosus.

ABC of Rheumatology, Fifth Edition. Edited by Ade Adebajo and Lisa Dunkley.
© 2018 John Wiley & Sons Ltd. Published 2018 by John Wiley & Sons Ltd.

Large-vessel vasculitis

Large-vessel vasculitis includes giant cell arteritis and Takayasu's arteritis. Giant cell arteritis is described elsewhere (Chapter 17). Takayasu's arteritis is uncommon and affects young adults, who initially present with a non-specific illness and later with loss of pulses, claudication (especially of the upper limbs) and stroke.

Medium-vessel vasculitis

Polyarteritis nodosa

A multisystem vasculitis characterized by formation of microaneurysms in medium-sized arteries. Patients present with a

Box 23.1 **Symptoms suggestive of vasculitis**

Systemic	Respiratory
• Malaise	Cough
• Fever	Wheeze
• Weight loss	Haemoptysis
• Myalgia	Dyspnoea
• Arthralgia	**Ear, nose and throat**
Skin	• Epistaxis
• Purpura (palpable)	• Crusting
• Ulceration	• Sinusitis
• Infarction	• Deafness
Gastrointestinal	**Cardiac**
• Mouth ulcers	• Chest pain
• Abdominal pain	**Neurological**
• Diarrhoea	• Sensory or motor impairment

constitutional illness, which is often associated with rash, mononeuritis multiplex, vascular hypertension and organ infarction. Polyarteritis nodosa may be confined to the skin. Angiography shows typical microaneurysms. Polyarteritis nodosa is associated with hepatitis B infection.

Kawasaki's disease (mucocutaneous lymph node syndrome)

An acute vasculitis that primarily affects infants and young children. It presents with fever, rash, lymphadenopathy and palmoplantar erythema. Coronary arteries become affected in up to one-quarter of untreated patients; this can lead to myocardial ischaemia and infarction.

Medium- and small-vessel vasculitis

This group includes the major necrotizing vasculitides: microscopic polyangiitis, granulomatosis with polyangiitis (Wegener's), eosinophilic granulomatosis with polyangiitis (Churg–Strauss), with involvement of both medium and small arteries. The symptoms depend on the size and site of vessel affected and on the individual diagnosis. They are associated with the presence of antineutrophil cytoplasmic antibodies (ANCA).

Granulomatosis with polyangiitis (Wegener's)

This is characterized by a granulomatous vasculitis of the upper and lower respiratory tracts and glomerulonephritis, but almost any organ system can be affected (Figures 23.1, 23.2). The lungs are affected in 45% of patients at diagnosis. Symptoms in the ear, nose and throat (such as epistaxis, crusting and deafness) particularly are associated with this condition, and they should be

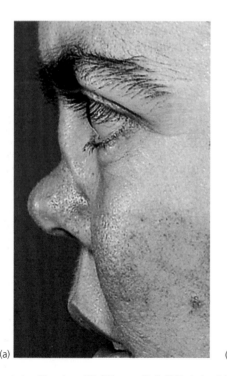

(a)

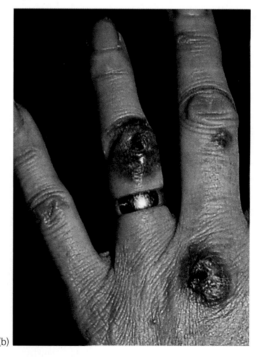

(b)

Figure 23.1 Granulomatosis with polyangiitis (Wegener's). (Left) Typical saddle nose deformity (reproduced with patient's permission). (Right) Vasculitic rash

sought in all patients with suspected vasculitis. Biopsy of affected organs shows a necrotizing arteritis, often with formation of granulomas.

Microscopic polyangiitis

This is characterized by a vasculitis that commonly affects the kidneys. Lung involvement usually presents with haemoptysis caused by pulmonary capillaritis and haemorrhage (pulmonary-renal syndrome). Biopsy of the kidney shows a focal segmental necrotizing glomerulonephritis with few immune deposits (sometimes called pauciimmune vasculitis).

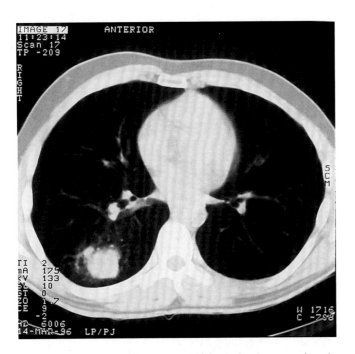

Figure 23.2 Computed tomography scan of thorax showing a granuloma in granulomatosis with polyangiitis (Wegener's)

Eosinophilic granulomatosis with polyangiitis (Churg–Strauss)

This syndrome is characterized by atopy (especially late-onset asthma), pulmonary involvement (75% of patients have radiographic evidence of infiltration), and eosinophilia in the tissues and peripheral blood ($>1 \times 10^9$/L). Such features can develop several years before the onset of systemic vasculitis.

Small-vessel vasculitis

Small-vessel vasculitis (leucocytoclastic or hypersensitivity) is usually confined to the skin, but it may be part of a systemic illness. The rash is purpuric, sometimes palpable, and occurs in dependent areas. The lesions may become bullous and ulcerate. Nailfold infarcts occur. Biopsy shows a cellular infiltrate of small vessels often with leucocytoclasis (fragmented polymorphonuclear cells and nuclear dust).

IgA vasculitis (Henoch–Schönlein purpura)

This is a form of small vessel vasculitis that occurs mainly in childhood and young adults. Patients present with rash, arthritis, abdominal pain and, occasionally, renal involvement (Figure 23.3). Deposits of immunoglobulin A can be detected histologically in the skin and renal mesangium.

Behçet's disease

Behçet's disease is a systemic vasculitis of unknown aetiology, characterized by orogenital ulceration. It is most common in Turkey and Japan. Ocular involvement occurs early in the disease course and affects 50% of patients. The pathergy phenomenon is characteristic and is a non-specific hyperreactivity in response to minor trauma.

Investigation

Investigation aims to establish and confirm the diagnosis, the extent and severity of organ involvement, and disease activity.

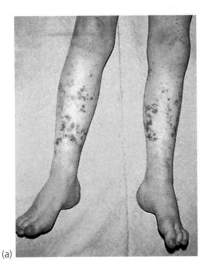
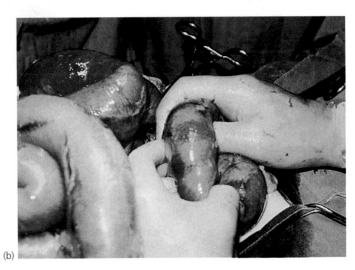

(a)　　　　(b)

Figure 23.3 Small-vessel vasculitis in IgA vasculitis (Henoch–Schönlein purpura). (Left) Affecting the skin. (Right) Affecting the gut

Urine analysis

This is the most important investigation because the severity of renal involvement is one of the key determinants of prognosis. Detection of proteinuria or haematuria in a patient with systemic illness needs immediate further investigation and the patient is a medical emergency.

Blood tests

Leucocytosis suggests a primary vasculitis or infection. Eosinophilia suggests eosinophilic granulomatosis with polyangiitis or a drug reaction.

Liver function tests

Abnormal results suggest viral infection (hepatitis A, B, C) or may be non-specific.

Immunology

Antineutrophil cytoplasmic antibodies are associated with the primary systemic necrotizing vasculitides. Cytoplasmic ANCA in association with proteinase 3 antibodies are highly specific (>90%) for granulomatosis with polyangiitis (Wegener's). Perinuclear ANCA associated with myeloperoxidase antibodies occur in microscopic polyangiitis and eosinophilic granulomatosis with polyangiitis (Churg–Strauss). Rheumatoid factors and antinuclear antibodies may indicate vasculitis associated with connective tissue disease.

Biopsy

Tissue biopsy is important to confirm the diagnosis before treatment with potentially toxic immunosuppressive drugs. The choice of tissue to biopsy is crucial.

Other investigations

Angiography can show aneurysms. Blood cultures, viral serology and echocardiography are important to exclude infection and other conditions that may present as systemic multisystem disease.

Differential diagnosis

Livedo reticularis

Livedo reticularis is characterized by persistent patchy reddish-blue mottling of the legs (and occasionally arms) that is exacerbated by cold weather (Figure 23.4). It may lead to ulceration and is associated with vascular thrombosis (Sneddon's syndrome) and the presence of antiphospholipid antibodies.

Bacterial infections

Direct bacterial infection of small arteries and arterioles infection causes a necrotizing vasculitis or thrombosis. *Neisseria meningitides* (Figure 23.5), *N. gonorrhoeae* (Figure 23.6) and *Streptobacillus moniliformis*, for example, may infect the vascular endothelium directly and cause maculopapular or purpuric skin lesions.

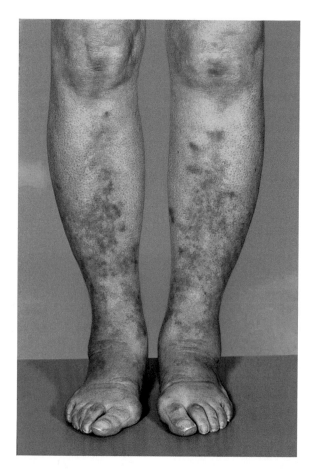

Figure 23.4 Livedo rash in cutaneous polyarteritis nodosa

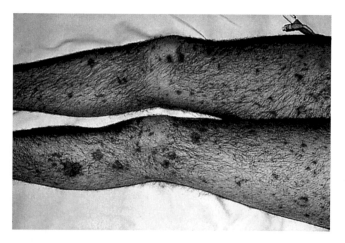

Figure 23.5 Haemorrhagic pustular rash in disseminated infection with *Neisseria meningitides*

Infective endocarditis

Several organisms – streptococci, staphylococci, Gram-negative bacilli and *Coxiella* – can cause endocarditis. Polyarthritis may be accompanied by splinter haemorrhages, Janeway lesions (red macules over thenar and hypothenar eminences; Figure 23.7), Osler's nodes (tender papules over extremities of fingers and toes) and clubbing.

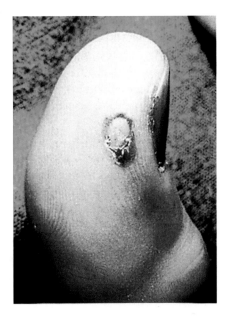
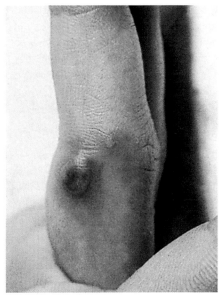

Figure 23.6 Gonococcal pustules in disseminated infection with *Neisseria gonorrhoeae*

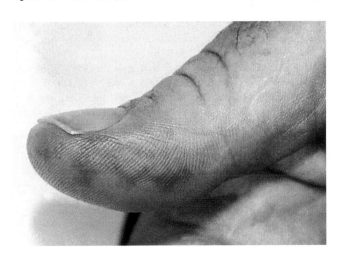

Figure 23.7 Janeway lesions in infective endocarditis

Cholesterol embolism

Cholesterol embolism may occur spontaneously or after trauma to the aortic wall during vascular surgery or angiographic procedures. Typical cutaneous manifestations are ischaemia of the digits, particularly the toes from abdominal atheroma, emboli and livedo reticularis.

Atrial myxoma

Cardiac myxomata are rare benign tumours found most often in the left atrium (90% of cases). Constitutional symptoms and systemic embolization may lead to a wrong diagnosis of vasculitis. Systemic manifestations seen in 90% of cases include fever, weight loss, Raynaud's phenomenon, clubbing, elevated acute-phase proteins and hypergammaglobulinaemia.

Antiphospholipid antibody syndrome

Antiphospholipid antibody syndrome may present as catastrophic widespread thrombosis, and this can mimic systemic vasculitis.

Livedo reticularis is the most typical cutaneous lesion and it occurs in association with thrombosis and recurrent fetal loss.

Cocaine abuse

Cocaine abuse can cause destruction of the nasal mucosa and septum, mimicking systemic vasculitis.

Prognosis

The natural history of untreated primary systemic vasculitis is of a rapidly progressive, usually fatal disease. The use of oral low-dose cyclophosphamide combined with prednisolone resulted in a significant improvement in the mortality of granulomatosis with polyangiitis (Wegener's), with a survival rate at 5 years of 82%.

Small-vessel vasculitis confined to the skin without necrotizing features has an excellent prognosis. Takayasu's arteritis has a good prognosis (3% mortality) but typically relapses.

Treatment

Treatment depends on the size of vessel involved. Guidelines from the British Society for Rheumatology and European League against Rheumatism are available and the management outlined here is based on them.

Takayasu's arteritis requires high-dose corticosteroids (oral prednisolone 40–60 mg/day), and additional immunosuppression with methotrexate or azathioprine. The dose of corticosteroid should be reduced rapidly according to clinical and laboratory parameters. Intravenous immunoglobulin is effective in the treatment of Kawasaki's disease.

For patients with generalized small vessel disease, cyclophosphamide is used for remission induction and can be given either as continuous low-dose oral therapy or intermittent pulse therapy. Both routes are equally effective at inducing remission, but pulse therapy is probably associated with a slightly higher relapse rate. The major toxicities of cyclophosphamide are haemorrhagic cystitis, formation of bladder tumours, infertility and infection. Toxicity depends on the cumulative dose, so pulse therapy is less toxic. Mesna may reduce the frequency of bladder toxicity with intravenous cyclophosphamide. The risk of ovarian failure depends on age and cumulative dose of cyclophophamide. Prophylaxis with trimethoprim-sulfamethoxazole should be considered to prevent infection with *Pneumocystis jiroveci*. Immunosuppressed patients should receive vaccination with influenza and polyvalent pneumococcal vaccination.

Corticosteroids are started at a dose of 1 mg/kg and the dose is reduced quite rapidly so that the drug can be discontinued at around 12 months. Intravenous methylprednisolone is often given with the first two pulses.

Once remission has been achieved with cyclophosphamide (usually after 3–6 months), azathioprine (or weekly oral methotrexate) is substituted for maintenance therapy. Cyclophosphamide should not be continued for more than 1 year because of the risks of toxicity. Survival has improved and remission can be obtained in most patients (85%) with cyclophosphamide, but many need prolonged immunosuppressive therapy (5–10 years), and the rate of relapse is still substantial (50% at 5 years).

Methotrexate may be considered in patients with no evidence of life- or organ-threatening disease as an alternative to cyclophosphamide.

Patients with life-threatening disease (pulmonary haemorrhage) or a creatinine >500 μmol/L should receive plasma exchange in addition to intravenous methylprednisolone.

Rituximab (anti-CD 20 B-cell depletion) has been shown in two trials to be an effective therapy for ANCA-associated vasculitis (AAV). There are two main situations where its use should be considered:

- the newly diagnosed patient who is at high risk of infection, who wishes to preserve fertility or is intolerant of cyclophosphamide
- the relapsing or refractory patient who has already completed one course of cyclophosphamide and further cyclophosphamide should be avoided.

The licensed regimen is 375 mg/m^2 weekly for 4 weeks, but many physicians use 1g for two doses at a two week interval. The optimum maintenance strategy using rituximab is unknown but probably the best strategy is regular retreatment at 4–6-month intervals for a 2-year period.

Regular assessment of disease activity is required and treatment is tailored accordingly. Minor relapses may require an increase in maintenance therapy. Major relapses will require a further course of cyclophosphamide.

Further reading

Ball GV, Bridges L (eds). *Vasculitis*, 3rd edn. Oxford University Press, Oxford, 2014.

Mukhtyar C, Guillevin L, Cid M *et al*. EULAR recommendations for the management of primary small and medium vessel vasculitis. *Annals of the Rheumatic Diseases* 2009; **68**: 310–317.

Mukhtyar C, Guillevin L, Cid M *et al*. EULAR recommendations for the management of large vessel vasculitis. *Ann Rheum Dis* 2009; **68**: 318–323.

Ntatsaki E, Carruthers DM, Chakravarty K *et al*. BSR and BHPR guideline for the management of adults with ANCA associated vasculitis. *Rheumatology* 2014; **53**: 2306–2309.

Smith RM, Jones RB, Guerry MJ *et al*. Rituximab for remission maintenance in relapsing ANCA-associated vasculitis. *Arthritis and Rheumatism* 2012; **64**: 3760–3769.

CHAPTER 24

Basic Immunology and the Biologic Era

John Isaacs[1] and Nishanthi Thalayasingam[2]

[1] Newcastle University and Newcastle upon Tyne Hospitals NHS Trust, Newcastle, UK
[2] Institute of Cellular Medicine, Newcastle University, Newcastle, UK

OVERVIEW

- Our immune system has evolved a network of mechanisms to effectively recognize, respond to and eliminate pathogens and their toxic products.

- The innate immune system provides a rapid, non-specific response within hours.

- The adaptive immune system is activated to produce a pathogen-specific response.

- Dysregulated activation of the immune system results in immunopathologies such as autoimmunity.

- Biologic therapies specifically target cells or mediators that have become inappropriately activated or produced.

Inflammation

The classic hallmarks of inflammation: calor (heat), dolor (pain), rubor (redness) and tumor (swelling), occur at sites of tissue damage. These changes are a consequence of blood vessel dilatation, increased capillary permeability, recruitment of innate immune cells such as polymorphonuclear leucocytes and monocytes from the bloodstream and subsequent release of proinflammatory mediators (Figure 24.1). The innate immune cells become activated and are important for phagocytosis of pathogens and subsequently for tissue repair.

Antigen-presenting cells (APCs) in the inflamed tissue also become activated, by 'danger signals' released by pathogens or by tissue damage itself. APCs include dendritic cells and macrophages, and act as the bridge between the two arms of the immune response. In health, this leads to an immune response against pathogens but in autoimmunity these processes become subverted and autoreactive lymphocytes are triggered, leading to an unregulated immune response against self. The mediators released (cytokines, chemokines, growth factors) lead to further immune cell influx,

new blood vessel formation plus the activation of resident tissue cells, resulting in further tissue damage (Figure 24.2).

Activation of the adaptive immune response

APCs internalize and digest (process) the pathogen, then migrate to local lymph nodes where they initiate an immune response by 'presenting' the processed antigen to lymphocytes.

Lymphocytes (B-cells and T-cells) express specialized receptors on their surface which recognize antigen. T-cells respond to antigenic fragments displayed on the surface of APCs, in association with major histocompatibility complex (MHC) molecules, whereas B-cells interact with intact antigens. Following antigen recognition, lymphocytes proliferate and differentiate into effector cells: cytotoxic and helper T-cells, and memory B-cells and plasma cells. A proportion remain in the lymphoid tissue but the remainder enter the circulation and migrate to areas of inflammation.

Cells of the immune system

T-cells

T-cells develop in the thymus. Helper T-cells express the CD4 co-receptor and are central to the co-ordination of immune responses. This involves cytokine release but they also provide help for B-cell maturation and antibody production via molecules such as CD40 ligand (CD40L).

Three factors are required for T-cell expansion and differentiation: recognition of the antigen by its specific lymphocyte receptor (signal 1), binding of co-stimulatory molecules (signal 2) and receipt of appropriate cytokine signals (signal 3) (Figure 24.3). CD80 and CD86 are key co-stimulatory molecules expressed by APCs, which bind to CD28 on the T-cell to provide signal 2. Once activated, T-cells upregulate CTLA-4, which competes with CD28 for CD80 and CD86, and conveys a negative signal, acting as a brake to T-cell activation.

KEY FEATURES
1. Vascular changes
   - vasodilatation
   - increased permeability
2. Leucocyte changes
   - recruitment
   - activation

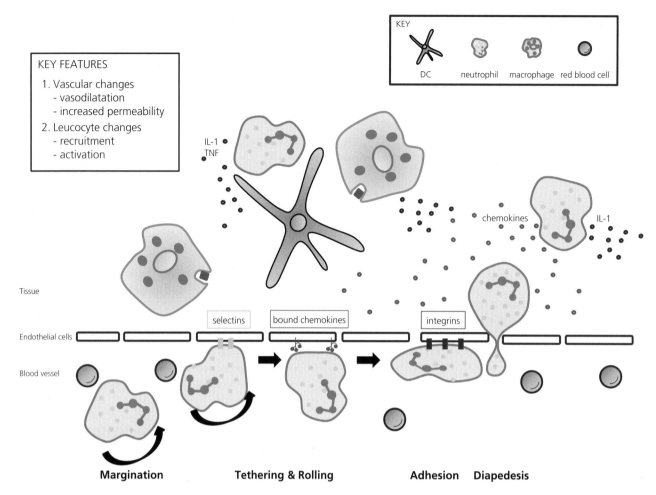

IL-1
TNF

chemokines   IL-1

Tissue

Endothelial cells

Blood vessel

selectins   bound chemokines   integrins

Margination   **Tethering & Rolling**   **Adhesion   Diapedesis**

Figure 24.1 Acute inflammation begins within seconds of tissue injury. The local blood vessels dilate and the increase in their permeability leads to the movement of fluid and proteins into the interstitial space. Proinflammatory cytokines upregulate the adhesion molecules, selectins and integrins, on the endothelial cell walls. Leucocytes, predominantly neutrophils, localize to the periphery of the blood vessel (margination). They bind loosely to selectins on the endothelium (tethering) and as these weak bonds are formed and broken, the cells roll along the endothelium. The leucocytes become activated and bind more tightly to integrins on the endothelium (adhesion), a process that is promoted by chemokines. These small, chemoattractant cytokines are produced at the site of inflammation and bind to molecules on the vascular surface of endothelial cells such as heparan sulphate. They thereby form a chemoattractant gradient that leads to activation and egress of leucocytes, which subsequently migrate between the endothelial cells and into the interstitial spaces (diapedesis)

The cytokine environment determines T-cell differentiation. Thus, transforming growth factor-beta (TGF-β) favours regulatory T-cells, gamma-interferon (IFN-γ) and interleukin (IL)-12 T_H1 T-cells, IL-4 T_H2 T-cells and a mixture of cytokines (IL-23, TGF-β and IL-6) T_H17 T-cells (see Figure 24.3). IL-6 and IL-21 are required for the differentiation of T follicular helper T–cells (T_{FH}), which guide B-cell differentiation. Disordered regulation of T_H1 and T_H17 responses are thought to underpin autoimmunity while abnormal T_H2 responses predispose to allergy. Regulatory T-cells limit the immune response and maintain tolerance. T_H17 cells are central in diseases such as psoriatic arthritis and ankylosing spondylitis.

B-cells

The multifaceted role of B-cells and the success of B-cell-focused therapies support a pathogenic role for B-cells in autoimmune diseases. There are three main mechanisms by which self-reactive B-cells may initiate and potentiate autoimmunity: the production of pathogenic autoantibodies, secretion of proinflammatory cytokines and by acting as APCs (Figure 24.4).

Terminally differentiated B-cells, plasma cells, secrete antigen-specific immunoglobulins into extracellular fluid where they bind their specific targets, activate complement and activate macrophages via Fc receptors (FcR) on their surface. Disease-associated autoantibodies mediate tissue damage in some autoimmune conditions but in others appear simply as biomarkers of a dysregulated immune response.

T_{FH} cells help B-cells to establish ectopic lymphoid structures in diseased tissue, resulting in local autoantibody production. There has been an increasing focus on B-cell subsets, in particular a regulatory subset which secretes IL-10 and which may therefore down-regulate the immune response. At present, B-cell-targeted therapies have focused on cell depletion and inhibition of survival factors.

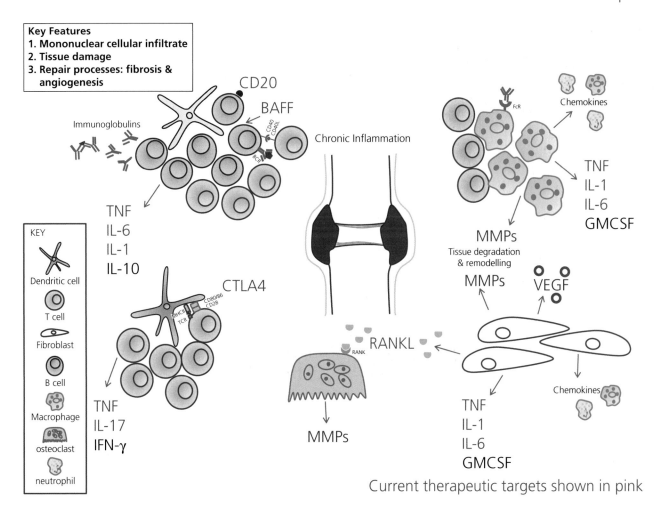

Key Features
1. Mononuclear cellular infiltrate
2. Tissue damage
3. Repair processes: fibrosis & angiogenesis

Current therapeutic targets shown in pink

Figure 24.2 Chronic inflammation. A key feature of chronic inflammation, shown here in an inflamed joint, is mononuclear cellular infiltration and the activation and proliferation of resident cells which leads to subsequent tissue damage. **T-cell activation** by APCs classically occurs in the lymph nodes but APCs are also present in the synovium. The T-cell response generated is dependent on the cytokine microenvironment. T-cells subsequently interact with macrophages and B-cells. **Macrophages** become activated following their interaction with T-cells or binding to immune complexes via their Fc-gamma receptors (FcR). The macrophage moves from its primary role in tissue of 'guarding' and 'scavenging' debris to secreting a wide range of substances: chemokines for leucocyte recruitment; cytokines; growth factors which, with cytokines, promote angiogenesis; and matrix metalloproteinases which lead to the breakdown of the extracellular matrix. **B-cell activation** leads to cytokine release and autoantibody production. The B-cells also interact bidirectionally with T-cells, receiving co-stimulatory help and acting as APCs. BAFF is essential to B-cell survival. In inflamed tissue, B-cells may be found in ectopic germinal centres, surrounding follicular dendritic cells. **Osteoclasts** accumulate in the inflamed synovium adjacent to bone, resulting in bone resorption and structural damage. Binding of RANKL to its receptor, RANK, promotes osteoclast differentation from monocyte precursors. RANKL is produced by activated T-cells and also from synovial fibroblasts under the influence of proinflammatory cytokines. **Fibroblasts** in RA are phenotypically different from those in the normal synovium and these changes are induced by the proinflammatory environment. They proliferate to form a 'quasi-malignant' pannus and secrete proinflammatory cytokines, chemokines, VEGF, which promotes angiogenesis, and MMPs which cause tissue breakdown. BAFF, B-cell activating factor; GMCSF, granulocyte macrophage colony-stimulating factor; IFN-γ, gamma interferon; MMP, matrix metalloproteinase; RANKL, receptor activator of nuclear factor kappa-B ligand; TNF, tumour necrosis factor; VEGF, vascular endothelial growth factor

Macrophages

Macrophages are long-lived cells which reside in most tissues. As part of the innate immune system, they phagocytose pathogens and other material at the site of damage. They can act as APCs but are also activated by the adaptive immune system to secrete proinflammatory mediators and to initiate repair mechanisms (see Figure 24.2).

Biologic therapies

Biologics were first introduced into rheumatology in the late 1990s and there is now a great deal of accumulated experience of treating patients with these agents. In contrast to chemically synthesized small molecules, which form the mainstay of drug therapy, biologic drugs are proteins generated from genetically

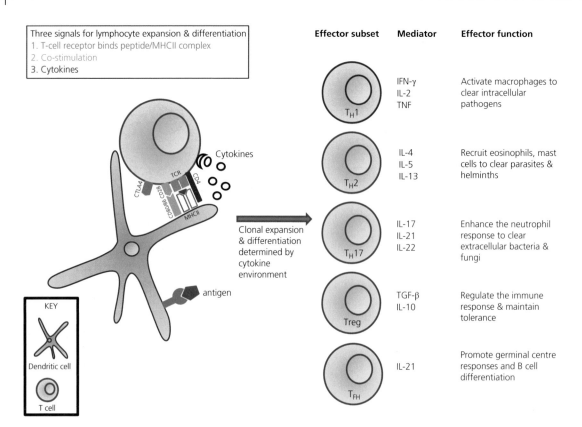

Three signals for lymphocyte expansion & differentiation
1. T-cell receptor binds peptide/MHCII complex
2. Co-stimulation
3. Cytokines

Effector subset	Mediator	Effector function
T$_H$1	IFN-γ IL-2 TNF	Activate macrophages to clear intracellular pathogens
T$_H$2	IL-4 IL-5 IL-13	Recruit eosinophils, mast cells to clear parasites & helminths
T$_H$17	IL-17 IL-21 IL-22	Enhance the neutrophil response to clear extracellular bacteria & fungi
Treg	TGF-β IL-10	Regulate the immune response & maintain tolerance
T$_{FH}$	IL-21	Promote germinal centre responses and B cell differentiation

Figure 24.3 T helper cell activation. Antigen-presenting cells (APCs), shown here as a dendritic cell, detect the pathogen, internalize it and present fragments of denatured proteins and peptides on class II MHC molecules to the T-cell receptor (TCR) on naive CD4 T-cells. Engagement of the TCR alone is not sufficient to stimulate the T-cell and two further signals are required. Signal 2 is provided by co-stimulatory molecules, e.g. CD28 binding to CD80 or CD86 which promotes T-cell expansion. Signal 3 is provided primarily by cytokines which direct T-cell differentiation into the different T-cell subsets, which each have distinctive cytokine profiles and functions. CD4 on the T-cell acts as a co-receptor for the TCR, binding to MHCII

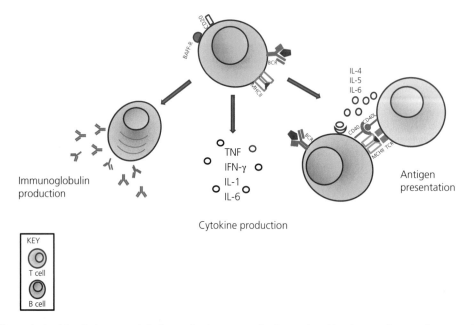

Figure 24.4 The multifaceted role of B-cells. **Immunoglobulin production:** autoantibodies produced by plasma cells can activate complement and effector cells, e.g. macrophages, ultimately leading to tissue damage. **Cytokine production**: the production of proinflammatory cytokines adds to the proinflammatory milieu. **Antigen presentation:** there is bidirectional communication between B-cells and T-cells. B-cells detect antigen using the surface immunoglobulin B cell receptor (BCR), then process and present antigen to the T-cell on MHCII molecules to activate them (see Figure 24.3). Co-stimulatory signals, shown as CD40/CD40L here, and cytokines enable the T-cell to provide 'help' to the B-cell, promoting proliferation and differentiation into antibody-producing plasma cells and memory cells

Table 24.1 Current biologic drugs and their targets

Biologic drug	Target
Etanercept	TNF
Adalimumab	TNF
Infliximab	TNF
Golimumab	TNF
Certolizumab pegol	TNF
Tocilizumab	IL-6 receptor
Sarilumab	IL-6 receptor
Anakinra	IL-1 receptor
Secukinumab	IL-17A
Brodalumab	IL-17 receptor
Ustekinumab	IL-12/IL-23
Belimumab	BAFF
Rituximab	CD20
Abatacept	CD80 and CD86
Denosumab	RANKL

BAFF, B-cell activating factor; IL, interleukin; RANKL, receptor activator of nuclear factor kappa-B ligand; TNF, tumour necrosis factor.

modified living cells. The biologic drug targets cytokines or cells which underpin the persistent inflammation and damage associated with autoimmunity (Table 24.1).

Structure

The most well-established biologic agents are full-length monoclonal antibodies but there are also fusion proteins and pegylated antibody fragments (Figure 24.5).

Biologic drugs are administered subcutaneously or intravenously to bypass the GI tract where they would be destroyed by digestive enzymes. Some are licensed as monotherapies but most are more effective when combined with methotrexate, at least in part reflecting reduced immunogenicity.

Cytokine-based treatments

The three most established cytokine targets are TNF, IL-1 and IL-6. Additional targets include IL-17, a survival factor for B-cells, known as either B-cell activating factor (BAFF) or B-lymphocyte stimulator (BLyS), which has a more cell-focused mode of action, and receptor activator of nuclear factor kappa-B ligand (RANKL) which is a central cytokine in bone metabolism.

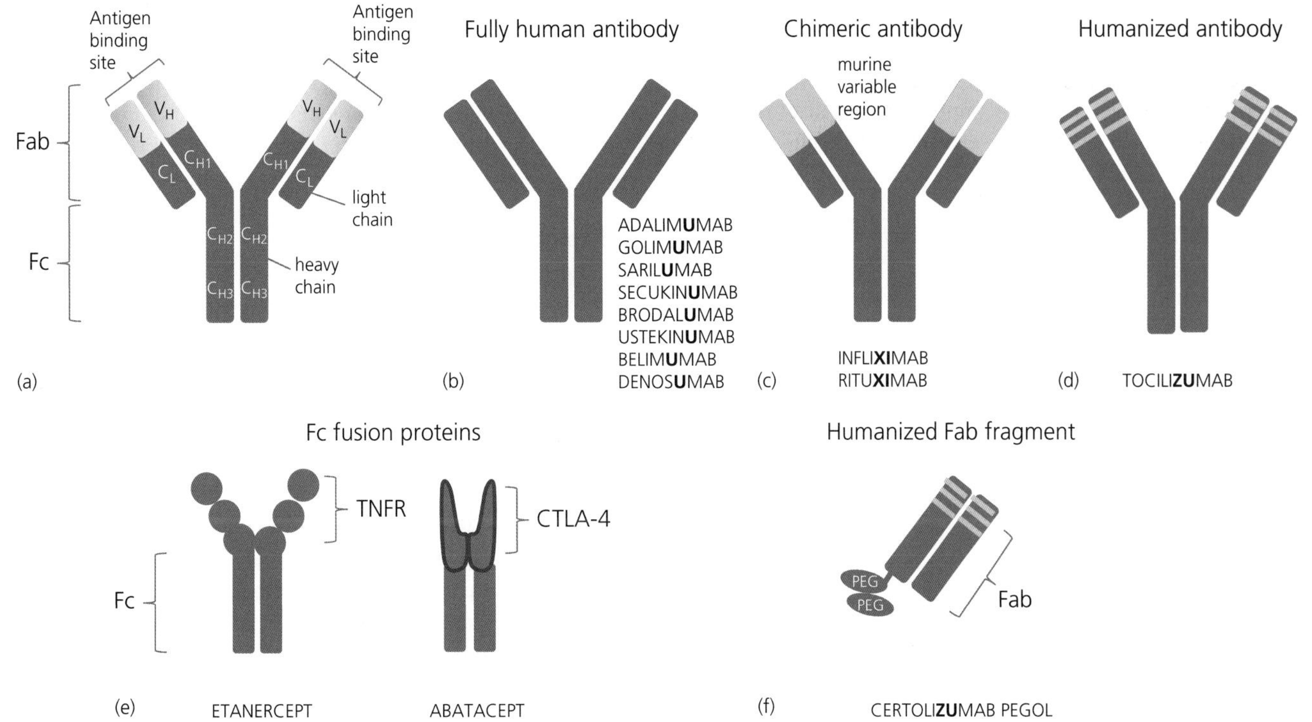

Figure 24.5 Structure of antibodies and biologic drugs. (a) The structure of an immunoglobulin molecule with two heavy chains and two light chains. Each chain has a variable region (V) and constant region (C). The Fab (fragment antigen binding) regions are composed of the variable region and a constant domain from each chain. The Fc (fragment crystallizable) or constant regions bind to cell surface receptors (FcR) and complement to mediate antibody function. (b–d) The different types of engineered therapeutic antibodies. The current nomenclature uses the ending 'mab' to denote a monoclonal antibody. If this is preceeded by 'u' this denotes a fully human antibody, 'xi' denotes a chimeric form with a human constant and mouse variable region, and 'zu' where only small sequences in the variable regions (the antigen binding site) remain murine in origin. (e) Etanercept is a chimeric protein genetically engineered by fusing the extracellular domain of human tumour necrosis factor receptor type II (TNFRII) to the Fc domain of human IgG1. Abatacept is composed of the Fc region of IgG1 fused to the extracellular domain of CTLA-4. (f) Certolizumab pegol is a recombinant, humanized antibody Fab fragment against TNF conjugated to polyethylene glycol (PEG)

Anti-TNF – TNF plays a crucial role in host defence and local injury but, in diseases such as rheumatoid arthritis (RA), excess local production in the joint leads to inappropriate inflammation and damage. There are currently five anti-TNFs available: the monoclonal antibodies infliximab, adalimumab and golimumab; a pegylated Fab fragment certolizumab; and the TNF receptor fusion protein etanercept. They reduce cellularity within the synovial membrane, mainly by reducing influx and increasing efflux of leucocytes.

IL-6 – High levels of IL-6 are found in rheumatoid arthritis and IL-6 is a key mediator of both local and systemic features of the disease, signalling via the IL-6 receptor (IL-6R), which exists in both a cell-bound and soluble form. Cell-associated IL-6R forms a heterodimer with transmembrane gp130 which transmits a signal to the cell interior. Soluble IL-6R can also dimerize with transmembrane gp130. The IL-6 pathway has been successfully targeted by tocilizumab and, more recently, sarilumab which bind to both soluble and cell surface IL-6R, preventing the engagement and signalling of IL-6 (Figure 24.6). Monoclonal antibodies targeting the cytokine itself are currently in development.

IL-1 – Blockade of IL-1 can be achieved using either anti-IL-1 monoclonal antibodies or a recombinant form of the naturally occurring IL-1 receptor antagonist, anakinra. Despite experimental evidence for a significant role of IL-1 in the pathogenesis of RA, anakinra demonstrated less robust efficacy than the other biologic drugs. Consequently, despite a licence for the treatment of RA, its use is not approved by NICE in the UK. However, IL-1 blockade has an important role in other rheumatic diseases, such as adult-onset Still's disease and the auto-inflammatory syndromes.

IL-17 – IL-17 is a potent, pro-inflammatory cytokine inducing chemokines which lead to immune cell infiltration, inhibiting chondrocyte metabolism and promoting osteoclast activation leading to joint damage. Monoclonal antibodies have been developed to target the IL-17 pathway: blocking the cytokine or its receptor or preventing T_{H17} differentiation. Secukinumab targets IL-17A, one member of the six member IL-17 cytokine family, and is approved for use in ankylosing spondylitis and psoriatic arthritis. Brodalumab is the first IL-17 receptor blocker and is used in the treatment of psoriasis, offering a broader blockade of IL-17 signaling than focusing on a single member of the cytokine family. Ustekinumab targets the p40 subunit shared by IL-12 and IL-23, thereby reducing T_{H1} and T_{H17} differentiation. It is currently used in the treatment of psoriatic arthritis.

BAFF (also known as BLyS) – B-cell activating factor is part of the TNF superfamily. BAFF levels are known to be elevated in certain autoimmune diseases, such as SLE. Belimumab selectively inhibits BAFF, removing a crucial B-cell survival factor, leading to B-cell apoptosis, a process that appears to affect newly activated B-cells more than memory and plasma cells.

RANKL – RANKL, a member of the TNF superfamily, binds to its receptor, RANK, promoting osteoclast differentation, activation and survival. Denosumab binds to and inhibits RANKL, mimicking the action of the endogenous RANKL inhibitor, osteoprotegerin, thereby inhibiting osteoclast-mediated bone resorption. It is licensed for use in postmenopausal women with osteoporosis and men who develop osteoporosis as a consequence of hormonal ablation therapy for prostate cancer.

Cell depletion

Rituximab, a cytotoxic anti-CD20 monoclonal antibody, was originally used for the treatment of B-cell malignancies but was later shown to be an effective treatment for rheumatoid arthritis that had not responded to anti-TNF treatment. CD20 is expressed on all B-cells from the pre-B-cell stage in the bone marrow but is absent from plasma cells. Nonetheless, secondary hypogammaglobulinaemia can develop after repeated cycles of treatment. Planned vaccinations should therefore be administered prior to treatment.

Rituximab kills cells by a combination of antibody-dependent cellular cytotoxicity (ADCC), complement-dependent cytotoxicity (CDC) and apoptosis. In ADCC, the monoclonal antibody binds its target and the Fc portion engages effector cells such as macrophages and natural killer cells via their cell surface Fc receptors.

The clinical use of rituximab has provided a unique insight into B-cell development and disease pathogenesis. B-cell depletion is not a guarantee of response, indicating that B-cells are not central to disease in all patients.

Co-stimulation blockade

Abatacept is a fusion protein of the extracellular domain of the CTLA-4 molecule and the Fc region of human IgG1. The molecule competes with CD28 for binding sites on CD80 and CD86, thereby preventing the second signal required for T-cell activation. In this way, it inhibits the activation of naive T-cells although the treatment may also impair the activity of previously activated T-cells.

Efficacy

Tumour necrosis factor blockade, IL-6R blockade, B-cell depletion and co-stimulation blockade are all licensed approaches for the treatment of RA. The efficacy of each approach is surprisingly similar. In established RA, about two-thirds of patients respond to treatment although, of these, only about a third achieve the highest quality of response.

Safety

Over a decade of registry data has shown biologic drugs, in particular anti-TNFs, to be well tolerated and safe. The main concern related to treatment is the propensity for serious infections, which is again similar across the approaches, amounting to 3–4 serious infections per 100 patient-years in clinical trial populations.

In addition, there are individual associations with particular modalities, such as reactivation of tuberculosis (TB) following TNF blockade, and progressive multifocal leucoencephalopathy due to JC virus reactivation as an extremely rare complication of rituximab. The aetiology of JC virus reactivation with rituximab is unclear. TNF is important for granulomata formation, and granulomas maintain tuberculosis latency following a previous infection, potentially many years beforehand. Consequently TNF blockade disrupts these structures, which can lead to reactivation of TB. Patients due to start biologic agents, particularly anti-TNF, are therefore screened for latent TB, which should be treated before initiation of therapy.

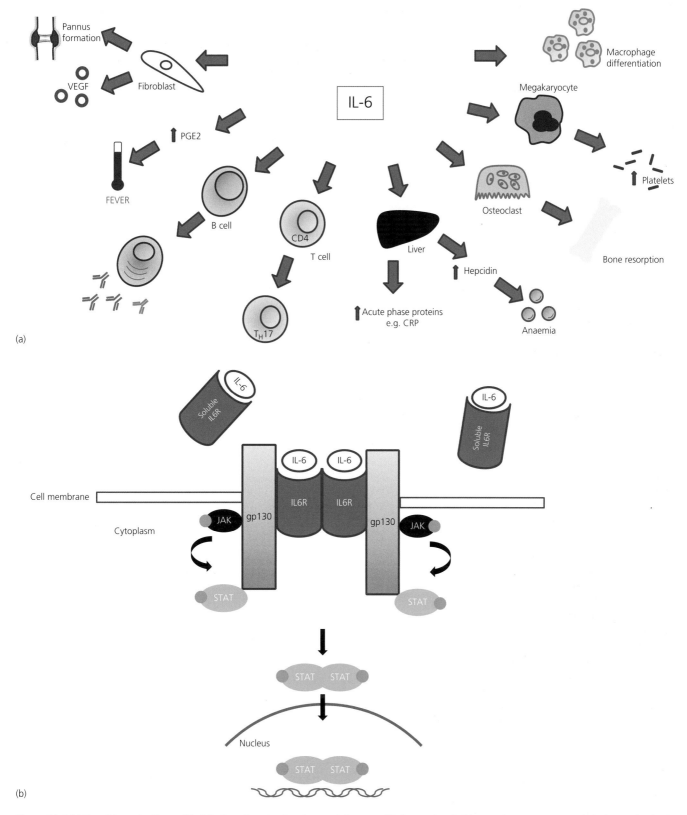

Figure 24.6 (a) The pleiotropic effects of IL-6. IL-6 mediates local and systemic features of inflammation. IL-6 is an endogenous pyrogen, inducing production of prostaglandin E2 (PGE2) which acts at the hypothalamus. IL-6 has a stimulatory effect on the immune system, promoting the differentiation of naive CD4 T-cells into T_H17 cells, the maturation and differentiation of B-cells into immunoglobulin-secreting plasma cells, and macrophage differentiation. In the liver, IL-6 activates hepatocytes to produce acute-phase proteins such as CRP, and induces the increased production of hepcidin, resulting in anaemia of chronic disease due to altered iron homeostasis. In the bone marrow, an increase in megakaryocyte differentiation leads to thrombocytosis. In the joint, IL-6 promotes the differentiation of osteoclasts, leading to bone resorption, and stimulates fibroblast proliferation and activation, thereby contributing to pannus formation and angiogenesis through the production of vascular endothelial growth factor (VEGF). (b) The **IL-6 signalling pathway** is an example of a JAK-STAT signalling pathway. IL-6 binds to its membrane-bound receptor, leading to the dimerization with the signal transducing gp130. This activates the Janus kinases (JAK1, JAK2) and tyrosine kinase 2 (TYK2) to autophosphorylate, then phosphorylate the signal transducer and activator of transcription proteins 1 and 3 (STAT1 and STAT 3), which dimerize and move into the nucleus to activate the transcription of their target genes. There is also a soluble form of the IL-6 receptor, which can bind IL-6, and subsequently binds to cells that express gp130 but not the membrane form of the IL-6 receptor (trans-signalling pathway). The anti-IL-6R antibody binds to both soluble and membrane forms of the receptor

To date, there is no evidence to associate biologic therapy with the development of malignancy, with the possible exception of non-melanoma skin cancer which is associated with most immunosuppressive treatments. The most commonly reported adverse events are localized injection site reactions with subcutaneously administered therapies, which tend to be self-limiting. Rituximab is associated with infusion reactions, which are linked to its cytotoxic mode of action, and can occasionally be severe.

Anti-drug antibodies

Biologic agents are proteins and so they sometimes provoke anti-drug antibodies (ADAs), which can neutralize efficacy and accelerate drug clearance. Clinically, patients may develop a secondary loss of effect, and sometimes side effects such as infusion reactions (e.g. with infliximab) and, rarely, hypersensitivity and anaphylaxis. The development of immunogenicity is influenced by the structure of the therapeutic antibody (e.g. a chimeric antibody is more immunogenic than a humanized antibody) as well as by the dose administered (e.g. the incidence of ADAs is lower with higher doses of infliximab), and the concurrent use of drugs such as methotrexate, which reduce the incidence of ADAs.

Biosimilars

As the patents expire on the original biologic drugs biosimilars have been developed. A biosimilar is highly similar to the original, reference biological product with no meaningful differences in terms of quality, safety or efficacy. However, it is not possible to generate identical copies of the reference product due to the complexity of the manufacturing process in living systems.

Regulatory bodies have developed clear guidelines for the evaluation and approval of these products which have the potential to improve affordability and accessibility. Once approved they are given similar clinical indications to the reference product but require ongoing pharmacovigilance and patient registers to monitor efficacy and safety. Biosimilars should not be automatically substituted for the reference product and should be prescribed by brand name to avoid any accidental substitution

Janus kinase inhibition

Janus kinases (JAK) are a family of four tyrosine kinases involved in the intracellular signalling pathways of many cytokines. They can be targeted by oral small molecule drugs but these are less selective than biologic drugs as they do not target a single cytokine pathway. Tofacitinib and baricitinib are currently licensed for use in RA.

Further reading

Electronic Medicines Compendium: www.medicines.org.uk/emc/

Murphy K and Weaver C. *Janeway's Immunobiology*, 9th edn. Garland Science, New York, 2016.

Singh JA, Wells GA, Christensen R *et al.* Adverse effects of biologics: a network meta-analysis and Cochrane overview. *Cochrane Database of Systematic Reviews* 2011; **12**: CD008794.

CHAPTER 25

Laboratory Tests

Marisa Fernandes das Neves[1], Rajendra Vara Prasad Irlapati[2] and David Isenberg[3]

[1] Medicine IV Department, Fernando Fonseca Hospital, Amadora; CEDOC - Chronic Diseases, Faculty of Medical Sciences, New University of Lisbon, Lisbon, Portugal
[2] Nizams Institute of Medical Sciences, Hyderabad, India
[3] Centre For Rheumatology, Department of Medicine, University College London, London, UK

OVERVIEW

- Abnormal laboratory tests occur frequently in patients with rheumatological disorders.
- Laboratory abnormalities suggesting non-specific inflammation are common and accompany many rheumatological disorders.
- Routine blood tests (haematology and chemistry) are useful to monitor known rheumatological diseases and may be helpful in diagnosis. Abnormalities may reflect adverse effects of medications or may indicate organ involvement from an underlying rheumatological disease.
- Immunological testing is primarily for diagnostic purposes and may help subsetting patients (e.g. patients with systemic lupus erythematosus who are anti-Ro positive are more likely to be photosensitive); however, the antinuclear antibody test is not diagnostic.

This chapter describes investigations that may be performed in a patient with a suspected or established rheumatological disorder. Abnormal haematology tests, particularly anaemia and platelet abnormalities, are commonly found. Biochemical abnormalities include raised protein and globulin levels and reflect a non-specific inflammatory response. Haematological and biochemical investigations are useful for both diagnostic and monitoring purposes, while most immunological investigations are mainly used to facilitate diagnosis.

Haematology investigations

A full blood count and erythrocyte sedimentation rate (ESR), although non-specific, are used to monitor disease activity, to assess the effects of drug treatment, to exclude factors such as dietary deficiency or haemolysis that may be contributing to the morbidity of a rheumatological disease, and (rarely) to exclude a primary haematological malignancy that can mimic various forms of arthritis (Table 25.1).

Anaemia

Anaemia of chronic disease (ACD) is the most common abnormality observed in rheumatic diseases. The cause for this is not clear, but likely causes include shortened red cell survival or impaired bone marrow response to erythropoietin. Another major contribution is from inflammation-induced activation of interleukin (IL) 6 and the hepcidin axis, which hampers iron absorption from gut and release from storage sites. It is sometimes difficult to distinguish iron deficiency anaemia from ACD as the smear in ACD can be normocytic or microcytic. Serum ferritin, which is an acute-phase reactant, may also be elevated due to the underlying rheumatic condition. Soluble transferrin receptor levels may help in such scenarios.

Autoimmune haemolytic anaemia (AIHA) is a rare complication in rheumatic diseases seen in SLE and related conditions such as antiphospholipid syndrome (APS) and Sjögren's syndrome. Evans' syndrome is AIHA with thrombocytopenia. A positive direct Coombs' test helps to identify AIHA. Non-immune haemolytic anaemias may be due to microangiopathic haemolytic anaemia in conditions like thrombotic thrombocytopaenic purpura (TTP) and catastrophic antiphospholipid syndrome (CAPS) or disseminated intravascular coagulation (DIC).

Macrophage activation syndrome (MAS) is a unique haematological complication seen in systemic-onset juvenile idiopathic arthritis (JIA) and SLE, characterized by pancytopenia, very high serum ferritin levels, rapid fall in ESR and elevated triglyceride levels.

Platelet abnormalities

Platelet abnormalities are common in rheumatic disorders. Mild to moderate thrombocytosis is one of the markers for acute or chronic inflammation. Platelet count is regulated by thrombopoietin, the synthesis of which is elevated in states of inflammation due to elevated IL-6. Platelets are often elevated in disease like rheumatoid arthritis (RA) and Still's disease when active. In the paediatric age group, thrombocytosis is often seen in systemic-onset JIA and Kawasaki's disease. A normal or low platelet count in a child with

ABC of Rheumatology, Fifth Edition. Edited by Ade Adebajo and Lisa Dunkley.
© 2018 John Wiley & Sons Ltd. Published 2018 by John Wiley & Sons Ltd.

Table 25.1 Anaemia and rheumatological disease

Type	Indices	Causes
Iron-deficient	↓Serum Fe ↑Serum TIBC Microcytosis, hypochromasia	NSAIDs ⎤ Peptic Corticosteroids ⎦ ulcer disease Disease *per se:* e.g. oesophagitis in scleroderma
Megaloblastic	Macrocytosis ↓Folate ↓B_{12} ↓TFTs	Azathioprine Methotrexate (↓folate) Pernicious anaemia
Haemolytic	Reticulocytes Haptoglobins Positive direct Coombs' test	SLE Drugs e.g. dapsone
Chronic disease	Normochromic, normocytic ↓serum iron, ↓TIBC, ↓ferritin	Multifactorial, ↓EPO, abnormal erythrocyte development, ↑cytokines e.g. IL-1, TNF-α

EPO, erythropoietin; IL-1, interleukin-1; NSAIDs, non-steroidal anti-inflammatory drugs; TFT, thyroid function test; TIBC, total iron-binding capacity; TNF-α, tumour necrosis factor alpha

suspected active systemic-onset JIA should raise the suspicion of underlying haematological malignancy or macrophage activation syndrome.

Thrombocytopenia, on the other hand, is often a manifestation of autoimmune rheumatic disease (ARD) and related diseases. An autoimmune thrombocytopenia (usually chronic but occasionally acute) occurs in up to 20% of patients with lupus and in patients with primary antiphospholipid antibody syndrome. Thrombocytopenia in APS is often mild, whereas it can be severe in SLE. In some of these patients, it has been possible to demonstrate the presence of antiplatelet antibodies. Approximately 15% of patients with 'idiopathic' thrombocytopenia later develop lupus, although identifying those patients prospectively remains a problem. Thrombocytopenia may also be seen in the subset of rheumatoid arthritis with Felty's syndrome (see below). Infections associated with arthralgia such as cytomegalovirus, hepatitis C and human immunodeficiency virus (HIV) can also be associated with thrombocytopenia.

Critically ill patients with multiorgan dysfunction and thrombocytopenia, with or without vascular manifestations, may be due to TTP, catastrophic APS and DIC. Thrombocytopenia in patients with cutaneous vasculitis excludes primary systemic vasculitis and secondary causes like lupus should be considered.

In patients under long-term follow-up, thrombocytopenia is an early marker for marrow suppression due to cytotoxic therapies like cyclophosphamide, methotrexate and mycophenolate mofetil.

White blood cell abnormalities

Felty's syndrome, the association of rheumatoid arthritis with leucopenia (predominantly neutropenia) and splenomegaly (and often leg ulcers), is rare. Leucopenia, particularly lymphopenia, is common in lupus. Most patients are asymptomatic but may be predisposed to infections. There are several causes for lymphopenia in SLE. Antilymphocyte antibodies are frequently found in patients with SLE; lymphocyte apoptosis is increased in active SLE and lymphocytes may be sequestered at sites of inflammation or lymphoid tissues. Lymphopenia may be associated with flares of disease activity.

Bone marrow suppression is a well-recognized complication of immunosuppressive drugs used to treat rheumatic disease such as azathioprine, methotrexate, leflunomide, sulfasalazine, cyclophosphamide and mycophenolate mofetil. Patients taking these drugs require regular haematological assessments to allow early detection of bone marrow suppression.

Systemic JIA characteristically has a severe neutrophilic leucocytosis. Mild to moderate neutrophilia is seen in RA and primary vasculitis. Leucocytosis is occasionally found in flares of lupus, but is more often a reflection of underlying infection or corticosteroid-induced demargination of neutrophils. Infections should be ruled out in all cases of leucocytosis, though it may be a marker for severe inflammation.

Eosinophilia is commonly seen in parasitic infections or secondary to drugs, but it is also characteristic of some rheumatic and inflammatory diseases such as eosinophilic granulomatous polyangiitis (formerly known as Churg–Strauss syndrome). A range of blood test abnormalities in rheumatological diseases is shown in Table 25.2.

Acute-phase response

This response defines a co-ordinated set of systemic and local events associated with inflammation, triggered by tissue damage. The term is misleading, as changes may occur in both acute and chronic inflammation. About 30 acute-phase proteins are known. Elevated serum concentrations of these proteins often last for several days after the initiating event, and their synthesis in the liver is triggered by cytokines, particularly IL-1, IL-6 and tumour necrosis factor alpha (TNF-alpha). These cytokines derive from activated macrophages that have been demonstrated at the site of the injury. Other types of cells such as fibroblasts and endothelial cells are also sources of cytokines. There is some specificity in the cytokine/acute-phase reactant interactions; for example, the synthesis of C-reactive protein (CRP) is dependent on IL-6, while haptoglobin production is influenced by the three cytokines mentioned above.

Measurement of the acute-phase response is helpful to ascertain inflammatory disease, as well as for the assessment of disease

Table 25.2 Blood test abnormalities in some rheumatological diseases

		RA	SLE	PMR	Crystals	Myositis	SSc	Osteoporosis	Osteomalacia
Anaemia	Chronic disease	++	++	+	–	–	++	–	–
	Microcytic/hypochromic	++	+	++	–	–	++	–	–
	Megaloblastic	++	–	–	–	–	–	–	–
Acute–phase response	ESR	++	++	+++	+/–	+	+	–	–
	CRP	+	–	+	+/–	–	–	–	–
Abnormal renal function		+	++	+/–	+	+/–	+	–	–
Abnormal liver function		+	+	–	–	–	–	–	–
Uric acid		–	–	–	+	–	–	–	–
Bone biochemistry	Alk phos	–	–	+	–	–	–	–	+/–
	Ca^{2+}	–	–	–	–	–	–	–	↓/–
	PO^{4-}	–	–	–	–	–	–	–	↓/–

Aik phos, alkaline phosphatase; CRP, C-reactive protein; ESR, erythrocyte sedimentation rate; PMR, polymyalgia rheumatica; RA, rheumatoid arthritis; SIE - systemic lupus erythematosus; SSc, systemic sclerosis

Table 25.3 Acute-phase reactants

Parameter	Measurement	Pathophysiology	Affected by
ESR	Distance in mm that RBC column falls in 1 hour	Dependant upon rouleaux formation (aggregation of red cells) and PCV. Indirect reflection of acute-phase proteins and immunoglobulins	Plasma proteins (i.e. fibrinogen. β2 microglobulin and immunoglobulins) Anaemia, ↓ in sickle cell anaemia
CRP	Immunoassay (mg/L)	Pentamenc protein released from liver under influence of IL-6 within 4 hours of tissue injury	↑↑ in infection, often normal in SLE

CRP, C-reactive protein; ESR, erythrocyte sedimentation rate; IL-6, interleukin-6; PCV, packed cell volume; RBC, red blood cell; SLE, systemic lupus erythematosus

activity, monitoring of therapy and the detection of intercurrent infection. It is impractical and unnecessary to measure all aspects of the acute-phase response; the most widely used measurements are the ESR, CRP and complement components, especially complement C3 (Table 25.3). ESR correlates with fibrinogen levels and CRP is linked to IL-6 activity. The ESR is the measure of the height of the layer of red blood cells that settle in a tube of anticoagulated blood in 1 hour (measured in millimetres per hour (mm/h)). Less common measurements include plasma viscosity, serum amyloid A (SAA) protein, haptoglobin and fibrinogen.

The disadvantages of ESR compared to CRP include variability with age and sex, it is slow to change with disease activity and can be affected by anaemia and raised immunoglobulin levels (both elevate the ESR). Other technical disadvantages are that it cannot be measured on a stored sample and is time consuming.

Tests for plasma levels of cytokines such as IL-6, IL-1 and TNF-alpha are not commercially available and are currently used solely as research tools. Other tests of potential use in the future are SAA protein and matrix metalloproteinase (MMP)-3; both may predict bone damage in early rheumatoid arthritis.

Characteristically, CRP is normal or low in SLE, except when associated with serositis and arthritis. An elevation should prompt search for underlying infection. High ESR and CRP in RA predict a poor outcome.

Serum procalcitonin, a prohormone of calcitonin, is a newly discovered acute-phase reactant. It has been shown to be a useful marker for invasive bacterial infections, especially in critically ill patients with SLE and other immune deficiency disorders. It does not rise significantly in non-infective inflammation. In the paediatric age group, it is shown to be more specific than CRP and correlates well with severity of infection.

Biochemical investigations

The majority of biochemical tests are useful in monitoring organ-specific complications of disease or in assessment of side effects of therapy.

Hepatic function

The most common liver abnormality in the context of autoimmune rheumatic diseases is an increase in enzyme activities. Importantly, these enzymes are not liver specific, which means that the clinician must bear in mind other organ origins (e.g. isolated alkaline phosphatase elevation in bone disease, aspartate aminotransferase (AST) elevation and accompanying creatine phosphokinase levels in muscle disease). Liver abnormalities in autoimmune diseases consist usually in mild elevations of liver transaminases or cholestasis. Frequently, hepatic function abnormalities occur as a consequence of hepatotoxic drugs, notably non-steroidal anti-inflammatory drugs, methotrexate, azathioprine, cyclophosphamide, sulfasalazine, leflunomide and the anti-TNF-alpha biologic therapies.

The recommended frequency of hepatic monitoring is dependent on the particular pharmacological intervention being used. However, a baseline assessment is generally recommended before initiating any of the drugs mentioned above. In addition to drug effects, other conditions that must be ruled out are concomitant viral hepatitis and alcohol abuse.

After excluding these common causes of raised liver enzymes, the differentials are between a concomitant specific liver disease and the systemic disease itself with liver involvement. The most important immune-mediated diseases that primarily affect the liver are primary biliary cirrhosis, primary sclerosing cholangitis and autoimmune hepatitis. Theoretically, any systemic autoimmune rheumatic disease can cause liver injury. The most frequently implied conditions are systemic lupus erythematosus, antiphospholipid syndrome, rheumatoid arthritis, Felty's syndrome, myositis, systemic sclerosis and Sjögren's syndrome.

Renal function

Abnormal renal function may be a component of a rheumatic disease or a consequence of treatment. The ARDs most frequently associated with renal impairment are SLE, vasculitis and systemic sclerosis. Rheumatoid arthritis can also affect the kidneys. Non-steroidal anti-inflammatory drugs are often implicated in renal dysfunction and may necessitate discontinuation of therapy. Dose reduction of renally excreted immune suppressants such as methotrexate may be required in the presence of renal impairment. Similarly, a dose reduction in allopurinol, a urate-lowering drug used in the management of gout, is required in the presence of renal impairment.

Measurement of plasma creatinine concentration is widely used as a test of renal function. However, it is not sensitive and requires a substantial loss of glomerular function before beginning to rise. The blood urea concentration is also an insensitive marker of renal function and is influenced by factors that include the rate of protein metabolism, adsorption of blood from the enteric tract, fluid balance and steroid use. An ideal filtration marker (e.g. inulin) can be used to determine glomerular filtration rate (GFR), but it is not available in everyday clinical practice. Instead, GFR is estimated through formulas based on serum creatinine levels, gender, weight, age and race.

Urinalysis is a simple method to detect renal disease. Patients with glomerulonephritis accompanying autoimmune rheumatic diseases will have active urinary sediment with protein and/or blood on dipstick testing and red cells and granular or cellular casts on light microscopy. Twenty-four hour urine collection, once thought to be the gold standard for quantification of proteinuria and to assess creatinine clearance, is now being replaced by a spot urine protein:creatinine ratio test, given its reliability and ease of determination. Serial estimations of urinary protein excretion are helpful to monitor treatment in rheumatological patients with renal involvement.

Bone biochemistry

The main diseases of bone presenting to rheumatologists are osteoporosis, osteomalacia and Paget's disease. The most commonly measured markers are serum alkaline phosphatase activity and serum calcium and phosphate concentrations. All three tend to be normal in osteoporosis, while a raised alkaline phosphatase activity of bone origin is the key biochemical feature of Paget's disease. Severe cases of osteomalacia are associated with hypocalcaemia, hypophosphataemia and increased alkaline phosphatase activity. Parathyroid hormone levels may be high, while vitamin D levels are usually low with this condition. Biochemical markers of cartilage and bone turnover consist of either collagen breakdown products (cross-linked collagen derivatives, pyridinoline, deoxypyridinoline and N-telopeptides) or non-collagenous matrix proteins and osteoclast-specific enzymes, respectively. These may be used to assess bone turnover in osteopenia and osteoporosis.

Other biochemical tests

Patients with chronic inflammatory diseases such as rheumatoid arthritis and lupus are predisposed to atherosclerosis independently of other risk factors. These patients should be screened for modifiable conditions such as diabetes, and dyslipidemia, which may confer increased atherosclerotic risk. In addition, abnormalities in lipid profile can be due to therapy in patients receiving tocilizumab, a monoclonal antibody against IL-6.

Muscle disease is associated with a rise in creatine phosphokinase (CK) activity. This enzyme occurs as three isoenzymes: CK MM originates from skeletal muscle, CK BB from brain and thyroid and CK MB from myocardium and regenerating skeletal muscle. Serial measurements of CK activity often reflect disease activity in myositis. However, in dramatic myositis with severe muscle wasting, CK levels can decrease to normal range, reflecting the loss of muscle fibres. Normal CK levels are higher in those of African origin. The interpretation of markedly elevated CK levels should include consideration of the effects of vigorous exercise and intramuscular injections, which can dramatically but temporarily raise enzyme activity. Levels of cardiac troponin I are typically absent in non-cardiac muscle disease and a negative troponin I will help to exclude a potential cardiac origin for an elevated CK.

Immunological tests

Autoantibodies

Autoantibodies are immunoglobulins that bind to self antigens. Virtually every molecule in the body can be an antigen and drive an autoimmune response, if the normal mechanisms of self-tolerance fail. Low concentrations of autoantibodies are present in the plasma of many normal individuals and have a higher prevalence in the normal elderly population. Autoantibodies may in some healthy people be anticipatory, that is, they may be found in the serum for months or years before the relevant disease manifests clinically. Examples include the appearance of rheumatoid factor years before rheumatoid arthritis becomes evident and anti-dsDNA antibodies previous to SLE developing. These antibodies are overexpressed in autoimmune conditions, and can also be involved in pathogenic mechanisms.

Table 25.4 Autoantibodies associated with some rheumatological diseases

	RF	CCP	ANA	dsDNA	Ro	La	Sm	RNP	ANCA	Jo1	Topoisomerase*	Cardiolipin
RA	+++	+++	+	–	+/–	+/–	–	–	–	–	–	–
SLE	+	–	+++	+++	++	++	++	++	–	–	–	++
Sjögren's	+	–	++	–	+++	+++	–	–	–	–	–	–
Myositis	–	–	++	–	–	–	–	–	–	+	–	–
SSc	–	–	++	–	–	–	–	–	–	–	+	–
APS	–	–	–	–	–	–	–	–	–	–	–	+++
Vasculitis	+	–	–	–	–	–	–	–	++	–	–	–

ANA, antinuclear antibody; ANCA, antineutrophil cytoplasmic antibody; APS, antiphospholipid syndrome; CCP, cyclic citrullinated peptide; dsDNA, double-stranded DNA; RA, rheumatoid arthritis; RF, rheumatoid factor; SLE, systemic lupus erythematosus; SSc, systemic sclerosis
*, also known as anti-Scl-70

Autoantibodies may be divided into those directed against organ-specific antigens (such as the acetylcholine receptor in myasthenia gravis or intrinsic factor in pernicious anaemia) and those that bind to more ubiquitous antigens such as DNA or the phospholipid component of cell membranes (such as cardiolipin). Relatives of patients with rheumatic diseases may show positivity for autoantibodies, reflecting a genetic tendency to autoimmunity; these antibodies are usually not organ specific. Detection of autoantibodies in rheumatic disorders (Table 25.4) is generally more useful for diagnosis than for monitoring disease activity. With the increasing use of rituximab, a monoclonal antibody against B-lymphocytes expressing CD20, in autoimmune diseases, autoantibodies have also been considered in the decision-making process.

Rheumatoid factors

Rheumatoid factors (RFs) are immunoglobulins (Ig) that bind the Fc (constant region) of IgG. Several assays are available, including the classic Rose–Waaler test, which relies on the ability of rheumatoid factors to agglutinate sheep erythrocytes coated with antisheep immunoglobulin, and the latex agglutination test, in which latex particles coated with human IgG aggregate in the presence of IgM RF. These tests identify only the IgM isotype. Detection of IgG and IgA RF by enzyme-linked immunosorbent assay (ELISA) is now widely available, but it is expensive and not widely used in practice. IgM RF is found in 70–80% of patients with rheumatoid arthritis compared to a maximum of 5% in healthy controls. It is also found, in increased prevalence as well as titre, in other autoimmune conditions, such as SLE, Sjögren's syndrome, cryoglobulinaemia and non-autoimmune conditions (most frequently chronic infections, notably tuberculosis, hepatitis B, hepatitis C, syphilis and leishmaniasis). The clinical specificity of IgA RF is not clear, but it has been found early in the course of rheumatoid arthritis. IgA RF, probably from the mucosae, is the most common isotype in Sjögren's syndrome. The development of low-titre RF also increases with age.

Antibodies to cyclic citrullinated peptides

Antibodies to proteins involved in epithelial cell differentiation, known as antiperinuclear factor, antikeratin, antifilaggrin and anticyclic citrullinated peptides, are found in patients with rheumatoid arthritis. Antibodies to cyclic citrullinated peptides (CCPs), found in 70–90% of rheumatoid arthritis patients, are 90–95% specific for rheumatoid arthritis. These antibodies are measured by ELISA, and have begun to replace rheumatoid factor in some hospitals.

Antinuclear antibodies

Antinuclear antibodies (ANA) were first demonstrated in SLE patients in 1948. ANAs are considered a hallmark of ARDs and are amongst the most commonly performed antibody tests worldwide. ANAs are immunoglobulins that bind to antigens in the cell nucleus, and are classically detected by immunofluorescence using murine liver or kidney cells, or a human epithelial cell line (HEp-2) (Figure 25.1). A titre of greater than 1:80 is usually considered positive, although autoimmune disease is generally associated with higher titres (>1:320). Newer assays using ELISA or fluorescent microsphere (bead) technology are increasingly utilized by commercial laboratories. The ANA indirect immunofluorescence (IIF) test using cell substrates is considered the gold standard assay for screening.

A positive test for ANA is not diagnostic of SLE, as an ANA may occur in several conditions, including other ARDs and hepatic, pulmonary, haematological diseases and malignancy. It occurs at significant titre in approximately 5% of the healthy population, and at low titre in up to 20% (more common in women and the elderly). In infectious diseases, the test tends to be positive only transiently, but in the right clinical context, a positive test is strongly suggestive of an autoimmune rheumatic disease.

Two aspects need consideration when interpreting an ANA test result by IIF: the titre at which the test is positive, as above, and the fluorescence pattern. The pattern of immunofluorescence varies according to which nuclear or cytoplasmic antigens are recognized (Table 25.5) and can narrow the spectrum of probable underlying disease. Some patterns, like centromeric, are pathognomonic. A fine dense speckled pattern is considered a normal variant.

Antibodies to DNA

Anti-DNA antibodies are typically detected by an ELISA, Farr assay or immunofluorescence test with the haemoflagellated organism *Crithidia luciliae* (Figure 25.2). Crithidia contains pure

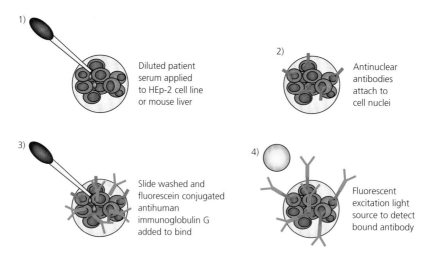

Figure 25.1 Indirect immunofluorescence for antinuclear antibodies. Serum from patients is diluted in serial doubling dilutions. A titre of 1:80 means that the patient's serum has been diluted by a factor of 80. The HEp-2 cell line is derived from human epithelial cells, which are cultured as a monolayer

Table 25.5 Antinuclear antibody staining patterns: associations with immunological disease

ANA staining patterns	Antigen	Disease associations
Homogeneous	DNA or histone proteins	SLE
Speckled	RNA, Sm, Ro and La proteins	Sjögren's syndrome, overlap syndromes
Nucleolar	Nucleolar proteins	Scleroderma
Centromere	Proteins in centromere	Limited scleroderma

ANA, antinuclear antibody, SLE, systemic lupus erythematosus

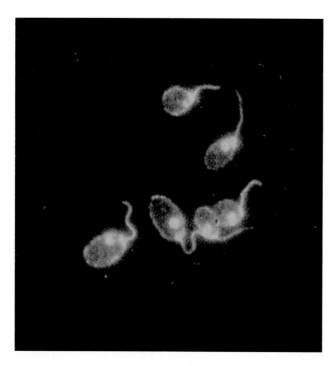

Figure 25.2 *Crithidia* staining

double-stranded DNA (dsDNA), and a positive assay is virtually specific for patients with lupus. Antibodies to dsDNA are often found in high titres in lupus and are especially likely to be found in patients with renal disease. These antibodies are monitored in lupus patients, as they may reflect disease activity, and a rising titre may be predictive of a flare, especially if associated with a falling C3 level. There are reports of the development of anti-dsDNA antibodies following treatment with TNF-alpha antagonists. These antibodies are predominantly of the IgM subtype and are rarely associated with a lupus-like syndrome.

Antibodies to extractable nuclear antigens

Antibodies to extractable nuclear antigens (ENAs) are directed against antigens such as Ro, La, Sm and ribonuclear protein (RNP). They were initially detected by counter-immunoelectrophoresis, a technique in which serum is tested against a saline extract of mammalian nuclei and compared with reference sera to determine a line of precipitation. More specific tests for each antigen (which consist of varying combinations of RNA and protein) are now available in many laboratories and are performed using immunoblot or ELISA.

The identification of antibodies to one or more antigens in a patient's serum can be helpful in the diagnosis of an autoimmune disease (see Table 25.4). For instance, antibodies to Sm are specific for lupus. Similarly, antibodies to Ro and La (also known as SS-A and SS-B) are often found in Sjögren's syndrome. Some antibodies relate to specific subtypes of disease; antitopoisomerase-1 (also known as anti Scl-70) is found in 25% of patients with systemic sclerosis with pulmonary and cardiac involvement, while anti-Jo-1 antibodies, which bind to tRNA histidyl synthetase enzyme, are specific to patients with myositis (polymyositis or dermatomyositis) and pulmonary fibrosis. However, as seen in Table 25.4, there is considerable overlap between expression of clinical disease and expression of particular antibodies. Longitudinal measurement of antibodies to ENAs is usually unnecessary, as there is no consistent association between titres and disease activity. However, the presence of high titres of ENAs in an asymptomatic subject may antedate the onset of clinical disease

Antiphospholipid antibodies

Antiphospholipid antibodies bind chiefly to negatively charged phospholipids such as cardiolipin. There are four tests available.

- The lupus anticoagulant test measures the ability of antiphospholipid antibodies to prolong clotting times (e.g. partial thromboplastin time, Russell's viper venom time) (Figure 25.3).
- Anticardiolipin antibodies (IgG, IgM or IgA) are detected by ELISA.
- Antibodies to beta-2 glycoprotein-I, a co-factor binding protein, also detected by ELISA.
- The Venereal Disease Research Laboratory (VDRL) test is used in the diagnosis of syphilis and utilizes a variety of phospholipids. Thus, false-positive results for syphilis can occur in the presence of antiphospholipid antibodies. This test is of limited diagnostic value for the detection of antiphospholipid antibodies.

Persistently raised concentrations of antiphospholipid antibodies (in at least two measurements 12 weeks apart) are a diagnostic criterion of antiphospholipid syndrome (APS). The IgG isotype of antiphospholipid antibodies confers the higher risk for thrombosis in APS patients. Apart from thrombotic phenomena (both arterial and venous), this syndrome is characterized by recurrent fetal loss, thrombocytopenia and various neurological disorders. APS may occur in isolation or in the context of an ARD, most commonly lupus. Antiphospholipid antibodies may occur in up to 20% of healthy individuals.

Antineutrophil cytoplasmic antibodies

Antineutrophil cytoplasmic antibodies (ANCAs) were initially identified by immunofluorescence, showing two main staining patterns: diffuse cytoplasmatic (cANCA) or perinuclear staining (pANCA). Different proteins are bound by cANCA and pANCA, that bind mainly but not exclusively to serine proteinase 3 (PR-3) and myeloperoxidase (MPO), respectively. Currently, the immunofluorescence aspects are integrated with the direct measurement by ELISA. ANCAs have a pathogenic role in the so-called ANCA-positive vasculitides: granulomatosis with polyangiitis (previously known as Wegener's), microscopic polyangiitis and eosinophilic granulomatosis with polyangiitis (formerly Churg–Strauss syndrome). In these diseases, circulating ANCAs constitute a diagnostic and monitoring tool. Granulomatosis with polyangiitis shows positivity to cANCA in 70–80% and pANCA in 10% of patients, microscopic polyangiitis has pANCA in 60% of cases and cANCA in 30%, and Churg–Strauss syndrome shows 30% of pANCA and cANCA each. Thus, the ANCA result must be integrated with the clinical aspects of the disease. Furthermore, pANCA can be positive in several other diseases, such as inflammatory bowel disease, lupus, autoimmune hepatitis and chronic airway infections.

Immunoglobulins

A polyclonal rise in immunoglobulins is common in inflammation. In Sjögren's syndrome, total IgG concentrations may be substantially raised, often up to 30 g/L or more. Quantification of immunoglobulins and determination of their subtype by protein electrophoresis should be performed in patients with Sjögren's syndrome, as these patients have an increased risk of developing lymphoma. One of the subtypes in particular (IgG4) is associated with a specific disease pattern (IgG4-related disease). Typically, there is lymphoplasmacytic tissue infiltration

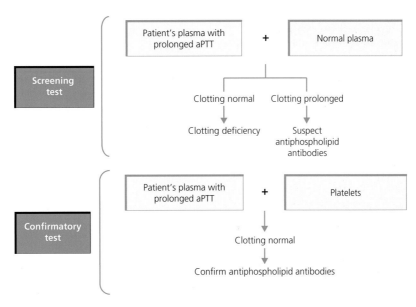

Figure 25.3 Detection of the lupus anticoagulant. Although the lupus anticoagulant is associated with thrombotic episodes *in vivo*, paradoxically the *in vitro* test relies on prolongation of the activated partial thromboplastin time. This is thought to be due to the interaction with the phospholipid portion of the prothrombin activator complex of the clotting cascade. When normal plasma is added to patient plasma, clotting factors are replenished and a clotting factor deficiency-related clotting prolongation will be corrected. However, if antiphospholipid antibodies are the cause of an abnormal test result, the clotting time will not correct. An excess of phospholipids may be added in the form of platelets, which should then correct the clotting prolongation. aPTT, activated partial thromboplastin time

Table 25.6 Changes in C3, C4 and/or CH50 in diseases

Change in C3, C4 or CH50	Characteristic conditions	Cause
↑↑	Bacterial infections Inflammatory diseases, including RA and seronegative arthritides	} Part of acute-phase response
↑		
↓	SLE, especially lupus nephritis, other vasculitides	Consumption by immune complexes
↓	Hereditary hypocomplementaemic syndromes	Hereditary

RA, rheumatoid arthritis; SLE, systemic lupus erythematosus

with a predominance of IgG4 plasma cells and T-lymphocytes, usually accompanied by fibrosis, obliterative phlebitis and elevated serum levels of IgG4.

Complement

Proteins of the complement cascade play a central role in cell lysis, opsonization of bacteria and clearance of immune complexes. C3 and C4 components are most commonly measured (and in some laboratories CH50, which is a measure of overall integrity of the complement pathway) and are useful in screening for complement deficiencies (Table 25.6). Complement degradation products, particularly C3d and C4d, are currently available as research tools as markers of SLE disease activity.

Genetic associations

Most rheumatic disorders are polygenic, and analysis of genetic markers is of limited value. Close human leucocyte antigen (HLA) associations are found with diseases such as ankylosing spondylitis and rheumatoid arthritis. In the former, 95% of patients possess an HLA-B27 allele. The frequency of B27 in the general population is around 10%. A thorough clinical assessment with appropriate haematological, biochemical, immunological and radiological investigations should lead to a definitive diagnosis. HLA haplotype determinations are not tests for specific diseases, because HLA haplotypes do not associate with individual rheumatological diseases. Furthermore, healthy family members of patients with rheumatic diseases (e.g. ankylosing spondylitis) may have a rheumatic disease-associated HLA and no clinical disease.

Microbiology

The differential diagnosis in any acute monoarthropathy must include septic arthritis. This is easily excluded by joint aspiration, with culture of synovial fluid and blood. It is necessary to inform the laboratory if tuberculosis or gonococcal infections are suspected, as specific culture media and techniques are required. Polyarthropathies may be associated with several viral and bacterial infections. Chronic hepatitis B or C or HIV infection may cause polyarthralgia. Acute rheumatic fever, which is rare in the Western world, is associated with streptococcal infection (i.e. positive antistreptolysin O titre or *Streptococcus* species in blood or throat cultures). The seronegative spondyloarthropathies may be related temporally to a diarrhoeal illness or to urethritis. Organisms often implicated in these diseases include *Salmonella*, *Yersinia*, *Campylobacter* and *Chlamydia*. Parvovirus B19 has been associated with a self-limiting polyarthritis similar to rheumatoid arthritis. Other viruses such as rubella and human T-lymphotropic virus may present with an arthralgia. Lyme disease is associated with a rash and polyarthropathy and the diagnosis depends on demonstration of antibodies to the spirochaete *Borrelia burgdorferi*.

Further reading

Hakim A, Clunie G, Haq I. *Oxford Handbook of Rheumatology*, 2nd edn. Oxford University Press, Oxford, 2006.

Playfair JHL, Chain B. *Immunology at a Glance*, 9th edn. Wiley, Chichester, 2009.

Warrell DA, Cox TM, Firth JD, Benz Jr EJ (Eds). *Oxford Textbook of Medicine*, 4th edition, Oxford University Press, Oxford 2003.

Watts RA, Conaghan PJ, Denton C, Foster H, Isaacs J, Muller-Ladner U. *The Textbook of Rheumatology*, 4th edition, Oxford University Press, Oxford 2013.

CHAPTER 26

Musculoskeletal Radiology

William R. Grant[1] and Richard J. Wakefield[2]

[1] Department of Rheumatology, Royal Hallamshire Hospital, Sheffield, UK
[2] Leeds Institute of Rheumatic and Rehabilitation Medicine, Chapel Allerton Hospital, Leeds, UK

OVERVIEW

- The diagnosis of rheumatic disease relies heavily on the clinical history and examination findings.
- The use of investigations such as imaging provides invaluable evidence to support the clinical diagnosis, as well as important additional information on disease severity and prognosis.
- In this chapter, we will cover the principal imaging modalities used in the assessment and monitoring of rheumatic disease.

Box 26.1 **Radiographic features of osteoarthritis**

- Osteophytosis
- Subchondral sclerosis
- Subchondral cysts
- Narrowing and loss of 'joint space'
- Bone remodelling

Plain radiography (X-ray)

Plain radiography remains the most widely used imaging modality in rheumatology practice. It is relatively safe and provides information on a broad range of different conditions affecting bones and joints. Its main limitation is that it provides little information on the soft tissues.

Osteoarthritis is an extremely common degenerative disorder of the joints, and is a major cause of morbidity worldwide. Its incidence increases with age, but is also influenced by a number of genetic, metabolic and occupational factors. The principal radiographic features of osteoarthritis are shown in Box 26.1. The earliest change is the development of osteophytes – bony outgrowths usually at the joint margins. Subchondral bone sclerosis and bone cysts also occur relatively early. In more advanced disease, cartilage compression and degeneration lead to narrowing and eventually loss of the 'joint space' (actually cartilage, being radiolucent and appearing black) – see Figure 26.1. Eventually, bone remodelling and attrition result in flattening or deformities of the articular bone surfaces.

As well as aiding with diagnosis, X-rays also provide information on severity. This is particularly useful in assessing the need for arthroplasty (joint replacement) – see Figure 26.2.

Radio-opaque loose bodies may also be seen and are a relatively common finding on plain radiographs of the knee. They represent fragments of cartilage or bone which have broken free within the joint. They characteristically cause the symptom of mechanical 'locking' of the affected joint. They can sometimes be removed by arthroscopy.

Chondrocalcinosis is the radiological finding of calcific deposits within cartilage, usually in older patients. Common sites include the knee (Figure 26.3) and the triangular fibrocartilage at the wrist. In the correct clinical context, the presence of chondrocalcinosis can help to confirm a diagnosis of calcium pyrophosphate deposition (CPPD) disease. However, it can also be an incidental finding and is not necessarily of clinical significance.

Rheumatoid arthritis is the most common form of inflammatory arthritis. If not adequately treated, it can be highly erosive and lead to significant joint damage and deformity. The radiographic features of rheumatoid arthritis are shown in Box 26.2. Early features include soft tissue swelling, juxta-articular (periarticular) osteopenia and the development of periarticular bone erosions (Figure 26.4). As with osteoarthritis, more advanced disease gives rise to narrowing and loss of the 'joint space' (cartilage). Ankylosis (fusion) of the joints may occur, most characteristically at the carpal bones. Joint subluxation leads to the classic deformities associated with

---

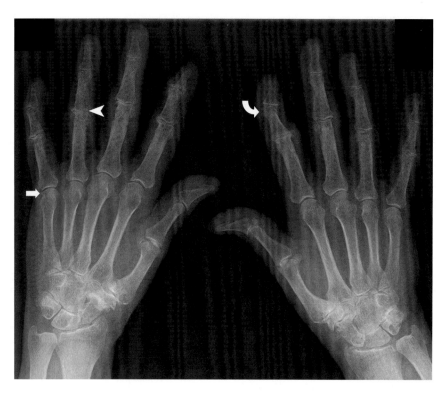

Figure 26.1 Osteoarthritis. The degenerative changes are most marked in the interphalangeal joints, first metacarpophalangeal and scaphotrapezoid joints. There are osteophytes (straight arrow), bone cysts (curved arrow) and loss of 'joint space' (arrowhead)

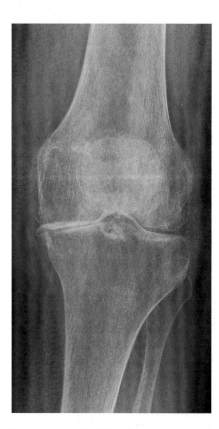

Figure 26.2 Severe osteoarthritis of the left knee in a patient awaiting arthroplasty. This weight-bearing film shows almost complete loss of 'joint space', most marked in the medial compartment. Subchondral sclerosis is also demonstrated

Box 26.2 **Radiographic features of rheumatoid arthritis**

Early disease:

- Soft tissue swelling
- Juxta-articular osteopenia
- Periarticular bone erosions

Advanced disease:

- Narrowing and loss of 'joint space'
- Ankylosis (fusion)
- Subluxation

rheumatoid arthritis (Figure 26.5). The most common patterns are radial deviation of the hand at the carpometacarpal joints and ulnar deviation of the fingers at the metacarpophalangeal joints.

Patients with suspected rheumatoid arthritis should undergo plain radiographs of both hands and both feet. The films of the feet are essential, even in patients who do not complain of foot symptoms. This is because the earliest erosive changes often occur in the joints of the feet (most commonly at the fifth metatarsophalangeal joint) and early inflammation may be subclinical.

Usually, serial radiographs are taken every 1–2 years, to ensure that there is no radiological progression. If new erosions develop, a patient's treatment may need to be reviewed even if their disease appears clinically controlled.

Fortunately, due to the modern approach of early diagnosis and aggressive treatment, as well as powerful novel therapies (tumour necrosis factor alpha inhibitors and other biologic agents), there are

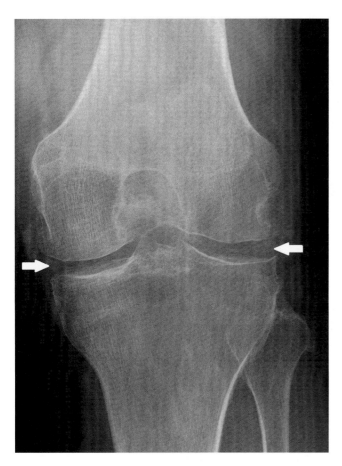

Figure 26.3 Chondrocalcinosis (arrows) within both menisci in the knee of a patient with calcium pyrophosphate deposition (CPPD) disease

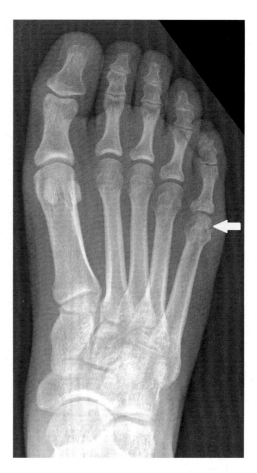

Figure 26.4 Early rheumatoid arthritis in a 22 year old woman. There is a single erosion (arrow) on the right fifth metatarsal head

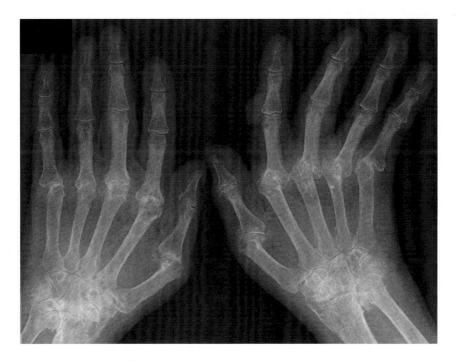

Figure 26.5 A 65 year old woman with more advanced, erosive RA. Note the loss of 'joint space' within each carpus and the marked subluxation at the MCP joints on the right

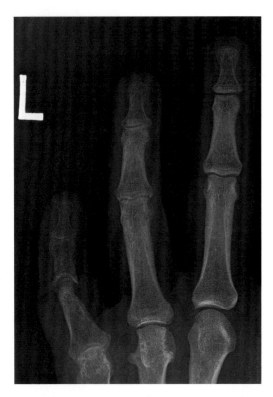

Figure 26.6 Arthritis mutilans in a patient with psoriatic arthritis. Note the 'pencil-in-cup' appearance at the proximal interphalangeal joint of the little finger, with associated telescoping of the digit

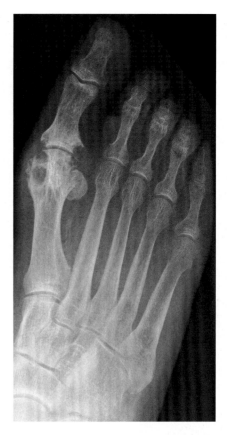

Figure 26.7 Gout. Note the para-articular erosions at the first metatarsophalangeal joint. (With thanks to David Moore.)

now very few patients with severe or disabling joint damage. It is likely that there will continue to be a small number of patients in whom this cannot be avoided, due to severe disease phenotype or medications being either contraindicated or poorly tolerated.

Psoriatic arthritis also has the potential to be highly erosive in some patients. The radiographic features of psoriatic arthritis are similar to those of rheumatoid arthritis, and in some cases the two diseases can be difficult to distinguish.

Arthritis mutilans is a rare but highly destructive small joint arthropathy which can occur in either rheumatoid or psoriatic arthritis. In arthritis mutilans, joint destruction is so severe that the joint architecture is completely lost, resulting in 'telescoping' of the affected digit. The plain radiograph shows a characteristic 'pencil-in-cup' appearance (Figure 26.6).

Gout is another potentially erosive arthropathy. In gout, erosions tend to be juxta-articular (para-articular) rather than within the joint itself (Figure 26.7). The most classic site for these changes is the first metatarsophalangeal joint (usually in patients who have suffered recurrent episodes of podagra) but gout can occur in any peripheral joint. Tophi are another radiographic feature of gout.

Plain radiography is also useful in the diagnosis of axial spondylarthropathy (ankylosing spondylitis and related disorders). The radiological features of axial spondylarthropathy are shown in Box 26.3. Axial inflammation often (but not always) starts at the base of the spine and progressively ascends. For this reason, patients are usually assessed initially via plain radiographs of the

Box 26.3 **Radiographic features of axial spondylarthropathy**

Spine:

• Vertebral squaring
• Romanus lesions ('shiny corners')
• Syndesmophytosis
• Ankylosis
• 'Bamboo' spine

Sacroiliac joints:

• Sclerosis
• Bone erosion
• Ankylosis

lumbar spine and sacroiliac joints (Figures 26.8a and 26.8b). Vertebral squaring is seen on lateral views of the spine and is the earliest abnormality, caused by erosions at the corners of the vertebral bodies. Bone sclerosis due to repair at these sites gives rise to a 'shiny corner' appearance (Romanus lesions). In more advanced disease, there is ossification of the longitudinal ligaments and the outer fibres of the intervertebral discs, resulting in the formation of syndesmophytes. Eventually, this process of progressive fusion (ankylosis) spreads to involve the entire spine. The 'bulges' seen radiographically due to syndesmophytosis at each intervertebral level give a characteristic 'bamboo' appearance.

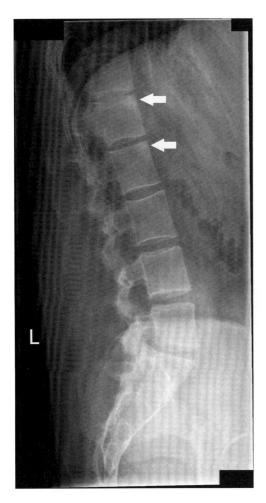

Figure 26.8a Lateral radiograph of the lumbar spine in a patient with ankylosing spondylitis. Note the vertebral squaring. There are Romanus lesions (arrows), particularly notable in the first and second lumbar vertebrae. (With thanks to David Moore.)

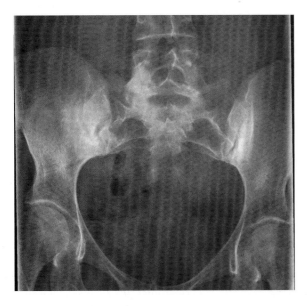

Figure 26.8b Radiograph of the sacroiliac joints in the same patient as Figure 26.8a. There is marked sclerosis around both sacroiliac joints. (With thanks to David Moore.)

Ultrasound scanning

Ultrasound (US) is a highly sensitive imaging modality for the assessment of soft tissues and bone. With the development of modern high-frequency transducers (which yield very high-resolution images, but to a limited tissue depth), US technology is ideally suited to musculoskeletal imaging. It is a very safe, low-cost and well-tolerated investigation. US is also dynamic, allowing direct patient interaction and movement to help demonstrate pathology during the scan. The use of US has spread far beyond the radiology department. Many rheumatologists and other healthcare professionals are developing skills in musculo-skeletal US and incorporating it into outpatient clinic settings. The portable nature of modern systems also makes US a viable investigation for point-of-care imaging in sports and military applications.

Whilst US is widely available, it is a highly operator-dependent modality and appropriate training is essential. Its use is also limited to areas to which the ultrasound beam can gain access. It is not suitable for areas obscured by bone, such as the spine or the full articular surface of a joint.

In rheumatology practice, a major use of US in recent years has been in the assessment of inflammatory arthritis, including rheumatoid arthritis. Many of the structural features of inflammatory arthritis are seen on grey-scale US (Figure 26.9a). However, a major development has been the evolution of Doppler US, which can detect abnormal synovial blood flow (Figure 26.9b). This has been shown to correlate with disease activity and the future risk of bone damage and flare of symptoms. Ultrasound (and MRI) have both been shown to detect inflammation and damage earlier than clinical examination and radiographs respectively. The sonographic features of inflammatory arthritis are listed in Box 26.4, though it is important to be aware that not all of these findings may be present. Tenosynovitis is another important manifestation of rheumatoid arthritis that is readily demonstrated by US.

Ultrasound is also highly useful in confirming common enthe-seal lesions, which may be primary mechanical disorders in their own right or may represent manifestation of an underlying inflammatory disorder, typically a spondylarthropathy such as psoriatic arthritis. In tennis elbow (lateral epicondylitis) and golfer's elbow (medial epicondylitis), US can demonstrate inflammation at the common extensor and flexor tendon origins at the elbow, respectively. Insertional Achilles tendinosis and plantar fasciitis are further forms of enthesopathy commonly seen in patients with spondylarthropathies, and well demonstrated by US.

Shoulder US is widely used for the assessment of the rotator cuff tendons, as well as giving information about the subacromial bursa and the glenohumeral and acromioclavicular joints.

Another important role of US is in the guided aspiration and injection of joints and other structures. Guided injections have been shown to be superior to 'blind' injections.

Ultrasound has also been used to investigate vasculitis. Superficial vessels such as the temporal artery are readily accessible. In the diagnosis of giant cell arteritis, US is thought to have a sensitivity comparable with that of temporal artery biopsy.

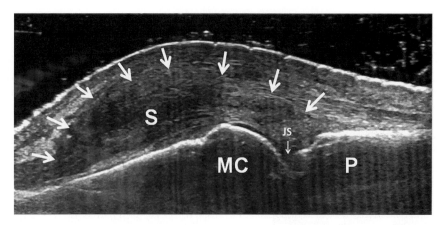

Figure 26.9a Longitudinal greyscale image through a metacarpophalangeal joint of a patient with rheumatoid arthritis. There is grossly thickened synovium (S), which is seen distending the joint capsule (white arrows). MC = metacarpal; P = proximal phalanx; JS = joint space

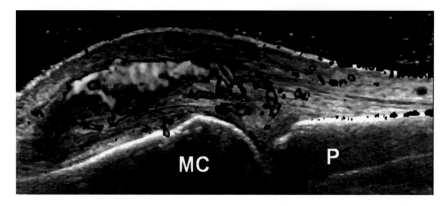

Figure 26.9b Superimposed Doppler image showing increased vascularity of the thickened synovium. This is indicative of active synovitis

---

Box 26.4 **Sonographic features of inflammatory arthritis**

- Synovial hypertrophy
- Joint effusion
- Tenosynovitis
- Increased Doppler activity
- Cartilage loss
- Bone erosions

Magnetic resonance imaging

Magnetic resonance imaging (MRI) provides high-resolution, three-dimensional imaging and is very safe, lacking the radiation exposure associated with other imaging modalities, including plain radiography and computed tomography (CT) scanning. MRI has the further advantage of providing detailed soft tissue imaging, in comparison with plain radiography. It can also visualize deeper and larger joints in greater detail than US, which loses resolution with increased tissue depth.

Magnetic resonance imaging remains relatively expensive, and imaging times are long compared with other modalities. It is also contraindicated in some patients, including those with pacemakers or metallic implants. Claustrophobic patients cannot usually tolerate

MRI, although sedation or general anaesthetic may be an option for some of these. For patients unable to undergo MRI, other imaging modalities such as US and CT scanning must be used.

In rheumatology practice, MRI is highly sensitive for the detection of synovitis in large and small joints, and is primarily used to assess inflammatory arthritis. Whilst plain radiographs provide a good assessment of established structural changes in axial spondylarthropathy, the use of certain MRI sequences provides additional information on current disease activity. This is useful in very early disease (in which radiographic features have not yet developed) or to help to differentiate between active and 'burnt-out' inflammation. Muscle MRI is used in the assessment of inflammatory muscle disease (polymyositis and dermatomyositis) and may be used to identify a suitable site for biopsy (Figure 26.10).

Computed tomography

Computed tomography scanning is not used frequently in rheumatology practice. Detailed musculoskeletal imaging can be achieved by US or MRI, which avoid radiation exposure. However, CT scanning does give excellent bone detail, and can usually provide the necessary information in cases where the safer imaging modalities are either unavailable or contraindicated. CT also has a role in imaging less accessible joints such as the sternoclavicular and costovertebral joints.

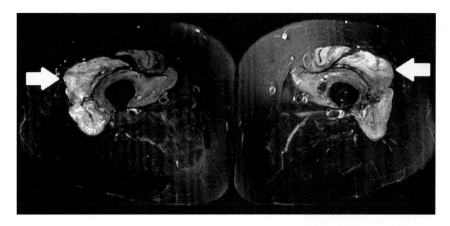

Figure 26.10 Transverse T2 weighted MR image showing increased signal in the thigh muscles (arrows) in a woman with polymyositis

One important application of CT is in fluoroscopically guided aspiration and injection of joints or bursae. As with US, this technique allows highly accurate needle placement.

Computed tomography or MR angiography is sometimes used in the assessment of vasculitis. For example, angiography of the coeliac axis may demonstrate microaneurysm formation in polyarteritis nodosa.

Bone scintigraphy

Bone scintigraphy (isotope bone scanning) is a nuclear medicine investigation in which a radioactive tracer (usually technetium-99 m) is injected intravenously and taken up by any bone tissue with excessive metabolic activity. This may be due to inflammation, degenerative change, infection or malignancy.

The main limitation of bone scintigraphy is that tracer uptake is non-specific and thus not usually diagnostic. For this reason, it is most often used to determine the wider distribution of a pathology already identified at a particular site, for example:

- bony metastases
- Paget's disease of bone (Figure 26.11)
- fragility (stress) fractures.

Another important limitation of bone scintigraphy is that it does not detect the lytic bony lesions of multiple myeloma; for this condition, a skeletal survey (systematic series of plain radiographs of the entire axial skeleton and long bones) is used.

Positron emission tomography

Positron emission tomography (PET) is a modern nuclear medicine investigation in which a radioactive tracer, attached to glucose, is injected intravenously and taken up by tissues. Positron emission is then detected by specialized equipment. PET is usually performed in combination with CT scanning to enable anatomical mapping. Increased tracer uptake is detected in tissues with excessive metabolic activity; again, this is most commonly due to inflammation, infection or malignancy.

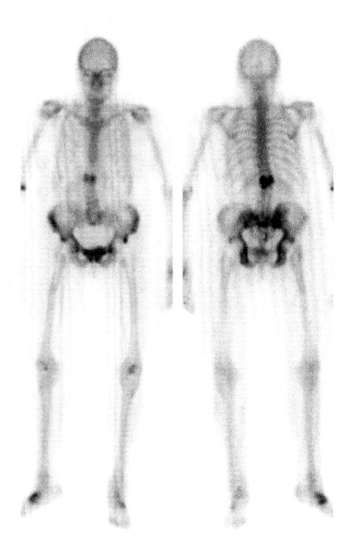

Figure 26.11 Bone scintigram showing the distribution of Paget's disease in a 79 year old woman, with tracer uptake throughout the pelvis and the first lumbar vertebra, where there is additionally an endplate fracture

In rheumatology practice, PET is most frequently used in the diagnosis of vasculitis. It is most useful for large vessel disease (such as systemic giant cell arteritis, affecting the aorta and its branches) – see Figure 26.12. Sometimes, PET may be used to assess a patient

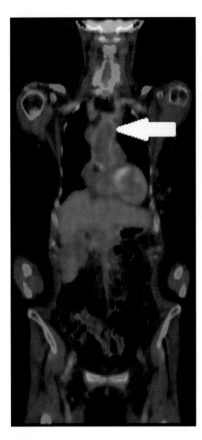

Figure 26.12 Coronal image from PET-CT of a 75 year old woman with large-vessel vasculitis. Intense tracer uptake is seen in the aorta (arrow) and arterial tree

The availability of PET (as well as radiologists with the necessary expertise in interpreting the images) is limited. PET-CT also carries a high radiation burden compared to other imaging modalities.

As with bone scintigraphy, a limitation of PET is that increased tracer uptake is non-specific and does not necessarily yield a diagnosis. Following an abnormal PET, patients may need to undergo further investigation (e.g. tissue biopsy) before a final diagnosis is reached. Another limitation of PET is that it gives little information about the heart and brain. These highly metabolically active tissues demonstrate high levels of tracer uptake in all subjects.

Dual energy X-ray absorptiometry

Dual energy X-ray absorptiometry (DEXA) is a specialized form of plain X-ray which is used to assess bone density. All patients at risk of osteoporosis should undergo fracture risk assessment and DEXA. This includes females aged over 65, those with a history of low-trauma fracture and those receiving glucocorticoid therapy.

Bone density is primarily assessed at the spine and proximal femur. The T-score at each of these sites is calculated as the number of standard deviations by which the subject's bone density lies above or below that of a healthy 30-year-old adult. A T-score of -2.5 or below is diagnostic of osteoporosis.

The assessment and management of osteoporosis are discussed in greater detail in Chapter 11.

Further reading

Conaghan PG. *Musculoskeletal Imaging*. Oxford Specialist Handbooks in Radiology. Oxford University Press, Oxford, 2010.

Grainger A, O'Connor PJ. *Grainger & Allison's Diagnostic Radiology: Musculoskeletal System*, 6th edn. Elsevier, New York, 2015.

with a pyrexia of unknown origin (PUO) and/or persistently elevated inflammatory markers, but in whom standard serological and imaging investigations have failed to yield a diagnosis. In such cases, PET may detect a vasculitis, occult infection or malignancy (such as lymphoma).

CHAPTER 27

The Team Approach

Louise Warburton[1] and Sarah Ryan[2]

[1] Shropshire Community NHS Trust; Keele University, Keele, UK
[2] Haywood Hospital, Stoke on Trent, UK

OVERVIEW

- Evidence for the effectiveness of the multidisciplinary team.
- Members of the team.
- Roles and responsibilities of the members of the team.
- Wider team members such as general practitioners.
- Charity organizations which offer additional support to the patient and MDT.

Many rheumatological conditions, including rheumatoid arthritis (RA), are not curable and the patient faces the challenge of learning to live with their symptoms on a daily basis. Input from a variety of team members can be required to help the patient maximize their physical, psychological and social function. Modern treatments such as combination disease-modifying antirheumatic drugs and anti-TNF drugs have improved the outlook for the patient with RA, and the patient lives *with* the disease, rather than the disease controlling the patient's life. Rheumatoid arthritis will be used as a model to illustrate how a team approach may work in practice.

The patient as a member of the multidisciplinary team

The multidisciplinary team is made up of many people (Box 27.1). Sometimes, the patient will require input from all the members of the team and sometimes very few. The approach needs to be flexible. Each member of the team will deal with a different part of the disease and have different skills and approaches to care. No single member of the team can function in isolation and a good team will allow the patient access to them whenever required.

In the United Kingdom, the National Institute for Health and Care Excellence (NICE) emphasizes that the patient is a pivotal

---

Box 27.1 Members of the multidisciplinary team

- General practitioners
- GPs with a special interest
- Consultant rheumatologists
- Nurse specialists
- Extended scope practitioners
- Physiotherapists
- Occupational therapists
- Podiatrists
- Chiropodists
- Orthotists
- Pharmacists

Box 27.2 Physiotherapy interventions

- Exercise
- Education
- Ice/heat therapy
- Low-level laser therapy
- Wax treatment
- Hydrotherapy

---

member of the team and that all treatment should be based on a discussion of the patient's needs and preferences, with patients having ongoing access to a multidisciplinary team to assess the effect of the condition on their day-to-day activities as well as their mood, social, work and leisure activities (Box 27.2).

A single member of the team, the 'named team member', should have overall responsibility for that patient's care, and be responsible for co-ordinating their care. This person should be accessible

---

ABC of Rheumatology, Fifth Edition. Edited by Ade Adebajo and Lisa Dunkley.
© 2018 John Wiley & Sons Ltd. Published 2018 by John Wiley & Sons Ltd.

quickly by the patient in case of flare management and other problems which require prompt attention.

It is important to involve patients in decisions about their care. There are now many resources available for clinicians and patients to use, to aid in making difficult decisions such as whether or not to start disease-modifying treatments in RA. The MDT should be aware of these clinical decision aids and incorporate them into their everyday care (Box 27.3).

Effectiveness of multidisciplinary team working

The evidence for the effectiveness of a MDT in rheumatology is slim. There is some evidence that patients with RA who were treated by a MDT reported lower levels of pain and increased knowledge of their condition and its management. There is a greater evidence base supporting the input of the MDT in other conditions, such as cancer. A national survey was completed by over 2000 members of cancer MDTs and at least 90% of team members agreed with a wide range of criteria which define effective team working. Respondents felt that team working resulted in improved clinical decision making, more co-ordinated patient care, improvement in overall quality of care, more evidence-based treatment decisions and improved treatments. However, they did acknowledge that MDTs require more time and resources than traditional care.

Roles and responsibilities of members of the team

A typical rheumatology MDT will consist of the following members.

Consultant and medical staff
The medical team is usually led by one or more consultants who have many years' experience in rheumatology and often general medicine as well. It is usually the doctors' role to assess and diagnose the patient and decide on a management plan, taking into account the severity of the disease and current guidelines on treatment.

Traditionally, regular review with the medical team happened every 3–12 months, depending on whether control of the condition had been achieved. Any issues with the disease and treatment were dealt with. Now, some of these regular review appointments may be undertaken by a rheumatology nurse or an extended scope practitioner.

Rheumatology nurse specialist
The rheumatology nurse specialist (RNS) will normally be a registered general nurse who has undertaken extra training in rheumatology. Following diagnosis, the patient will often be referred to a RNS to commence disease-modifying antirheumatic drug therapy and receive ongoing psychological support as the patient commences the process of adapting to living with a long-term condition

Rheumatology nurse specialists have a large role to play in the education of the patient about their disease and the drugs which are used to control it. Being told that you have a life-long disease such as rheumatoid arthritis can be devastating for patients and they are often not receptive to information about the disease when first diagnosed. Follow-up appointments with clinical nurse specialists allow the patient to be educated at a more comfortable pace.

The RNS is usually the named team member, who is easily accessible by the patient in times of difficulty. She or he will often therefore run a rheumatology telephone helpline and try to deal with problems as they arise.

Nurses often undertake assessments of patients, including the Disease Activity Score (DAS) to evaluate the effectiveness of drug treatment, and will make referrals to other members of the team when, for example, physiotherapy or occupational therapy will be of benefit to the patient.

Some RNSs will have extra skills in administering intra-articular joint injections, prescribing disease-modifying drugs and obtaining funding for biologic drugs from the health authority, health management organization or other relevant commisioners of health.

Inpatient care in rheumatology is becoming much less common because of the effectiveness of modern treatments. However, there are still some inpatient rheumatology wards and nursing staff are involved in the care of patients in this setting as well.

Occupational therapist
Occupational therapists (OTs) are responsible for helping the patient to embrace a full role in their lives, both in leisure and work activities. They are often involved in patient education. Many OTs have received training in psychological assessment and can deliver cognitive behaviour-type interventions to help patients overcome anxiety and depression. Depression can co-exist with RA but is frequently overlooked. Occupational therapists can screen for depression and offer early intervention.

Occupational therapists are also trained to improve the functioning of joints and advise patients about joint protection. This involves the use of splinting and avoiding using inflamed joints for heavy or repetitive tasks. OTs and physiotherapists often deliver treatment such as wax baths to improve hand function.

Occupational therapists also improve patient function by advising about aids for daily living and devices to make certain tasks around the home easier. Examples include cutlery with extra-large handles which are easier for the patient to grip.

Helping the patient to remain at work once they are diagnosed with an inflammatory arthritis is also an important part of the OT's job. Many patients give up work because of their arthritis, but there is plenty of evidence that work is good for both mental and physical health. The following are statements from patients with rheumatoid arthritis.

'Working has helped boost my self-esteem. I truly believe that if I wasn't working, my RA would have progressed faster and I would be in a worse state than I am now.'

'The visit [OT work assessment] was a turning point in my life … with the adjustments that followed I could continue to support my family … and achieve a measure of success in the workplace.'

National Rheumatoid Arthritis Society, *I Want to Work: A Self-Help Guide for People with RA* (2007)

Physiotherapist

When joints are inflamed, the muscles around the joint tend to atrophy through lack of use. Moving a swollen joint is painful, so it is only natural that patients will stop using their inflamed joints. If joints are not regularly taken through their normal range of movement, they can become very stiff and eventually contractures of the soft tissues around these joints occur, making it even more difficult for the patient to use that joint in its normal manner.

Physiotherapists are able to offer a range of interventions (see Box 27.2), and have a role in moving and manipulating joints to take them through a normal range of movement, even if the patient is unable to do this themselves. They will also show the patient exercises to maintain strength and proprioception in the muscle groups around inflamed joints, to prevent atrophy and joint damage. It is imperative to begin physiotherapy early in the disease process to prevent many of the common joint problems which develop as the disease progresses. Therefore, the physiotherapist is a very important part of the team.

Some physiotherapists will have extended roles involving intra-articular injections, diagnostic ultrasound scanning and interventional ultrasound where joints and soft tissues can be imaged and injected using ultrasound control.

Podiatrist

The foot is often involved extensively in inflammatory arthritis, but frequently overlooked. Pain and changes in foot structure can severely affect gait and mobility. The use of foot orthoses and specialist therapeutic footwear are recommended by NICE which also advocates that people with RA should have access to foot health assessment and management early in the disease process.

Orthotics (appliances) such as insoles or supports are used to take the load off one part of the foot and prevent further damage and reduce pain (Figure 27.1). Podiatrists will provide advice about the styles of footwear that can accommodate both the foot and the orthoses.

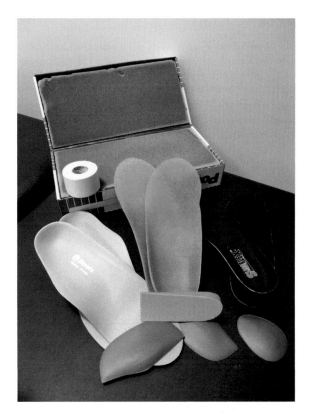

Figure 27.1 A series of podiatry items; selection of insoles and foam to produce impressions of feet for custom orthoses

Specialist podiatrists are involved in the management of significant structural change, vasculitis, neuropathy, bacteria and fungal infections and ulceration, and can carry out nail surgery for persistent nail deformity and infection

Other members of the MDT

It is important to remember that the family or general practitioner is part of the MDT and is often the first person who will see the patient if they develop a problem. The GP will prescribe any disease-modifying drugs as part of a shared care agreement between primary and specialist care. The shared care agreement lays out the expected responsibilities of the patient, GP and specialist in the provision of this drug treatment and the monitoring which is required. Other members of the primary healthcare team will also be involved, such as practice nurses.

Where biologic drugs are prescribed, these are often supplied to the patient by home care organizations. These organizations will deliver the drugs directly to the patient's home and can also teach patients how to self-administer their drugs by injection.

Charity organizations

Charity organizations provide helplines and many sources of advice for patients with inflammatory arthritis. The National Health Service could never have the resources to provide all this care and support and these charities form an integral part of the MDT (see Box 27.3).

Further reading

Ahlmen M, Sullivan M, Bjelle A. Team versus non-team outpatient care in rheumatoid arthritis. A comprehensive outcome evaluation including an overall health measure. *Arthritis and Rheumatism* 1988; **31**(4): 471–479.

National Institute for Health and Care Excellence. *Rheumatoid Arthritis in Adults: Management*. Clinical Guideline 79. Available at: www.nice.org.uk/guidance/cg79 (accessed 20 November 2017).

National Rheumatoid Arthritis Society. *I Want to Work: A Self-Help Guide or People with Rheumatoid Arthritis*. NRAS, London, 2007.

Taylor C, Munro AJ, Glynne-Jones R *et al*. Multidisciplinary team working in cancer: what is the evidence? *BMJ* 2010; **340**: c951.

CHAPTER 28

Epidemiology of the Rheumatic Diseases

Anna E. Litwic and Elaine M. Dennison

MRC Lifecourse Epidemiology Unit, University of Southampton, Southampton General Hospital, Southampton, UK

OVERVIEW

- Globally, all musculoskeletal disorders combined account for over 20% of the total years lived with disability, second only to mental and behavioural problems.

- In this chapter, we review the epidemiology of the most common rheumatic diseases, highlighting the incidence of each condition, along with known risk factors for development.

Globally, all musculoskeletal disorders combined account for over 20% of the total years lived with disability, second only to mental and behavioural problems. Each year, 20% of the UK general population consult a GP with a musculoskeletal problem. The most common rheumatic diseases are osteoarthritis (OA) and gout (Figure 28.1). These diseases become more prevalent with age; since it has been estimated that the proportion of over-65s in the population will increase three-fold in the next 30 years, this demographic change will significantly increase the burden on healthcare systems from musculoskeletal disorders.

Osteoarthritis

Osteoarthritis (OA) is the most common form of arthritis and a leading cause of disability. OA may develop in any joint, but most commonly affects the knees, hips, hands, facet joints and feet. The prevalence of OA varies greatly depending on the definition used (radiological, clinical or self-reported), age, sex and geographical area studied. OA of the hips and knees tends to cause the greatest burden to the population as pain and stiffness in these large weight-bearing joints often lead to significant disability requiring surgical intervention. Psychological distress is more frequently experienced by patients with OA compared to patients with other chronic diseases.

A radiographic case definition of OA results in the highest reported prevalence. Interestingly, individuals with early clinical OA may be free of radiographic changes and, conversely, those with severe radiographic changes may be entirely asymptomatic, although there is a correlation between the severity of radiographic disease and symptoms. The incidence of hand, hip and knee OA increases with age, and women have higher rates than men, especially after the age of 50 years. It is estimated that each year, over 2 million people in the UK visit their GP with OA symptoms.

There are a number of systemic and local risk factors associated with OA (Box 28.1). Genetic factors are important, and OA in some families displays classic mendelian inheritance. The heritability of cartilage volume, as a marker of degeneration, has been estimated at over 70%. Congenital joint deformities may increase the stress on the cartilage and contribute to OA development.

The increase of obesity in the population is one of the major factors associated with both the development of knee OA and progression of the disease; having a high body mass index has been associated with up to nine-fold increased risk of knee OA.

Joint injury can also increase the risk of OA. This may be due to direct cartilage damage or a result of increased stress on the cartilage due to the injury. Workers in certain occupations are at increased risk, for example jobs that require excessive knee bending and farming.

Recent studies have shown that a low vitamin D intake can increase the risk of OA, and a high vitamin C intake may reduce the risk.

Musculoskeletal pain

The majority of chronic pain experienced by older adults is musculoskeletal in origin. The severity of symptoms and their impact on the patient's life vary greatly. The pain can be generalized or affect one region. The most commonly reported localized pain is sited in the lower back, knee, neck, foot and shoulder (Figure 28.2).

Low back pain

Low back pain (LBP) is a symptom, not a disease. Despite several potential causes for LBP (Box 28.2), it is often difficult to establish

---

ABC of Rheumatology, Fifth Edition. Edited by Ade Adebajo and Lisa Dunkley.
© 2018 John Wiley & Sons Ltd. Published 2018 by John Wiley & Sons Ltd.

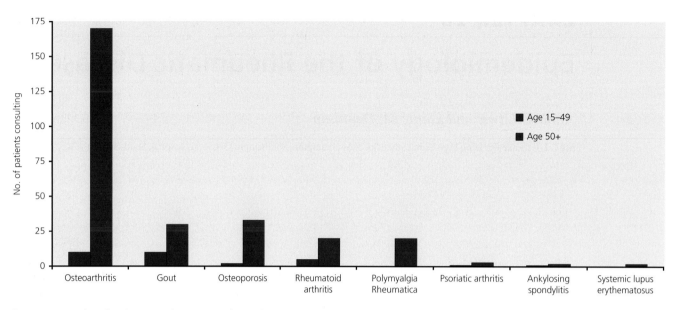

Figure 28.1 Number of patients consulting in 1 year by condition in a practice of 10 000

Box 28.1 **Risk factors for OA**

Systemic	**Age**
	Gender
	Ethnicity
	Genetics
	Obesity
	Diet
	Bone metabolism
Local	Muscle strength
	Physical activity/occupation
	Joint injury
	Joint alignment
	Leg length inequality

Box 28.2 **Causes of back pain**

Mechanical causes

Degenerative conditions

Inflammatory conditions

Infective causes

Neoplastic causes

Metabolic bone disease

Referred pain

Psychological distress

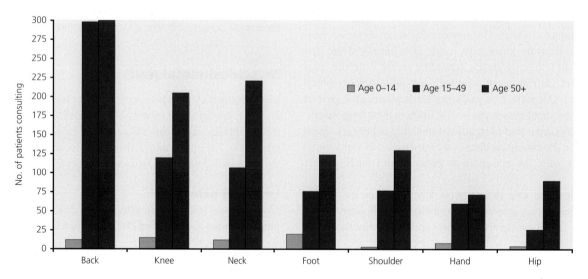

Figure 28.2 Number of people consulting for problems in selected regions by age in a practice of 10 000

a single underlying cause. Every year, around 7% of the adult UK population present in general practice with LBP. Back pain tends to be episodic and the majority of episodes settle within 6 weeks. However, back pain is also recurrent and back pain in the past is one of the strongest predictors for back pain in the future. The lifetime incidence of back pain ranges between 58% and 84%. A number of studies have suggested that fewer than 20% of back pain episodes are brought to medical attention. LBP is generally more common in women and the prevalence increases with age.

A number of risk factors are implicated with LBP, including poor posture, occupation, poor job satisfaction, smoking, obesity, previous LBP episode and lower social class (Box 28.3). The prevalence of back disability is thought to be increasing faster than any other form of disability. According to the Labour Force Survey, the prevalence of work-related musculoskeletal disorders mainly affecting the back was reported to be 800 per 100 000 in 2007, and estimated to result in the loss of 4.1 million working days.

Neck pain

Neck pain is common in the general population and causes substantial disability and economic cost. The global reported prevalence of neck pain is 4.9%. Neck pain is more prevalent among women, at 5.8%, than in men, at 4%. The prevalence of neck pain increases with older age, peaking in the middle years and declining in later life. There is also some geographical variation: age-standardized prevalence in 2010 was reported to be highest in North America, at 6.5%, followed by western Europe, 6.3%, and lowest in South Asia, at 3.3%. Reported incidence depends on neck pain definition and cause of pain and ranges from 0.055 per 1000 person-years (disc herniation with radiculopathy) to 213 per 1000 person-years (self-reported neck pain).

There are several risk factors implicated with neck pain, including age, gender, genetics, smoking and psychological health. Furthermore, there is consistent evidence that previous neck pain or trauma is predictive of both incident and prevalent neck pain, suggesting that neck pain often follows an episodic course similar to low back pain.

Chronic widespread pain and fibromyalgia

Fibromyalgia is a common condition of middle-aged adults characterized by widespread musculoskeletal pain, symptoms of fatigue, lack of refreshing sleep and cognitive dysfunction. The diagnostic criteria for fibromyalgia were originally published in 1990 and emphasized chronic widespread pain with a number of tender points. In the more recent American College of Rheumatology criteria from 2010, tender points are not required and patients are assessed by the widespread pain index and symptoms severity score. Depending on the diagnostic criteria used, the prevalence of the condition ranges from 2% to 8%. More common in women, with a female:male ratio of 2:1, fibromyalgia can develop at any age. There appears to be no difference in prevalence between developed and developing countries, different cultures and ethnic groups.

Patients developing fibromyalgia commonly have life-long histories of chronic pain throughout their body. Patients with fibromyalgia often have a history of other medical complaints, including headaches, dysmenorrhoea, chronic fatigue and irritable bowel syndrome. Risk factors reported as possible triggers for fibromyalgia include genetic factors, as well as environmental factors including infection and trauma and psychological stress. It has been reported that siblings of patients with fibromyalgia have a 13.6-fold increased risk of developing the condition compared with the general population.

Fibromyalgia can be thought of as a centralized pain state and psychological and social factors can contribute to this central amplification mechanism. Population studies have shown an association of such factors with the initiation and persistence of fibromyalgia. Fibromyalgia has a high impact on the quality of life, loss of productivity, unemployment and disability. Consequently, this puts a strain on involved healthcare and non-healthcare resources.

Gout

Gout is a crystal arthropathy caused by monosodium urate monohydrate crystals. The prevalence varies globally, with a high reported disease burden in developed countries. Extremely high rates are found in Pacific countries, particularly among Polynesians (up to 10% in New Zealand Maori males), whereas gout is less commonly found in African populations, although robust data are lacking for large parts of the world. In UK general practices, gout has an overall reported prevalence of 1.4%. It is more common in men with a male:female ratio of 3.6:1. The incidence and prevalence of gout are both strongly age related, with a prevalence of >7% in men and >4% in women over the age of 75 years. Several studies suggest that the prevalence and incidence of gout have risen in recent decades.

Hyperuricaemia is the single most important risk factor for developing gout. This most often results from impaired renal function. Other risk factors for hyperuricaemia include genetic factors, dietary factors, high alcohol consumption, metabolic syndrome, hypertension, obesity and diuretic use. Dietary consumption of meat and seafood is associated with an increased risk of gout, whereas consumption of dairy products and higher total vitamin C appears to be protective.

Rheumatoid arthritis

Rheumatoid arthritis (RA) is a symmetrical inflammatory polyarthritis. Classification criteria for RA were first proposed by the ARA in 1958 and were revised in 1987 and again in 2010.

Box 28.3 **Risk factors for low back pain**

Age

Number of children

Previous episode of low back pain

Obesity

Smoking

Fitness

Occupation (heavy lifting, prolonged sitting)

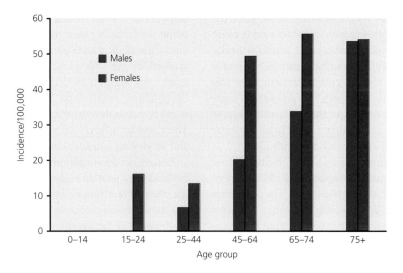

Figure 28.3 Incidence of RA by age and gender in 2011

The annual incidence of RA has been reported to be around 40 per 100 000 adults per year (Figure 28.3). The disease prevalence is about 1% in Caucasians but varies between 0.1% (in rural Africans) and 6% (in Pima, Blackfeet and Chippewa Indians). Women are affected 2–3 times more often than men, and the disease most commonly presents in the sixth and seventh decades.

A number of genetic and environmental factors have been linked with the risk of developing RA. Some factors increase the risk, whereas others are thought to offer a protective role in disease development. Data from national twin studies have shown concordance rates of 15–30% between monozygotic twins and 5% among dizygotic twins, suggesting that 50–60% of RA cases are due to genetic factors. Among the genetic factors linked to RA susceptibility are differences in human leucocyte antigen (HLA)-DRB1 alleles, especially in patients who are positive for rheumatoid factor or anticitrullinated protein antibody. Other genes have also been identified as being involved, including PTPN22 and TRAF5. The TRAF1 genetic region conferring susceptibility to RA has also been associated with radiological damage.

Gene–environment interactions have been observed. Specifically, population-based case control studies have demonstrated that the genetically defined risk factor HLA-DRB1 is strongly influenced by smoking. Various other environmental factors, albeit with weaker effects, have been implicated in the aetiology of RA, including exposure to ultraviolet light, climatic differences, exposure to pollutants and silica and lifestyle factors, such as diet and exercise.

Several studies have implicated hormonal factors in RA, although the results have been conflicting. The higher incidence in women may suggest a hormonal influence on disease onset. A consistent finding is that current or ever use of the oral contraceptive pill has a protective role. RA onset is also reduced by 70% during pregnancy, but there is a five-fold increased risk in the postpartum period. Infectious agents have been implicated as a risk factor for RA. Both pet ownership and prior blood transfusion have been shown to increase the risk of RA five-fold. There is

an association between Epstein–Barr virus and RA, an observation that has been recognized for over 25 years, although the mechanism is not clear

Spondyloarthritis

Spondyloarthritis (SpA) is an umbrella term applied to a group of rheumatic diseases with features in common with and distinct from other inflammatory arthritides, particularly rheumatoid arthritis. SpA encompasses ankylosing spondylitis, reactive arthritis, psoriatic arthritis, inflammatory bowel disease-related arthritis and undifferentiated SpA

Ankylosing spondylitis

Ankylosing spondylitis (AS) is three times more common in males than females, and the peak onset is between 20 and 40 years of age. The mean AS prevalence per 10 000 was recently reported as 23.8 in Europe, 16.7 in Asia, 10.2 in Latin America and 7.4 in Africa. The causes of the disease are still unknown, although a strong link with HLA-B27 has been established, with the frequency of the gene in white AS patients at around 90%. There is an increased risk of the disease in relatives of probands, and results of twin studies show concordance rates of 50–75% in monozygotic twins. Infection may play a part in the disease, but the data are conflicting despite several decades of study. A possible link between AS and periodontitis has been made, mirroring observations previously made with RA.

Psoriatic arthritis

The absence of universally accepted criteria for this condition has hampered epidemiological studies. Psoriatic arthritis (PsA) has a prevalence of around 0.1–0.2%, and there is little difference in the rate between genders or age bands. It has been reported that up to 30% of patients with psoriasis develop PsA. There is significant geographic variation, with the reported prevalence varying from 0.1/million in Japan to 23.1/100 000 in Finland. Collectively, compared to the Americas and Europe, Asia has a lower incidence and prevalence of PsA. Risk factors for the disease include family history, and there is some evidence that the disease is linked to HLA alleles. There are also a number of environmental triggers associated with PsA. The disease is known to start after HIV infection, and prior trauma has also been associated with disease onset.

Connective tissue disease

Systemic lupus erythematosus

Systemic lupus erythematosus (SLE) has a reported prevalence of between 10 and 250/100 000. It is more common in women than men, with a peak onset between 35 and 50 years of age. It is noticeably more prevalent in African-American, Asian and Afro-Caribbean populations than in white populations. There is strong evidence for a genetic cause for the disease, and first-degree relatives of patients are at up to nine-fold increased risk of disease development. Twin studies also show a high concordance rate, supporting a genetic contribution for the disease. Associations with HLA have been reported, but these vary between populations. Despite the high female excess, so far no hormonal link to the disease has been found, and there is limited support for environmental risk factors, although infectious agents and chemical exposure have all been studied. A recent meta-analysis has suggested that smoking increases the risk of SLE, though effects are less marked than for RA.

Scleroderma

Scleroderma is a rare disease; it usually presents between the ages of 35 and 55, with an up to eight-fold female excess. Population prevalence studies estimate the prevalence of scleroderma to be between 30 and 1130/million – the wide variation is due to the lack of population studies, as the disease is rare and classification problematic. Improved survival has contributed to recent reports of higher prevalence; allowing for variation in case definition, the reported prevalence is consistently higher in the USA and Australia than Japan and Europe. In Europe, a north-south divide has been observed, with lower rates reported in northern European countries. There have also been reports of geographic clustering, including a high prevalence (150 cases/million) in three areas close to two major UK airports. To date, the highest prevalence has been reported in a group of Choctaw Indians living in Oklahoma, USA (469/100 000 in full-blooded Choctaws and 66/100 000 in all Choctaws, against 9.5/100 000 in the region generally). Several studies have reported a higher prevalence in black populations, and these patients are more likely to have severe disease than white patients.

It is unlikely that a single genetic or environmental trigger is responsible for the condition. Familial clustering has been observed; in population-based registries, a family history of the condition is associated with a 13–14-fold increase in relative risk for a first-degree relative. So far, only a weak association between HLA and

scleroderma has been found, although stronger links have been found with specific autoantibodies. The most extensively studied environmental factors include organic solvents and silica.

Polymyalgia rheumatica and giant cell arteritis

Polymyalgia rheumatica (PMR) and giant cell arteritis (GCA) are related disorders that usually present in the over-50s. Prevalence over the age of 50 is between 0.2 and 2.2/1000 for GCA and 5.5 and 10.9/1000 for PMR. Both diseases are more common (2–3-fold higher) in women than men. Both diseases increase with age, peaking at around 70 years with a decline after that. The conditions are more common in western countries, particularly in Caucasian individuals of Scandinavian descent. A north-south gradient has been observed, with reported rates of 20 new GCA cases/100 000 in northern Europe compared with 10 cases per 100 000 in southern Spain. The incidence of GCA and PMR is lower in Hispanic, Asian and African-American populations.

There is some evidence that there is a genetic link between HLA alleles and PMR/GCA, but results have not been consistent in different populations. Reports suggest that both diseases may be seasonal in incidence, but again the results have been inconsistent. There are a number of reports that suggest infectious agents may be a risk factor for these diseases, and increased incidence has followed outbreaks of *Mycoplasma pneumoniae*, human parvovirus B19 and *Chlamydia pneumoniae*.

Osteoporosis

Osteoporosis represented by low bone mineral density was included in the Global Burden of Disease 2010 report for the first time as one of the 67 risk factors studied. It has been estimated that 10 million Americans >50 years old have osteoporosis and a further 34 million are at risk of the disease. There are an estimated 1.5 million fragility fractures each year. While most American women under the age of 50 have normal BMD, 27% are osteopenic and 70% are osteoporotic at the hip, lumbar spine or forearm by the age of 80 years.

Epidemiological studies from North America have estimated the remaining lifetime risk of common fragility fractures to be 17.5% for hip fracture, 15.6% for clinically diagnosed vertebral fracture and 16% for distal forearm fracture among white women aged 50 years. Corresponding risks among men are 6%, 5% and 2.5%. Data from the UK General Practice Research Database has indicated that the risk is similar in the UK. The lifetime risk of any fracture was found to be 53.2% at age 50 years among women, and 20.7% at the same age among men. Thus, one in two women and one in five men who are 50 years of age will have an osteoporotic fracture in their remaining lifetime. Among women, the 10-year risk of any fracture increased from 9.8% at age 50 years to 21.7% at age 80 years, while among men the 10-year risk remained fairly stable with advancing age. Osteoporotic fracture is more common in Caucasian and Asian populations than in African populations.

Index

abaloparatide 70

abatacept 79, 100, 134, 165–6
  see also biologic drugs

Achilles insertion enthesopathy 48

Achilles tendinopathy 48

Achilles tendon 46, 47–9, 50, 82–5, 86, 96, 181

acromioclavicular and sternoclavicular joint
  disorders 16, 18, 19

acupuncture 16, 18, 21, 29, 40, 53

acute gout 10, 50, 61, 64–6
  see also gout

acute synovitis, feet 45–6

acute-phase response, laboratory tests 170–1

adalimumab 78–9, 87, 100, 165–6
  see also biologic drugs

adaptive immune system
  see also B-cells; immune system; macrophages;
    T-cells; white cells
  background/concepts 161–8

adenosine 99

adhesive capsulitis (frozen shoulder) 13, 16,
  18–19, 114

adolescents 103–11
  see also children; younger people

aerobic exercises 58, 60, 153

aetiopathogenesis 132

Africa
  ankylosing spondylitis 192
  gout 61–2, 191

African-Americans
  giant cell arteritis (GCA) 193
  osteoarthritis 56
  systemic lupus erythematosus (SLE) 120,
    144, 193

age statistics
  ankylosing spondylitis 81, 190, 192
  giant cell arteritis (GCA) 113, 193
  gout 61–2, 189–90, 191
  neck 191
  osteoarthritis 56, 60, 189–90

osteoporosis 67–9, 190, 193
polymyalgia rheumatica (PMR) 113,
  190, 193
rheumatoid arthritis (RA) 73–4, 190, 192
sports 150
systemic lupus erythematosus (SLE) 190, 193

Aircast boots, feet 45

alcohol, gout 63, 65, 191

alcoholics 7, 48, 63, 70, 172

alkaline phosphatase activity 172

allopurinol, gout 65, 172

alopecia 120–7, 130

American College of Rheumatology (ACR) 51,
  90, 99, 114, 120–1, 129, 191

American Rheumatology Association 120

amitriptyline 16, 54, 86

amyloidosis 8, 80, 95

anabolic agents, osteoporosis 69, 70–2

anaemia 75, 94, 97, 124–5, 167, 169–71

anakinra 79, 95, 100, 165–6
  see also biologic drugs; interleukin-1

analgesics 11, 13, 14–16, 17–18, 20–1, 28–9,
  31–5, 37, 39–42, 52, 53, 58, 62, 65–6, 106,
  126, 151
  see also aspirin; drugs; NSAIDs; opioids;
    paracetamol

anatomy 5–6, 13–14, 23–5, 37, 43–4, 152
  see also individual topics

angiotensin 125–7, 130, 134, 135

angiotensin-converting enzyme (ACE) inhibitors
  125–7, 130, 134, 135

ankle deep tendon reflexes 27

ankles 27, 32, 43–50, 55, 64, 86, 91–2, 94,
  96–100, 152
  see also feet

ankylosing spondylitis 25, 32, 33, 41–2, 49, 68,
  81–3, 86–7, 93, 97–8, 139, 155, 162, 176,
  180–1, 190, 192–3
  see also spondyloarthropathies
  age statistics 81, 190, 192

background/concepts 81–4, 86–7, 162, 176,
  180, 181, 190, 192–3
Bath Ankylosing Spondylitis Disease Activity
  Index (BASDAI) 83
clinical assessment 83
diagnosis 81–3, 97, 176, 180, 181
ethnicity statistics 192
gender statistics 81, 192
imaging studies 81–4, 180, 181
incidence 81–2, 190, 192–3
investigations 81–3, 176, 180, 181
modified New York criteria 81–3
symptoms 81–3, 97–8, 180, 181
treatments 81, 86–7

anorexia 41, 68, 97, 105, 121

anterior knee pain syndrome 39–40

anterior metatarsal soft tissue pad
  inflammation 46

anti-CCP (ACPA) 73, 75, 76, 173

anti-drug antibodies (ADAs), biologic drugs 168

anti-dsDNA method 120–6, 141–3, 145,
  172–5, 185

anti-inflammatory drugs 10, 16, 17, 28–9, 40–2,
  46–50, 86–7, 99, 121
  see also NSAIDs

anti-inflammatory gels 7, 9, 40, 46

anti-RNA polymerase III ANA (ARA) 131–6,
  143–7

antibiotics 11, 21, 34–5, 42, 95, 110, 126, 135–6
  see also infections

antibodies 52, 65, 73–6, 78–80, 90, 91, 93–4,
  95–100, 109, 119–27, 132–6, 141–7, 161–8,
  169, 172–6
  see also auto…; immune system
  background/concepts 141–7, 161–8, 172–6
  cyclic citrullinated peptides 173

antibody-dependent cellular cytotoxicity
  (ADCC) 166

anticoagulants 124, 125, 126–7

antidepressants 16, 29